HIGH PRAISE FOR
HEALING MIND, HEALTHY WOMAN:

"REQUIRED READING FOR EVERY WOMAN'S HEALTH AND WELL-
BEING."—Herbert Benson, M.D., president, Mind/Body Medical Institute,
author of *The Relaxation Response*

"THIS BOOK IS A TREASURE TROVE OF INFORMATION AND
PROVEN EXERCISES THAT CAN LEAD TO HEALING, PEACE OF MIND,
AND THE AWAKENING OF THE COMPASSIONATE HEART THAT IS AT
THE CORE OF WOMEN'S WISDOM."—Joan Borysenko, Ph.D., president,
Mind/Body Health Sciences, Inc., author of *Minding the Body, Mending the Mind*

"AN INSPIRING BOOK THAT SHOWS HOW TREATING THE WHOLE
WOMAN CAN REALLY MAKE A DIFFERENCE."—Steven E. Locke, M.D.,
chief of behavioral medicine, Harvard Pilgrim Health Care

"A VERY WISE BOOK, GROUNDED IN BOTH SCIENCE AND SPIRIT.
AS WE ENTER A NEW MILLENNIUM, THIS IS A FITTING MANIFESTO
FOR WOMEN'S HEALTH. HIGHLY RECOMMENDED."—Larry Dossey,
M.D., author of *Prayer Is Good Medicine* and *Healing Words,* executive editor,
Alternative Therapies

"AN IMPORTANT BOOK . . . A VALUABLE RESOURCE
FOR WOMEN."—*Upfront*

HEALING
MIND,
HEALTHY
WOMAN

· · · · · ·

ALICE D. DOMAR, PH.D.,
AND HENRY DREHER

HEALING
MIND,
HEALTHY
WOMAN

◆ ◆ ◆ ◆ ◆ ◆ ◆

Using the Mind-Body Connection

to Manage Stress and

Take Control of Your Life

Delta
Trade Paperbacks

A Delta Book
Published by
Dell Publishing
a division of
Bantam Doubleday Dell Publishing Group, Inc.
1540 Broadway
New York, New York 10036

ISBN: 0-385-31894-4

Reprinted by arrangement with Henry Holt and Company, Inc.

Manufactured in the United States of America
Published simultaneously in Canada

September 1997

10 9 8 7 6 5

To Dave
A.D.D.

In memory of my mother,
Rose Dreher
H.D.

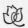

Contents

◆ ◆ ◆ ◆ ◆

Part II · *Women's Conditions, Women's Treatments*

Authors' Note

. . . .

*A*lthough *Healing Mind, Healthy Woman* is a collaborative effort by Alice Domar, Ph.D., and Henry Dreher, for the sake of clarity and simplicity we decided to use the pronoun *I,* for Dr. Domar, throughout, particularly because the scientific findings and case histories herein are a product of her research and clinical work. The names and identifying details of the patients discussed in this book have been changed to protect anonymity.

The sections in this book on mind-body medical techniques are offered as health recommendations, not as substitutes for conventional medical therapies for disease. We recommend that you utilize these approaches only in conjunction with—not instead of—mainstream medicine. Consult your physician about any symptom or illness you may have, and inform him or her about any treatments you embark upon.

Acknowledgments

◆ ◆ ◆ ◆ ◆ ◆ ◆ ◆ ◆ ◆ ◆

I would like to thank so many people for sharing their knowledge and experience with me throughout my training. These individuals include Ed Yeterian, Ph.D., for introducing me to the field of Health Psychology; Gil Levin, Ph.D., Charlie Swencionis, Ph.D., Andy Razin, M.D., and Alan Goldstein, Ph.D., for their guidance and support in graduate school; the late Joel Noe, M.D., for his assistance with my Ph.D. thesis; and Bruce Masek, Ph.D., and Dennis Russo, Ph.D., for their clinical wisdom during my postdoctoral fellowship.

My colleagues in the Division of Behavioral Medicine have been exceptional in their willingness to share new ideas, their sense of humor, their dedication to the best possible patient care, and their creation of the wonderfully caring atmosphere in the department. I would like to especially thank Joan Borysenko, Ph.D., and Steve Maurer, M.A., for providing me with my clinical training in mind-body techniques and Tricia Zuttermeister, M.A., and Richard Friedman, Ph.D., for their contributions to my research efforts, but all of my colleagues have had a role, either directly or indirectly, in the development of this book. I thank them all for their friendship.

Herbert Benson, M.D., has been a true mentor, colleague, and friend throughout my eleven years in the division. I thank him for his continuous support, loyalty, and his belief in the importance of this work.

I would also like to thank my husband, Dave Ostrow, for his love, patience, and understanding, which enabled me to take the time I needed to write this book. And I could not have succeeded in any of these endeavors without the love and encouragement of my parents, Carola and Evsey Domar.

Finally, I would like to thank my patients, who have taught me so much and who trusted me to try to help them at times when they were feeling very vulnerable.

—*Alice D. Domar, Ph.D.*

I wish to thank a few individuals whose support was invaluable during this project. I am grateful to Dr. Barbara Miller and Dr. Yan Wu for their healing gifts, humor, and perspective. I am not entirely certain I could have completed my work on this project, or at least not without a significant toll on mind and body, without their assistance.

I am also grateful to my wife, Deborah Chiel, who remained steadfastly supportive throughout this intensive process, and whose suggestions were unfailingly on target. I could not ask for a better adviser, not to mention a better partner.

I wish to thank Dr. Elizabeth Tyson, who shared her personal story with me. I am especially grateful to all of Dr. Domar's patients who took time out for personal interviews. Every woman revealed aspects of her medical history and emotional life, and I appreciate their trust and candor. They were an enormously courageous and life-affirming group of individuals. By offering the gift of their own stories, I believe that they have made contributions to alleviating the suffering of other women with medical conditions.

—*Henry Dreher*

We would both like to thank those colleagues of Dr. Domar who helped us greatly with key parts of this book, including Margaret Caudill, M.D., Ph.D., Margaret Ennis, M.A., Richard Friedman, Ph.D., Judith Irvin, Ph.D., Cynthia Medich, R.N., Ph.D., Dixie Mills, M.D., Ann Webster, Ph.D., and Tricia Zuttermeister, M.A.

We wish to thank Therese Brown of Speed of Light Word Processing in New York, without whom we could not possibly have written or delivered this book while retaining our sanity. Her efforts and support went beyond the proverbial call of duty.

Our gratitude to our agent and friend Chris Tomasino is enormous. She has been an ardent supporter whose help, judgment, and multileveled talents have been invaluable at every stage of this project.

We deeply appreciate the support, wisdom, and skill of our wonderful editor at Henry Holt and Company, Cynthia Vartan. We also thank everyone at Holt—too many to name individually—who has been behind this project from the outset, and whose enthusiasm has never waned.

We are also grateful to our respective spouses, Dave Ostrow and Deborah Chiel, whose smart and savvy suggestions about the manuscript were extraordinarily helpful.

Introduction

♦ ♦ ♦ ♦ ♦ ♦ ♦

THE BLOOMING ROSE

During my graduate training, I had an experience that presaged my later life's work. I was enrolled in the Health Psychology doctoral program at Albert Einstein College of Medicine in New York. By our third year, we were required to choose a medical specialty on which to concentrate. I was interested in women's health, so I chose obstetrics and gynecology. I was the first student in the program's history to select this specialty, which showed how little attention was being paid to the mind's role in women's health. The head of OB/GYN agreed to let me participate in the medical student rotations in obstetrics and gynecology, as long as I kept quiet that I was from Health Psychology. He didn't want the medical team to view me any differently.

On the third day of the rotations, we were attending to a woman undergoing a difficult delivery. She was being given an episiotomy, in which a surgical incision is made to widen the vaginal opening and ease the birth process. All of the medical students were down by the expectant mother's pelvis, observing the episiotomy and its aftermath. But I was up by her head, asking questions about the experience: How are you feeling? Do you have any pain? I comforted her until her baby was born, and she was clearly relieved to have a health professional who cared as much about her emotional state as her physical state.

I wondered if my behavior with the expectant mother had blown my cover. When I persisted in spending more time by women's heads than their pelvises, I knew the jig was up. Instead of resenting me for concealing my department of origin, the other students recognized my particular skills and put them to good use. Whenever a patient was anxious about a surgical procedure, medical test, or examination, I became responsible for attending to her mental state.

It became clear to me that my evolving role was no sideshow in the theater of high-tech medicine. I saw how profoundly the patients benefited from psychological support, whether they were in the hospital to give birth, have a hysterectomy, receive cancer therapy, or undergo treatment for endometriosis. I recognized that women's minds had to be treated along with their reproductive organs. Almost every condition affecting women carries its share of emotional upset. A body of scientific evidence, and my own observations, pointed toward the same conclusion: psychological suffering can impede physical healing. I believed passionately that a mind-body approach to women's health was needed. That was the contribution I wanted to make.

Over the past decade, I have been fortunate to realize my dream of developing mind-body methods to help women with their most common health concerns. Today I direct the women's health programs in the Division of Behavioral Medicine at the Deaconess Hospital in Boston, one of Harvard Medical School's major teaching hospitals. Our division is led by Herbert Benson, M.D., a pioneer in the field more commonly known as mind-body medicine. To my knowledge, there are no similar programs anywhere in the country. (I am also a senior scientist at the Harvard-affiliated Mind/Body Medical Institute, which Dr. Benson founded and directs as a research and training facility for mind-body medicine.)

My patients share a form of suffering all too frequently associated with female conditions: they feel anxious, isolated, and out of control. Their doctors, who offer medicines and surgical procedures, treat their physical conditions but rarely offer remedies for their emotional distress. Our programs provide the needed psychological medicine: powerful techniques enabling women to relax, transform negative thought patterns, express emotions, and develop strong sources of social support. I have found that these methods also help healthy women to stay healthy, by defusing the impact of stress on their bodies.

When our patients adopt these methods, they not only feel better, they often get better more rapidly. By themselves, our mind-body methods are not cures for physical problems; they must be combined with traditional medicine. But they are essential components of a medicine that treats women as whole beings rather than as machines whose reproductive parts need fixing.

In my women's health programs, I have seen patients overcome the aggravating symptoms of PMS, the hot flashes of menopause, and the despair of infertility. In a series of published studies, my colleagues and I have documented these benefits. Our data have been published, and we're being funded by the federal government to expand our research on mind-body medicine for women's health.

Two of my studies showed that a surprising number of women who enter mind-body treatment for infertility become pregnant. With the help of a five-year research grant from the National Institute of Mental Health, my colleagues and I are conducting the first controlled clinical trial of mind-body therapy for infertility, comparing our approach to two different control groups. This study will provide a definitive answer to a tantalizing question: Could mind-body methods help infertile women to have babies?

At Harvard's Division of Behavioral Medicine, we've also had success using mind-body techniques to treat patients with pelvic pain, breast cancer, gynecologic cancers, and the eating disorders that disproportionately affect women. Moreover, mind-body methods have been shown to relieve the anxiety and depression that often accompany women's physical illnesses.

The mind-body medicine we practice at Harvard Medical School is not based on magical thinking, wishful theorizing, or unproven assertions. Our work is based on hard biological and behavioral science. *The efficacy of our methods has been demonstrated in our research.*

I treat my patients in both individual and group sessions. In these sessions, and in workshops I've conducted nationwide, I teach women that their hearts and minds can—and should—be engaged in their healing endeavors. My patients instinctively understand that hope, a sense of control, and human connections are strong medicine for mind and body.

In our groups, women reach out to others going through the same travails. These connections are so empowering that many women complete our programs with a revitalized sense of meaning and joy, as though they've had an emotional transfusion. A woman named Marion who participated in one of my infertility groups got pregnant within weeks of starting the program. But soon thereafter, she miscarried. It was a devastating loss for her; she had tried so hard and for so long to become a mother. She received warm phone calls or cards from every single one of her fifteen fellow group members. Marion said it was the most overwhelming outpouring of love and support she had ever experienced.

We've all known women whose spirits have been broken by bouts with cancer, infertility, multiple miscarriages, severe pelvic pain, eating disorders, or the symptoms of menopause. Yet I have seen women who not only protect their spirits during such crises, they discover ways to let their spirits soar. They actually *gain* strength, awareness, and a capacity for self-care.

Their sense of humor seems to return from its hiding place. The fun re-enters their marriages, partnerships, friendships. I have acted as a kind of midwife to this process for many of the women in my programs. In this book, I provide guidance on how you can turn a medical crisis into a positive turning point in your life.

I have written this book to provide you with an experience as close as possible to actual participation in one of my individual or group sessions. I tell stories of patients whose struggles, I expect, are much like your own. These are women who've found relief from their symptoms and their suffering by following the same program of relaxation, emotional healing, and medical self-care I describe in this book. I hope you will be inspired by their transformations and triumphs. Regardless of the severity of their conditions, my patients come to recognize that they *can* cope and they *can* get on with their lives.

I provide my patients with a whole new range of options to be used alongside conventional medicine to treat and prevent women's conditions. I offer you these same options. Each of them is an opportunity to use your mind to take control of your well-being. All of them are skills of empowerment in the realm of mind-body health, and they are as useful for health maintenance as they are for the alleviation of symptoms and suffering.

The mind-body methods I teach are richly varied. The "relaxation response," our inborn capacity to reduce internal stress, is central to our work with women. But we can elicit the relaxation response in many ways, including meditation, mindfulness, yoga, body scan, progressive muscle relaxation, and autogenic training. You may not be familiar with all these terms, but each method is a tool for achieving peace of mind and body. The positive physiologic effects of relaxation have been proven by Dr. Benson. Now we're seeing evidence that a calm mind can promote a healthy reproductive system. I customize relaxation techniques for the specific female conditions you may be coping with or trying to prevent.

I also teach "cognitive restructuring," a technique of cognitive therapy that enables you to accentuate the positive without denying the unhappy aspects of your experience. You begin to reclaim control over your life when you replace the negative thoughts that normally have control over *you*. Cognitive restructuring enables you to cast off the mental shackles of tyrannical (and usually baseless) beliefs, such as "I'll never feel good about my body," "I'm a lousy mother," "I'll never have a decent career," or "I'll never get well."

We have come to accept that emotions affect our physical health. But emotions, no matter where they fall on the negative–positive spectrum, ought not to be shelved or suppressed in the name of "positive attitude" or even "health." Anger in particular has been a phantom emotion for many women who've been trained from their earliest years to be nice at all costs. In terms of emotional and physical well-being, women benefit most by acknowledging the full palette of their emotions, from anger and sadness to pleasure and joy. Here, I provide guidelines to help you explore and express emotions in a safe, constructive manner.

You don't have to participate in a support group to mobilize sources of loving support. I offer guidance on how to create a fabric of nurturing relationships in your own life, woven of old friends, new acquaintances, and family members. For those of you who've suffered any disorder in isolation, or who've hidden your pains from loved ones, social support is powerful medicine.

Throughout, I describe scientific research showing that all these mind-body methods—relaxation, cognitive therapy, emotional expression, and social support—yield measurable physical and psychological benefits. At Harvard's Division of Behavioral Medicine, we've demonstrated that combining these mind-body methods with mainstream therapies produces results far superior to those achieved using either approach alone.

The mind-body methods I teach are not difficult to learn. They require commitment, but they don't require you to adopt an arcane philosophy of healing. I offer skills you can adapt to your own lifestyle, personality, philosophy, and spiritual beliefs. How is this possible? Overall, our program is designed to cultivate inner peace, self-esteem, joy, supportive relationships, and a sense of control over your life. My patients, with widely differing backgrounds and personalities, can embrace all these aims, because each goal is an essential element in our quest for wholeness—a nearly universal phenomenon. None of these goals forces us to don limiting straitjackets of thought or feeling. When we develop inner peace, self-esteem, joy, supportive relationships, and a sense of control, we allow our utterly unique selves to flourish in the world.

In this book, you won't find a compendium of information on such alternative medicines for women as homeopathy, acupuncture, aromatherapy, and massage. That has been done. Nor will you find comprehensive information on every mainstream medical option for a given disorder. That, too, has been done. But you will find mind-body methods tailored to your life stresses or medical conditions—methods you can combine with mainstream and alternative approaches for the best possible outcomes.

Although mind-body methods are the basis of this text, the book is bound together by principles that go beyond techniques. It's about women achieving new heights of psychological and physical well-being. Emerging fields of research teach us that mind and body are inseparable. Therefore, medical self-care means taking care of your emotional needs at every level. And the mind-body connection means something specific for women, because our physiology, our emotional makeup, and our cultural influences are distinct. For instance, I have found that many of us meet the needs of our significant others (and sometimes even our insignificant others) long before we tend to our own. I teach my patients how to treat themselves with the same loving concern they so readily give their husbands, partners, children, parents, and coworkers.

How much time each week do you devote to activities geared strictly toward your own pleasure and fulfillment? Many of my patients, regardless of their medical conditions, count the answer in minutes rather than hours. At first, they are astonished when I explain that this lack of time for themselves is a potential health risk. However, once they take a hard look at how they're living, they recognize the risk. Perhaps the time count for pleasurable activities should become a medical litmus test as significant as your cholesterol count.

Why is time for ourselves so crucial to health and well-being? In today's world, we are often overwhelmed by the dueling pressures of career and family life. Many of us are caught in a generational vise, in which our teenage children and elderly parents stretch our caretaking capacity to its limit. Inundated by the media and sometimes by our families with messages that our self-worth depends upon our "superwoman" status, we extend ourselves beyond our capabilities. The result is exhaustion, helplessness, or a low-lying anger that threatens to erupt at any time. Some of us become numb to just how bad we feel. We don't need scientific studies—though they exist in abundance—to tell us that chronic fatigue, depression, and anger contribute to physical illness. We understand this connection on a gut level.

That is why I teach women that self-care means more than regular breast self-exams, mammograms, and Pap tests, as critical as these are. Self-care also means taking time each day for activities with only one purpose: the nourishment of body and soul.

When we neglect our needs, it's because we lack a sense of deservedness. We must accept that we have the right, even the responsibility, to be good to ourselves. I have therefore devoted an entire chapter to the healing art of self-nurturance. I describe a combined mind-body approach that enables women to uncover that inner sense of deservedness, which, for so many, has long been in hibernation. We must get in touch with our body's needs, reject punishingly negative thoughts, and use communication skills to satisfy our relationship needs. We can learn to care for ourselves as lovingly as we care for others.

Indeed, building self-esteem is a health behavior, just as important as nutrition and exercise. In her book *Revolution from Within*, Gloria Steinem argues that damaged self-esteem has blocked women from realizing their personal and political potential. Research from the mind-body field suggests that damaged self-esteem also blocks us from achieving optimal health. In differing ways, every method described in this book is designed to build self-worth. The program as a whole enables you to feel more confident, more entitled to care, and more capable of meeting your needs.

How do these changes play out in real life? Jill was one of my patients whose story illustrates the transformation that often occurs in women in our mind-body programs. When she entered the ten-week Mind-Body Program for Infertility, she had been riding a roller coaster of high expectations and dashed hopes for four years. Jill and her husband had tried every high-tech fertility option offered by their specialist, all to no avail. When I met with Jill for a preliminary interview, she cried the whole time. When she joined her first group session, she cried the whole time.

Jill was on the edge of clinical depression. But she stuck with our program, and neither she nor the other group members would have predicted the payoff. From the start, Jill was surprised when the other members were not irritated by her continuous weeping. Rather than judging her, they embraced her. They understood exactly what she was feeling, and told her so. Jill was warmed by their compassion.

By the second session, Jill cried less often. The skills she was learning enabled her to quiet her fretful mind and alter her self-negating beliefs. During the third session, she cracked a joke. Week after week, Jill emerged as a hilariously funny woman, capable of breaking up the group with her stories and witticisms. Her vibrant personality, which had been hibernating for years under the stress of infertility, gradually surfaced.

The ninth session was an all-day affair attended by the women's partners. During that session, Jill's husband stood up and thanked the entire group for "giving me back my wife."

At the end of that memorable session, I told Jill that her emergence reminded me of a blooming rose, with its tightly compressed petals that slowly unfold to reveal the flower's magnificence. Jill's unfolding had delighted the group, as it delighted her husband and herself. On the tenth and final session, Jill brought in roses for each one of her fellow group members. Two months later, she called me with news: she was pregnant. Today, Jill's daughter, Susan, is a healthy, energetic six-year-old.

It required courage for Jill to enter our group, and it required commitment for her to stick with our methods, but the results surpassed her highest expectations. We can't be certain that she became pregnant as a result of her participation, but we can be certain that she recaptured her joyful spirit after years of feeling demoralized.

Jill's story illustrates the underlying purpose and process of mind-body medicine for women. Women who are suffering can find inner peace. They can reach out for the support of other women and the men in their lives. They can find their moorings again, and revive their ability to experience pleasure in daily events, no matter how minor.

By following the book's program, you can create similar experiences for yourself, whether or not you join a formal group. Like Jill, you can rediscover your true nature, which often gets lost in the turmoil of illness, tragedy, or just plain everyday hassles.

When you take up the challenge this book presents, your psychological well-being will certainly be enhanced. According to our research, you're also likely to experience fewer symptoms of stress-related illness. You stand an excellent chance of reducing PMS, menopausal hot flashes, and chronic pain. The potential for physical improvements even extends to cancer, as research by Dr. David Spiegel of Stanford University and Dr. Fawzy I. Fawzy of UCLA now suggests.

Despite all of these potential benefits, the focus of this program is *emotional* well-being. If your eyes remain fixed on the prize of an elusive "cure," you can get trapped by inflated expectations. Your mental state ebbs and flows with yesterday's diagnosis, today's symptoms, or tomorrow's test results. When that happens, you no longer relax for the sake of relaxing or build self-esteem for its intrinsic rewards. Your efforts lose their focus and their authenticity when the only reason you're changing is to get rid of a health problem.

Mind-body medicine works well as a complement to pills and other prescriptions, but it can't be used the same way they are. No reputable mind-body clinician will ever say, "Do your relaxation and call me in the morning."

You benefit most from mind-body medicine with your eyes trained on the prize of emotional health. In that way, you're not calibrating all your efforts toward medical results. When the physical benefits come—and they most often do—you accept them as a wondrous by-product of your commitment to living your life fully and joyfully.

We've written this book for those of you who wish to prevent illness and optimize your health. We've also written it for those of you with specific health problems or illnesses. Each chapter in Part I, "Mind-Body Medicine for Women," discusses one mind-body method—what it is and how you can use it. These chapters are for all readers: women who want to optimize their health and prevent disease as well as women who want to use mind-body techniques to treat specific conditions.

In Part II, "Women's Conditions, Women's Treatments," we devote one chapter each to seven conditions that commonly affect women. These chapters describe how you can combine mind-body methods into an integrated program for the treatment of your specific condition. You'll hear the voices of women who share your same symptoms, fears, and hopes, and you'll learn how to benefit from a comprehensive mind-body approach.

When you use mind-body medicine to take control of your well-being, you will never be a "victim" of disease. We echo the words of mind-body practitioner Rachel Naomi Remen, M.D., who said, "Every victim is a survivor who doesn't know it yet."

You can avoid victimhood by recognizing the remarkable healing and regenerative powers that lie within. Yes, you absolutely need traditional medicine to heal serious illnesses, and you need proper nutrition and exercise to maintain peak performance and energy. But our message, one that has yet to be fully heard or understood, can be summed up simply: the mind is at the heart of women's health.

Part I

· · · · ·

MIND-BODY MEDICINE FOR WOMEN

One

• • •

WOMEN, STRESS, AND
MIND-BODY MEDICINE

*A*t the end of *The Wizard of Oz*, the classic in which Dorothy's odyssey is driven by her desire to return home, the Good Witch reveals to our young heroine that she had the power all along to get back to Kansas. The power didn't lie with wizards or witches; all she had to do was close her eyes and click her heels. This parable captures an essential truth about mind–body medicine for women: much of our emotional and physical suffering can be alleviated by powers that reside within. It may not be as easy as a click of our heels, but by drawing upon our innate capacities for emotional well-being and inner peace, we can return home to a place of wellness and well-being.

Unlike the proclamations of the Good Witch, however, the claims that mind–body medicine can "get us home" are more than wishful thinking. For a decade, I have conducted research and clinical practice using mind–body medicine for women, while investigators from other institutions and parts of the country have also carried out studies. We now have strong evidence that mind–body medicine alleviates the suffering of infertility. It calms the symptoms of PMS. It ameliorates the discomforts of menopause. It promotes the well-being of breast cancer patients and may even extend their lives. It reduces chronic pain in patients with endometriosis and other pelvic conditions. It helps women beset by eating disorders. It liberates women from the disabling emotional and physical consequences of chronic anxiety.

Indeed, mind–body approaches can ease suffering among women with almost any medical condition. Mind-body medicine may also help to prevent conditions that exclusively or predominantly affect women.

What explains the vast potential of a mental approach to physical ills? One reason is clear. The stress in our lives, and the internal distress it causes, can wreak havoc on our bodies. Our hearts get overstimulated, our hormonal output becomes imbalanced, and our immune systems—those inner networks of healing and defense—are weakened. We now have evidence that women's reproductive systems can be affected by stress and ongoing emotional upset.

When we learn to manage stress and free ourselves from chronic unhappiness, we alter our physiology in favor of health. Mind-body methods can remove the albatross of stress from all our biological systems, including our reproductive systems. For women, this may mean fewer and less severe symptoms of the disorders that commonly afflict us.

Mind-body medicine is not a panacea. On its own, it is rarely a cure for disease. But used carefully in combination with traditional medicines, it is an essential aspect of health and wellness for women. The logic is simple: if outer stress and inner distress can exacerbate illness, then we must manage that stress and heal our psychological wounds. Otherwise, our medical programs—no matter how smart and scientific—are missing a vital piece.

What exactly is mind-body medicine? It is any method in which we use our minds to change our behavior or physiology in order to promote health and recovery from illness.

These include:

- Any technique that elicits a state of relaxation, such as meditation, yoga, mindfulness, and deep breathing.
- "Cognitive therapy," on an individual and group basis. This approach, which helps us to challenge and replace thought patterns that make us depressed and anxious, has been shown to enhance physical as well as psychological health.
- The teaching of coping skills, such as self-nurturance, seeking support, problem-solving, emotional expression, and journaling, which are effective forms of stress management.
- Assertiveness training and communication skills that empower us to develop and sustain a nurturing network of relationships.
- Biofeedback and hypnosis, which tap mental capacities to treat conditions such as irritable bowel syndrome, migraine headaches, and many others. (This book does not dwell on biofeedback and hypnosis, primarily because they are not techniques you can readily practice on your own.)

The underlying logic of mind-body medicine is not complicated. Since mind and body are intertwined, then our efforts to heal the mind will have a positive effect on the body. Some would say this is a leap of faith, but it's a faith born out in many scientific studies.

Mind-body medicine is more important now for women than ever before. Stress is a fixture in our lives, one that looms larger as society becomes more complex and our roles and responsibilities expand. I don't counsel stress *avoidance*, because who can sidestep stress without becoming a shut-in? Living in the world means living with stress. And we've finally come to recognize that certain types of stress are positive—the ones that challenge us to find creative solutions, stretch our capabilities, and elicit strengths we never knew we had. But when the demands placed on us are overwhelming, we need all the coping skills we can summon.

That is why I teach stress *management*. And that means coping. As I do for my patients, I offer you a variety of methods—I call them a "bag of tools"—that enable you to handle life's inevitable stresses with greater calm, grace, self-acceptance, and conviction. With these tools, you can gain a sense of control over your life and health. That "sense" quickly translates into reality: your actual quality of life and health improve as you regrasp the reins of control.

In action, mind-body medicine is a dynamic process. I teach the various techniques in individual sessions as well as in mind-body groups. Such groups, which are rapidly springing up in hospitals and other health-care facilities throughout the nation, have certain typical features. They are generally led by physicians, psychologists, nurses, or social workers who specialize in mind-body interactions. They are frequently (though not always) composed of people experiencing the same symptom, illness, or disorder. For instance, I have directed groups specifically for women at menopause, women with infertility, and women undergoing high-tech procedures for infertility such as IVF (in vitro fertilization). But I have also run groups for people with a variety of problems, from PMS to pelvic pain to irritable bowel syndrome.

These groups foster a sense of support, and they encourage members to confide their thoughts and feelings. But unlike a standard support group, they concentrate on teaching empowering techniques. Sometimes groups break into smaller subunits so that people can share their experiences or practice certain methods together. I have structured this book as a re-creation of my teaching methods, as practiced on both an individual and group level.

I strongly believe that daily practices of mind-body medicine—ranging from relaxation to emotional expression to simply being good to yourself—are no different than sound nutrition and regular exercise. They are genuine forms of health maintenance, with the potential to treat illnesses as well as to prevent them from developing in the first place. But can mind-body medicine fit into the mainstream?

My colleague and mentor, Herbert Benson, M.D., is not only a pioneer in the field of behavioral (a.k.a. mind-body) medicine, he is an impassioned advocate for its integration into the mainstream. To explain this integration, Dr. Benson uses the metaphor of a three-legged stool to represent the proper balance needed in medicine. One leg is pharmaceuticals, the use of drugs to prevent and treat diseases. The second leg is surgery and related medical procedures. The third leg is psychological and behavioral care—mind-body medicine.

Dr. Benson asserts that mainstream medicine has, for numerous reasons, neglected the third leg of mind-body medicine. As a result, the "stool" that is medicine is badly imbalanced. In the real world, that imbalance is easily perceived in patients with chronic stress-related conditions who, for lack of psychological care and self-help strategies, never get better. When stress is a factor in ill health—whether the condition is migraines, back pain, PMS, or hot flashes—drugs or surgery may still be necessary, but they won't be sufficient. As a result, countless patients suffer with stubborn symptoms, and the economic costs are incalculable. Effective treatments for stress-related illnesses would save our health-care system billions of dollars. In recent years, mind-body medicine has been shown to improve outcomes for a vast variety of difficult-to-treat chronic conditions.

Mind-body approaches have also been shown to humanize the practice of medicine. As it stands, when we are diagnosed with an illness, we are too often left to fend for ourselves. We may get inadequate information from our doctors, and even less emotional support. Of course there are marvelous exceptions, but our health-care system isn't set up to assist us with the psychological aspects of disease. My patients often come to me feeling alone. Their loneliness abates when they discover, firsthand, how many others feel the same confusion, fear, or shame. Mind-body groups, and the methods they impart, can transform the entire experience of being ill.

Imagine that the stories in this book are of women you could meet, women you could know. Let them be reminders that you are not alone with your particular condition. Nor are you alone in your confusion, fear, or shame. If you can, find a support group of others who share your condition. But if you can't, allow the voices here to resonate, knowing that these are real women who shared their stories in the hopes that other women—like yourself—would experience the connectedness that heals.

At a time when women seem to be more stressed-out than ever, the need for mind-body medicine—both for the prevention and the treatment of common conditions—could not be greater.

Stress: Women's Number One Concern

*W*hen Tania joined one of my mind-body groups several years ago, she was in a state of overload. Her rheumatoid arthritis was flaring up, causing severe pain in her knees and hands. She had tried every arthritis drug but had not gotten sufficient relief. Not until she joined our group did she realize how stress worsened her condition, and how mind-body methods could help control her symptoms.

Stress was present in every corner of Tania's life. She had worked for thirty years at the same job with a demanding boss who did not treat her with respect. Her husband had died when the oldest of her three children was nine years old, so she'd been a single parent for the better part of their lives. Now, at age fifty-seven, she had two children in trouble—one with divorce, the other with addiction. They both returned home for support and unconditional love, which for Tania was a painfully mixed blessing. She loved the time with her daughter's children but felt overwhelmed by the problems facing both her daughter and her son, who were now competing for space in her home and her heart.

The first thing Tania learned in our program was to breathe naturally. With her accumulating stresses, she'd long since lost the art. She practiced relaxation techniques I describe in the next chapter, and a sense of calm and control returned to her. Tania then took on one problem at a time, each with a new frame of reference. Cognitive restructuring (see chapter 5) changed her outlook. "One morning I left the house and discovered I had a flat tire," she recalled. "Before, I'd have said to myself, 'This is the beginning of another bad day.' Instead, I said, 'That was a bad fifteen minutes.' It may seem minor, but that shift made all the difference."

She brought that new perspective with her as she confronted circumstances far more challenging than the flat tire. Using assertiveness skills she learned in our program, she spoke plainly to her boss for the first time. She let him know she wanted better treatment and a pension plan comparable to that of other workers. His response was better than she'd imagined.

Tania's next challenge was to stop letting guilt pigeonhole her into a rigid caretaker role with her grown children. "I'm too old for this," she remarked. She refused to "enable" her son in his addiction and shepherded him into recovery. With considerable pain but also courage, she asked him to leave her house. At the same time, motivated by love, she traveled with him across the country to participate in a weeklong recovery program for families. Both learned a great deal about their family dynamics and about each other. Tania received a medallion after completing the program. "I carry that medallion with me all the time," she said. Tania also gave her divorced daughter, who'd been living with her for more than a year, a deadline to leave the house. Ultimately, her actions improved her relationships with her children, sustaining her contact with them and her beloved grandchildren.

In all these efforts, Tania received unquestioning support from the other members of our group. She says that our support "buoyed her spirits," and she's kept in touch with her fellow group members to this day.

Over time, Tania's symptoms of rheumatoid arthritis abated. She still has an occasional flare-up, but the pain is no longer severe and disabling as it was before. She sees a direct correlation between her use of mind-body medicine and her physical improvement. "The mind-body group was the best present I've ever given myself," she said.

Tania is like countless other women. For years she endured the double load of breadwinning and child-rearing responsibilities. She experienced on-the-job stress due to a difficult and unappreciative employer. She'd been taught from an early age to take on a caretaking role without complaint, and her grown children returned home once again to bask in her nurturance. And she suffered with an autoimmune disease—rheumatoid arthritis (RA)—that strikes women three times as often as men. Though stress does not likely cause RA, it's been shown to exacerbate the disease.

Tania's case exemplifies how stress affects women's lives and health. It also illustrates how a mind-body approach can empower women to confront stress. Often, the result is a wondrous side effect: relief from physical suffering.

In 1994, Labor Secretary Robert Reich released findings from a U.S. Department of Labor survey of 250,000 working women. Sixty percent of these women said that their number one problem was stress—ranked first on the overall list of daily difficulties.

And it is no wonder. Today's women have taken on multiple roles to adapt to the pressures and demands of a changing society. We continue to raise children and maintain homes while pursuing work and creative activities. Over the past few decades women have entered the workforce in

droves. The rigid 1950s culture in which men worked and women tended to home and hearth is but a wispy memory. In our families we're often the prime movers who nourish broader social connections. We make plans, maintain contact with relatives, throw parties, create social events. Certainly many of us have male partners who embrace equality and act accordingly: they cook, clean, socialize, and take care of the kids every bit as skillfully as we always have. Yet gaps can remain, because some men are unable or unwilling to meet us halfway. This is not to lay blame; work and financial pressures rob them of precious time, or social conditioning blunts their awareness. In any event, women remain saddled with more than they can handle.

Although many women have indeed been victimized, we should try not to see ourselves as victims, and we cannot slough off our newly acquired roles. In other words, we can't turn the clock back to a distant past, we can only make a better present and future. A mind-body approach asks us to change our perceptions of hard realities, to view our newfound roles as challenges rather than threats to our well-being.

I therefore counsel my patients to handle stress by taking time every day for both relaxation practice and sheer pleasure. I also teach empowerment: assertiveness training to deal with demanding people on the job and in the home, and communication skills to get their needs met. I demonstrate how they can procure needed help from coworkers and loved ones, help that enables them to juggle many balls at once without undue suffering of mind and body. This book will show you how to manage daily pressures with aplomb, balance, and strength.

To Fight or to Flee: That Is the Question

You perform a breast self-examination, as you've been taught to do. You discover a lump you've never felt before, and you can't help but be worried. It seems larger than lumps you've felt in the past, which you later found out were garden-variety cysts. This one seems different.

You call your gynecologist and make an appointment. During the three days you wait to see her, your fear grows like the thump-thump of a beating drum that only gets louder. You get to the office for your appointment, and wait forty-five minutes to see her. By now, the beating drum is so loud you feel it pounding in your body. Your heart is racing, your temple is throbbing, your stomach is churning. A light sweat breaks out on your forehead, arms, and torso.

Finally, you get to see your doctor. She examines you, then takes a mammogram. The drumbeat grows louder still as you sit waiting for results. Finally she calls you back into her office. "You have another cyst," she says. "It's nothing to worry about." She suggests that you cut back on coffee and chocolate and consider taking vitamin E.

You leave her office and step out into the sunny light of day. The thump-thump has receded. Your stomach feels better, as if you'd scarfed a few antacids. Your head feels fine now, but you haven't taken any aspirin. All that's left of your perspiration are the telltale splotches on your blouse. You heave a mighty sigh of relief.

What you've experienced is known to stress researchers as the fight-or-flight response. Threatening situations are registered in the brain, which triggers a veritable cascade of messenger molecules, traveling from one glandular source to another. The messages lead to the synthesis and release, by our adrenal glands, of stress hormones such as adrenalin and noradrenalin. In extreme circumstances, the fight-or-flight trigger is like lighting the end of a long fuse on a bundle of dynamite: the flame zips quickly toward its goal, and the end result is a small explosion of hormones into our bloodstream. These hormones—adrenalin in particular—have marked effects on the body, jacking up our heart rate, blood pressure, breathing rate, and muscle tension.

It's called fight-or-flight because our brains interpret this entire sequence to mean one thing: "Danger! Fight or flee!" The stress hormones prepare our bodies to act swiftly and powerfully, whether that action involves a struggle or a quick getaway from the scene. Prehistoric men and women, our evolutionary ancestors, needed to fight or flee from dangerous animals during their hunting forays. In the modern world we're rarely faced with such nakedly physical dangers. But everyday psychological dangers—like waiting in the gynecologist's office—can stimulate many of the same physical changes.

How powerful is the fight-or-flight response? Powerful enough to help us survive horrendous threats. The surging adrenalin of the caveman being chased by a saber-toothed tiger enabled him to run far more swiftly than usual. Let's not forget the cavewoman, either, who presumably faced down animals and tribal interlopers who threatened her and her children.

Today we face mortal danger far less frequently than our prehistoric ancestors. But the same abilities remain hard-wired into our sympathetic nervous systems, the branch responsible for the fight-or-flight response. I've heard stories from patients that underscore the lifesaving aspect of fight-or-flight, especially when it kicks in during an immediate crisis.

Maryann remembered the time she was playing in her backyard pool with her two-year-old daughter and their new babysitter. She went back into her house, and then turned around to face the babysitter, who'd followed her inside. In a flash she realized that her daughter had been left alone in the pool. "I did not *run* back to the pool," recalled Maryann. "I flew." Maryann wasn't fast to begin with, and the sudden burst of speed took her completely by surprise.

Fight-or-flight can protect us during all manner of dangerous encounters. A young woman at one of my workshops recounted a frightening experience on a New York subway. A man followed her off the car at her stop and grabbed her buttock. "The next thing I knew," she said, "the guy was literally sailing through the air, and my foot hurt like hell." The adrenalin surge enabled her to kick a large man with such controlled force that he became airborne on a New York subway platform!

Thus, fight-or-flight is a mechanism for self-protection, one that can save women's lives. We rarely need such bursts of adrenalin, since in the modern world we rarely confront mortal dangers, yet we often respond to daily hassles with the same primordial intensity.

We're late getting to work. One of our kids flunks a course in school. We're angry at our mate for forgetting to make the bed. Our boss criticizes our work on an important project. We lose a job and wonder where we'll get the money for next month's rent. How often have we reacted to such circumstances with sweaty palms, acid stomachs, tense foreheads, or rubbery legs? All these physical manifestations of anxiety are instances of the fight-or-flight response.

By one estimate, Americans experience fifty brief fight-or-flight episodes every day. For many of us, the first one occurs the moment our alarm clock goes off in the morning. That awful, intrusive buzz or burst of music triggers a spurt of stress hormones and a domino effect of anxious thoughts about the day ahead.

Why do we respond to unpleasant situations as if they were life-threatening? Why do we experience an irritable husband or a nasty boss as if they were saber-toothed tigers? We don't know all the answers. But clearly, our nervous systems are not terribly deft at distinguishing between physical threats, when we *really* need to fight or flee, and psychological threats, when we really need to think and speak clearly.

One reason for the prevalence of fight-or-flight has to do with our culture's information explosion. Our highly evolved brains allow us to interpret complex information regarding events that might be dangerous only in the distant future. The woman who finds a lump during a breast self-examination will experience the fight-or-flight response only because she learned about such examinations—and the implications of such a lump— through media reports. Although this woman will be anxious the moment she feels the lump, her reaction is useful: it will propel her to the doctor. Other information-age anxieties are not so useful; people overexposed and oversensitive to the media's endless crime stories may come to believe that muggers and murderers lurk around every corner. Such individuals will have few calm moments out of doors, even on the safest streets of their towns or cities.

Along with information-age anxieties, women's expanding roles in the modern world cause many of our fifty daily bursts of tension. Stress associated with work is a major factor, causing episodes of anger and anxiety, emotions that herald fight-or-flight. The examples are legion: A professional woman in a meeting has her judgment criticized because she isn't granted the same esteem as male colleagues. A mother, already late to pick up her son at day care because she was forced to stay late at work, is greeted by bumper-to-bumper traffic. A bank teller is confronted daily by a coworker who's made inappropriate sexual advances. A waitress is harassed by several customers at once, until she loses her usual cool entirely.

"Stressors," or stressful events, can be placed in two broad categories: instances like the above, which aren't directly linked to health issues, and those that are related to health. The fear of breast cancer is a health-related stressor. In fact, any informed woman with a family history of breast cancer will probably experience fight-or-flight when she goes for a mammogram. So will a pregnant woman with a history of miscarriages whenever she enters a bathroom, out of fear of seeing blood spots that could signal an end to her pregnancy. As will a woman struggling with infertility who awaits the results of a pregnancy test. Even the most normal pregnancy presents women with a host of stressors: medical tests, profound bodily changes, a painful delivery, sleep loss, and all the radical changes in lifestyle ushered in by the presence of a newborn.

Individual psychological factors can also cause unnecessary fight-or-flight. Those of us who've experienced childhood traumas or who suffer from anxiety disorders may misread current circumstances to be more dangerous than they are. A woman who was humiliated by her father during childhood may react to minor slights by a male boss with the same flood of stress hormones as she did when she was young. Our nervous systems overreact to everyday events when we map experiences from a disturbing past onto a relatively benign present.

Whatever their causes, our daily stress responses take their toll on mind and body. We certainly need fight-or-flight to jump out of the path of an oncoming car, or to chase after our young child who's run across the street. But our spirits are depleted and our bodies enervated by all-too-frequent bursts of stress hormones. Ongoing fight-or-flight overstimulates the heart and weakens the immune system. Research from the emerging field of mind-body science—known as psychoneuroimmunology—shows that the stress hormones can dampen our immune cells, the body's disease-fighting sentries.

Now we recognize that excessive fight-or-flight harms not only our hearts and immune systems. It can also disrupt women's hormonal balance and disregulate our reproductive systems, contributing to many of our most common health problems.

The Effect of Stress on Women's Bodies

In 1986, while I was doing postdoctoral work with Dr. Benson at Harvard Medical School, I was invited to hear him speak to residents and attending physicians in OB/GYN at Boston's Beth Israel Hospital. He remarked that the fight-or-flight response begins in that walnut-sized nugget of brain tissue called the hypothalamus. Our "relaxation response," which I will describe shortly, also originates in the hypothalamus.

The then-head of Beth Israel's infertility program, Machelle Seibel, M.D., was present during Dr. Benson's talk. He stood up and said, "You know, every aspect of reproduction is also mediated by the hypothalamus. Might that indicate a link between stress and reproduction? And what about the potential effects of relaxation?"

Lights, bells, whistles, you name it, went off in my head. I spoke with Dr. Benson and Dr. Seibel. We planned research on the potential of relaxation and stress management in the treatment of infertility, research that will be described later.

If stress altered reproductive functions, then the ramifications would go beyond even fertility. Especially intriguing was the fact that the hypothalamus regulates both our stress responses and our sex hormones. Stress—and its opposite, relaxation—might therefore play a significant role in a host of women's conditions. Why? Because our reproductive organs respond, with exquisite sensitivity, to the ebb and flow of estrogen, progesterone, prolactin, and other sex hormones. The balance of these hormones in our bodies may be a factor in PMS, menopausal symptoms, menstrual irregularities, breast cancer, and uterine cancers. If stress influences the balance of these hormones, perhaps it influences every one of these conditions as well.

Research before and since 1986 tends to bear out this theory. Stress and unresolved emotions have been shown to disrupt hormonal balance and menstrual rhythm. Stress can cause tubal spasms, a factor in some cases of infertility. In one study, excess adrenalin, a clear sign of fight-or-flight over-drive, was associated with menstrual irregularities. Stress has also been cited as a contributor to complete shutdown of ovulation, a condition known as anovulatory amenorrhea.

We're beginning to understand just how stress, anxiety, and other nega-tive emotions can disrupt reproductive functions. Take, for example, the role of one class of stress hormones, the corticosteroids. Our reproductive cycles are themselves orchestrated by a symphonic dance of sex hormones, some commonly known by their lettered abbreviations (LHRH, LH, FSH), others more readily pronounceable, such as estrogen and prolactin. The corticosteroids, secreted by our adrenal glands when we're stressed, can block or inhibit the effects of all these sex hormones, including estrogen. Indeed, our chances of normal ovulation are reduced when stress causes a continuing outflow of corticosteroids.

Prolactin is a hormone released by the pituitary gland when we're under extreme emotional or physical stress. Stress expert Robert M. Sapolsky, Ph.D., made this comment about prolactin: "It is extremely powerful and versatile; if you don't want to ovulate, this is the hormone to have lots of in your bloodstream." Prolactin may be the link in the correlation between strenuous exercise and ovulatory shutdown, which has often been observed in female athletes.

Animal studies have verified the link between chronic stress and the loss of estrogen. Jay Kaplan, Ph.D., and his colleagues at Bowman-Grey Medical School showed that subjecting female monkeys to stressful social conditions suppressed their estrogen levels to that of females who had their ovaries surgically removed.

Estrogen deficiency will certainly interfere with normal ovulation. It may bring on premature menopause, which has been known to occur among women undergoing extreme stress or emotional trauma. Not only that, estrogen loss contributes to hot flashes, osteoporosis, and heart disease in vast numbers of postmenopausal women. Studies have already shown that hot flashes are indeed worsened by stress. New studies will confirm whether stress-induced loss of estrogen plays a significant role in postmenopausal bone loss and heart disease.

Stress may influence other conditions that commonly strike women—conditions that, at least superficially, are not rooted in our reproductive organs. Among them are the autoimmune diseases, in which our bodies' immune systems mistakenly attack our own tissues. Most autoimmune diseases are far more prevalent among women. As mentioned in Tania's story, rheumatoid arthritis, an often crippling disease of the joints, is three times more common among women than men. Multiple sclerosis, now considered an autoimmune disease, afflicts twice as many women as men. And lupus, a disorder with many vexing symptoms that can be life-threatening, is nine times more prevalent among women.

Though we have little hard evidence that stress directly *causes* autoimmune disease, traumatic events and strong negative emotions can exacerbate these conditions. In the case of rheumatoid arthritis, some data suggest that certain personality types—people who don't express emotions and assert themselves—are more vulnerable.

Why are autoimmune diseases so much more common in women? One theory blames estrogen imbalances, though the evidence remains incomplete. We do know, however, that stress can perturb both our sex-hormone balance and our immune systems. Conceivably, stress alters the outflow of sex hormones, which in turn send inappropriate "messages" to our immune cells. These messages instruct immune cells to attack our body's own tissues, with terrible consequences. While genetic factors undoubtedly influence autoimmune disease, for many patients stress is also a contributor.

I find it remarkable that a list of medical disorders common among women is also a list of medical disorders with a proven stress component. Take, for instance, migraine headaches, those agonizing episodes of pain that can be utterly disabling. Three times as many women as men are afflicted with migraines. (Here again, estrogen balance may play a part.) Approximately one in five women suffers from them, and stress has been shown to trigger such episodes.

Oddly, many diseases with three-letter acronyms are both stress-related and predominant among women:

- *Irritable bowel syndrome* (IBS), a catchall term for chronic gastrointestinal symptoms such as stomach pain, gas, and diarrhea, is also exacerbated by stress. IBS appears to be more prevalent in women who have experienced early sexual or physical abuse. Overall, IBS strikes twice as many women as men.
- *Mitral valve prolapse* (MVP) is a relatively benign heart condition that

can cause irritating symptoms such as chest pain and palpitations. MVP, which occurs in twice as many women as men, is notoriously sensitive to emotional states: symptoms tend to occur more often when a person is extremely upset.

- *Temporomandibular joint syndrome* (TMJ): a disorder of the joint where the jawbone is attached to the skull, causing severe pain. About 60 to 80 percent of the 10 million Americans with TMJ are women. The role of stress in TMJ has been accepted.

IBS, MVP, and TMJ are chronic conditions in which the prevalence among women cannot readily be explained. Theories abound, however. Women could be more susceptible to MVP because of subtle anatomical differences in the folds of the mitral valve. We might be prone to TMJ due to estrogenic effects on bones, namely, a softening of bone that could predispose us to problems in the temporomandibular joint. But there is still a stress component in IBS, MVP, and TMJ, and women with these conditions can benefit from mind–body medicine.

What about the influence of psychological factors on life-threatening conditions, like breast cancer? I'll address this issue more fully in chapter 15. But Sandra Levy, Ph.D., formerly of the National Cancer Institute, discovered that breast cancer patients who rarely complained, were listless and apathetic, and had poor social support had more cancerous lymph nodes than others. They also had weaker "natural killer cells," immune cells that may be able to stop the spread of cancer in our bodies. Although the issue remains unresolved, a woman's emotional responses—or lack of them—may influence her immune system's ability to fight breast cancer.

Three decades ago, peptic ulcers, a condition notoriously linked to stress, occurred in twice as many men as women.* During these past decades, we've entered the workforce in great numbers, and now we get just as many ulcers as men. I doubt we had this goal in mind as we tried to catch up with our male counterparts in the workaday world!

We know that heart disease—the nation's number one killer—is caused partly by genetic, environmental, and dietary risk factors. But three decades of research have demonstrated that stress, low social support, and chronic hostility also contribute to heart disease risk. Heart disease has always been

---

* Although a bacteria, *H. pyloraia,* has been implicated as a causal factor in ulcers, stress has not been ruled out as a co-factor, especially since most people infected with this bug do not get ulcers.

thought of as a man's disease, but it kills even more women each year than men. Part of the problem is that on average, heart disease strikes women about ten years later than men (due to the loss of heart-protecting estrogen after menopause), and older women have traditionally gotten short shrift from many physicians.

Cardiovascular diseases cause 240,000 deaths among American women each year—six times more than does breast cancer. While the death rate for heart disease has dropped over the past forty years, it has come down more significantly for men than for women. Undoubtedly, massive social changes and accumulating pressures have taken their toll on women's hearts.

Although we know that stress, and our reactions to stress, contribute in some measure to all of the diseases I have mentioned, we don't know precisely how much they contribute. But we are beginning to understand how stress and emotions influence our bodies, and the more we learn, the more it becomes evident that mind-body factors are significant in many of these common afflictions.

One key to understanding this link is the distinction between acute and chronic stress, something we all intuitively grasp. When we experience acute stress, as we do during, say, a mugging or a car accident, fight-or-flight goes into full throttle. Chronic stress is different. It develops in the crucible of everyday life: pressures at work, a slowly progressing illness, ongoing marital conflicts, or caretaking a sick parent. Such circumstances become harder to manage when they pile up one upon the other. We may not feel our hearts pumping or our blood pressure rising, but chronic stress takes a gradual toll. It overheats our nervous systems, keeping us in a constant state of mental and physical hyperresponsiveness. Our constant, low-level anxiety will either erupt in angry outbursts or get turned inward, causing fatigue, depression, or physical symptoms. When chronic stress does contribute to illness, this state of affairs only gets worse. As one mind-body expert has said, "Stress causes illness causes more stress causes more illness." This tight, vicious cycle is both a psychological and physiological reality, and it can play a role in many conditions and diseases.

There might appear to be no escape from such vicious cycles, no way to untie knots of tension built up over years of fight or flight. But there is a way. We have a mechanism to counter fight-or-flight, and it's as close at hand as Dorothy's ruby slippers. The mechanism, which resides within us, is an intrinsic capacity called the relaxation response. This inborn response, and the methods used to activate it, are at the heart of mind-body medicine for women.

Two

• • •

THE RELAXATION RESPONSE
AND OTHER COPING SKILLS

*T*he relaxation response is nature's balancing act against excessive fight-or-flight. During the stress response, danger in the environment sets off a series of psychological and physiological alarm bells. The relaxation response enables us to turn off these warning systems when they're no longer needed. Through conscious effort, we can calm our racing minds and soften our tense bodies.

I've described the fight-or-flight scenario, in which the hypothalamus orchestrates a swift passage of stress hormones throughout the body, causing rapidly elevating heart rate, breathing rate, blood pressure, and muscle tension. The relaxation response scenario is like running the film backward: breathing and heart rate slow, blood pressure drops, muscles slacken. By cooling down our overheated nervous systems, the relaxation response returns us to a set point of true physiologic relaxation.

In the late 1960s, Harvard cardiologist Herbert Benson, M.D., was approached by practitioners of transcendental meditation (TM), who thought they could lower their blood pressure by meditating. Eventually, Dr. Benson agreed to run a series of physiologic tests on them. To his surprise, the tests showed that by simply sitting quietly and giving their minds a focus, the meditators' physiology changed markedly. Their metabolism decreased, heart and respiratory rates slowed, and their brain waves took on a distinctive pattern.

Benson studied other meditators until he realized that this phenomenon was real, and that it occurred when people practiced all sorts of relaxation methods. (The TM practitioners had no corner on the market.) He named this unique set of psychological and physiological changes the relaxation response. He saw it as an inborn mechanism we all have to counterbalance fight-or-flight.

The relaxation response is not a technique. It is a coordinated series of internal changes that occur when mind and body become tranquil. But a vast number of techniques can be used to elicit this inborn mechanism: deep breathing, meditation, mindfulness, yoga, repetitive prayer, body scan, progressive muscle relaxation, autogenic training, visual imagery, qi gong, and more. In widely differing ways, all of these methods have the same ultimate effect of cooling down our nervous systems, helping us to achieve a tranquil state of mind and body.

Although relaxation practices differ, the physiologic changes do not. Regardless of the method employed, once a person elicits the relaxation response the bodily transformations are roughly identical: heart rate, breathing rate, muscle tension, and oxygen consumption fall below resting levels. Normal waking brain wave patterns shift to predominantly slower patterns. In some individuals, blood pressure decreases.

The relaxation response differ markedly from sleep. Once we fall asleep, our metabolic rate, as reflected in the amount of oxygen we consume, gradually decreases over the course of one to five hours. During meditation, for example, the same decrease occurs within three to five minutes. The brain wave patterns seen during meditation also differ markedly from those observed during sleep. The physiology of the relaxation response is also substantially different from that seen with simple resting. Vegging out in front of the TV simply won't do.

How we get peace of mind—the technique we use—is less important than simply getting there. This gives us great latitude in choosing a method or methods for relaxation that work best for us. Freed from the dogma that there is only one path to inner peace, we can select paths that meet our needs, suit our personalities, and reflect our core beliefs. In the next chapter, I offer you choices for relaxation.

In a series of scientific studies, Dr. Benson and his colleagues at Harvard Medical School's Division of Behavioral Medicine have shown the extraordinary benefits of eliciting the relaxation response. Given its calming effects on the cardiovascular system, regular relaxation can help patients with angina, atherosclerosis, and other heart diseases. But relaxation can also be used to treat a range of stress-related conditions.

My colleagues at the New England Deaconess Hospital have demonstrated the powerful and wide-ranging clinical uses of the relaxation response:

- Psychologist Gregg Jacobs, Ph.D., has shown that insomnia patients who elicit the relaxation response fall asleep four times more rapidly, and their brain wave patterns slow. Many patients return to completely normal patterns of sleep.
- Physician Margaret A. Caudill, M.D., Ph.D., demonstrated that chronic pain patients who practice the relaxation response and other behavioral treatments decrease their doctor visits by an average of 36 percent.
- Dr. Benson and Eileen Stuart, R.N., M.S., showed that practicing the relaxation response can lower blood pressure by 5 to 10 millimeters of mercury in patients with hypertension. The greatest benefits accrue to patients whose high blood pressure is clearly exacerbated by stress.
- Psychologist Ann Webster, Ph.D., teaches the relaxation response and other mind–body treatments in group settings to people with cancer and AIDS. She's shown that these techniques reduce anticipatory nausea and vomiting in patients undergoing chemotherapy.

All of these advances have relevance to women. The hot flashes and related symptoms of menopause often cause insomnia, which in turn brings on fatigue, stress, and even more symptoms. Chronic pain is an immense problem for women with endometriosis, menstrual cramps, headaches, rheumatoid arthritis, TMJ, fibromyalgia, and unexplained pelvic discomfort. Hypertension and related cardiovascular disorders are on the rise among women. Women with breast and gynecologic cancers are often faced with chemotherapy and its unpleasant side effects.

Scientists at other institutions have confirmed the utility of the relaxation response in all these conditions, and many more, including Raynaud's disease, a vascular condition in which fingers and toes become cold and painful; irritable bowel syndrome; migraine headaches; and anxiety disorders. All these health problems occur far more frequently among women.

Now, consider the following scientific findings from our research, which support the use of relaxation techniques in the treatment of specific women's conditions:

- Judith Irvin, Ph.D., and I conducted a study of thirty-three menopausal women who experienced persistent hot flashes. Eliciting the relaxation response reduced the frequency and intensity of hot flashes by 50 percent. Members of a control group who either read or simply monitored their symptoms did not realize such benefits. Two studies by other scientists have demonstrated similar results.

- Along with myself and Dr. Benson, the late Irene L. Goodale, Ph.D., showed that eliciting the relaxation response resulted in a 58 percent reduction of symptoms among women with severe PMS. Relaxation was significantly more effective than simply reading or charting symptoms. The most recent, highly touted study of Prozac for PMS showed a 52 percent reduction of symptoms in patients taking this antidepressant drug.
- Two studies have shown that my Mind-Body Program for Infertility, in which relaxation training is an essential element, significantly reduced depression and anxiety in women with infertility. Six months after the program, one third of the participants, who averaged three and a half years of infertility, had become pregnant.
- I led a study of breast cancer patients taking tamoxifen, a drug that blocks estrogen and may prevent recurrences. The drug can also induce hot flashes similar to those of menopause. Our preliminary findings show that the relaxation response reduces by 37 percent the frequency of these drug-induced hot flashes, a significantly better result than we observed in a control group.

One likely reason why the relaxation response is so broadly applicable to women's conditions is the considerable impact of stress on women's bodies. And we now have greater insight into the effect of stress on our physiology. In an important study, Dr. Benson and the late Dr. John Hoffman showed that the relaxation response reduces end-organ sensitivity to the stress hormones adrenalin and noradrenalin. In other words, when we regularly practice relaxation, we continue to release adrenalin and noradrenalin when stressed, but these hormones no longer have the same overstimulating effect on our tissues, muscles, and organs—including, we now believe, our reproductive organs.

What does this mean for the clinical treatment of women? The above-listed studies tell us: Eliciting the relaxation response reduces menopausal hot flashes without the hormone replacement pills that could possibly increase breast cancer risk for some women. It alleviates PMS at least as effectively as Prozac, the antidepressant drug that can produce side effects. It helps ease distress among women with infertility, distress that may worsen hormonal imbalances, tubal spasms, and ovulatory irregularities. It relieves pain, medical side effects, and anxiety among women with breast, ovarian, and other gynecologic cancers. When used in a comprehensive behavioral program, it helps women manage their eating disorders.

We still don't fully understand every mechanism behind these marvelous effects for women. But we do know they occur. And the evidence to date suggests that relaxation blocks the negative effects of excessive fight-or-flight on our endocrine systems and reproductive organs.

Healthy Control: A Key to Women's Health

*E*ver since the birth of her son, Karen had struggled with a host of symptoms. It began with a serious bout of postpartum depression and moved on to physical complaints: vaginal infections, skin rashes, and neck spasms. Worst of all were the ongoing anxiety attacks that prompted her to seek psychiatric help. Although medication alleviated some of her anxiety, Karen continued to suffer in mind and body.

Like so many women in their mid-forties, Karen led a many-tentacled life. She was a preschool teacher, a professional artist, and the mother of a six-year-old son and a fourteen-year-old daughter. She enjoyed all these facets of her life, but also felt pressure to accomplish too much, having come from an intense, achievement-oriented family. She played the family caretaker role, tending to siblings when they were in trouble, no matter how overwhelmed she was. Karen had also suffered her share of grief. In the prior decade, a younger brother and sister had died under tragic circumstances.

Karen's symptoms stressed her out even more, which fueled the classic vicious cycle. As she became ever more upset, her vaginal infections, skin rashes, and neck spasms got worse. During this period, a friend told her about our Mind–Body Clinic at the Deaconess Hospital. "It was really a low point in my life," recalls Karen. "It was just fortuitous that I had dinner with someone who'd been to the Mind–Body Clinic."

When Karen entered my program, she felt as though she had no control over her health or her life. She took to the relaxation practices immediately, practicing deep breathing and mindfulness meditation on a daily basis. Karen discovered that she could relieve her own depression and anxiety by eliciting the relaxation response.

"I began to realize I could stave off the anxiety attacks," she says. "I had tools to combat them, when before they were overwhelming and quickly got out of hand. The relaxation practice would short-circuit an anxiety attack in progress."

In Karen's case, the physiologic effects of relaxation broke the vicious cycle and relieved her spasms of anxiety. But Karen's psychological revelation was just as crucial: she had found a lever of control. "Getting a handle on my anxiety through breathing and relaxation has been like a miracle," she said. Not only did Karen's anxiety attacks cease almost altogether, her skin rash cleared up. Her vaginal infections became far less frequent. Her neck spasms disappeared.

A sense of control is vital to our well-being. When we think we've lost control over our lives and health, we become vulnerable to all manner of mental and physical ills. We don't always need actual control. We primarily need to *believe* we have control. Robert M. Sapolsky offers a perfect example from everyday life: "Airplanes are safer than cars, yet more of us are phobic about flying. Why? Because, despite the fact that we're at greater risk in a car, most of us in our heart of hearts believe that we are above-average drivers, thus more in control. In an airplane, we have no control at all. My wife and I, neither of us happy fliers, tease each other on flights, exchanging control: 'Okay, you rest for a while, I'll take over concentrating on keeping the pilot from having a stroke.' "

As we travel through life, some of us feel like airplane passengers. It's a potentially dangerous trip; we could tumble from the sky at any minute. What's worse, we can't possibly affect the outcome since we're not in the cockpit. To stop feeling helpless and frightened, we need a different mode of transportation—a life in which our actual or perceived degree of control is greater. In work, relationships, and creative endeavors, we can occupy the driver's seat, where, no matter how adept, at least we have that perception of control.

Studies have shown that people who feel helpless to change stressful conditions may be at increased risk of heart disease and immune system disorders. Numerous animal studies have proven that rodents helpless in the face of stress—say, a shock delivered to their tails—have suppressed immune systems. They are even more susceptible to the growth of tumors.

A sense of control allows us to handle daily stressors with fewer physical breakdowns. If we do break down, the stress of the physical condition itself, which may be chronic or life-threatening, calls upon our sense of control. In my clinical practice, I've found that women with conditions of the reproductive organs feel especially out of control. From a psychological standpoint, it's one thing to suffer an injury to an arm or leg, or a disease of an organ (e.g., the liver) that normally does its job in the quiet anonymity of our viscera. It's another thing altogether when illness affects a woman's reproductive organs. Not only is she intimately familiar with their workings, they are inextricably bound with her sexual identity. Pain or dysfunction in these organs, or sex hormone imbalances that cause physical problems, can make women feel helpless, insecure, even ashamed.

For part of each month, a woman with severe PMS feels that her body and emotions are no longer her province. The infertile woman whose hopes for a viable pregnancy rise and fall with each new high-tech treatment loses her sense of control. The menopausal woman whose mood shifts and hot flashes hit with no warning feels like a ship captain who is helpless to navigate through stormy seas. The patient with breast or ovarian cancer, faced with the loss of organs she associates with her sexuality, not to mention with a life-threatening invasion of wayward cells, feels out of control.

When my patients, regardless of their condition, notice how relaxation changes their physiology and makes them feel better, they instantly experience renewed control. Even when they can't rid themselves of a condition, they can diminish feelings of panic that ruin their quality of life.

How do we know that a psychological sense of control is good for our physical health? A body of research offers powerful evidence. Consider the phenomenon called "patient-controlled analgesia." Patients with pain— whether from severe burns, spinal injuries, surgery, or cancer—are not only saddled with agonizing discomfort, they are dependent on others for their pain medication. And they can't control the dosages. Hospital nurses know all too well the anguished cries of pain from patients beseeching them for more medication than has been prescribed by doctors.

In the late 1970s, a group of researchers came up with a novel idea that some considered outrageous: Why not let patients administer their own pain medications? Skeptical onlookers were convinced that patients would either become addicts or overdose victims. In several studies of cancer patients and postsurgical patients, the skeptics were proved wrong. The patients were literally handed the painkillers and told to self-medicate. They not only didn't overdose or become addicted, the total amount of painkillers they used actually *decreased*.

If you've ever experienced severe pain, or can just imagine lying in a hospital bed uncertain whether you're going to get enough medication to relieve your agony, you can easily understand how much suffering is caused by the loss of control. Giving patients the power to self-medicate instantly eased their uncertainty; they never had to fear the prospect of being left alone with their pain. Freed from their helplessness, the patients' physical pain became instantly more manageable.

Can a sense of control help people stay healthy under stress? Psychologist Suzanne Ouellette, Ph.D., thinks so, and she's staked her twenty-five-year career on the notion. In the late 1970s, Dr. Ouellette (then Kobasa) was at the University of Chicago, where she conducted research on hundreds of telephone company executives at Illinois Bell, which was at the time undergoing the most sweeping reorganization in corporate history. Needless to say, these workers were undergoing extreme stress: job descriptions and responsibilities were quickly shifting under their feet, and pink slips were being handed out in large numbers.

With her colleague Salvadore R. Maddi, Ph.D., Dr. Ouellette tracked 259 of the company's executives for two years. She discovered that a group of executives remained healthy under stress while others succumbed to a variety of illnesses. The healthy workers could be distinguished from the others by their high scores on a personality trait called *hardiness*. In fact, when hardy executives confronted extreme stress, they were only half as likely to get sick.

What is hardiness? According to Dr. Ouellette, who developed the concept and a questionnaire to measure it, hardiness consists of three components: commitment, control, and challenge. The healthy workers were committed to their work and relationships; had a sense of control over the stressful conditions they experienced; and had a sense of challenge in the face of change. They were proactive types who assessed problems, devised creative solutions, and carried out plans of action. Despite the swirl of change around them, these workers maintained a belief in their own personal power.

Dr. Ouellette and other scientists since have found that people with commitment, control, and challenge stay healthier under stress, regardless of their occupation, class, or national origin. Many of these studies, including the original Illinois Bell study, involved exclusively male subjects. What about hardy women? Did they stay healthier? Dr. Ouellette distributed her hardiness questionnaire to hundreds of women in their gynecologists' offices. "We've found that those who were more helpless than hardy have developed more illnesses, both mental and physical," writes Dr. Ouellette.

Though control is only one facet of hardiness, it is a critical one. Many experts believe—and I concur—that the success of any mind-body technique depends, in part, on how it bolsters control. Biofeedback is a perfect example. Patients who receive biofeedback therapy are hooked up to monitors that translate their physiologic functions—heart rate, blood pressure, skin resistance, muscle tension, or brain wave activity—into sounds or video images they can easily interpret. The biofeedback trainer teaches the patient to use mental means to control his or her physiology. Whether patients practice relaxation techniques or simply focus their concentration, the "biological feedback" guides them as they attempt to calm and balance their bodily functions. Biofeedback has been successfully used to treat patients with spinal injuries, hypertension, irritable bowel syndrome, and migraine headaches, to name a few.

The lesson patients learn from biofeedback is control. The patient who succeeds in changing her physiology and quieting her symptoms discovers that she has leverage over her body. As with the chronic pain patients, that measure of control yields enormous emotional and physical benefits.

Biofeedback is a wonderful tool, but, as Dr. Benson has emphasized, we can regulate aspects of our physiology without a lot of fancy instruments. The relaxation response is a fundamental skill that gives us a degree of control over our biologic systems. So do the other mind-body methods I teach, all of which relieve anxiety and calm our jazzed-up nervous systems. Though more research is needed, we may someday learn that mind-body methods work primarily *because* they enhance control. Preliminary studies have shown that committed meditators have an "inner locus of control," a social scientist's term for a sense of control.

For women, the concept of control can be tricky. Some of us are taught from a young age to strive for complete control over everything—our bodies, jobs, husbands, kids, social events, ad infinitum. That is not the healthy control I wish to engender.

A woman who believes in absolute control will blame herself for any bad thing that happens. If she loses a job due not to her performance but to organizational downsizing, she'll think, "I was fired because I wasn't good enough." If she experiences the painful breakup of a relationship, she'll decide that she "should have been able to hold him."

Perhaps the most pernicious self-blame may occur when a woman blames herself for the onset or progression of an illness. She'll feel responsible for her breast cancer: "I should not have eaten so much fatty food." "I shouldn't have repressed my emotions." Or she excoriates herself for infertility: "If only I had tried to get pregnant when I was younger." These comments are insidious traps, because there may be a bit of truth to each one. But they are self-negating beliefs based on a concept of control that leaves no room for human error. The "I should haves" suggest that total control is not only possible—which it isn't—but mandatory. Even if our behaviors play some part in our medical conditions, the notion that we are to blame is unrealistic and horrendously unfair.

Can we take more responsibility for our health and well-being? Of course. Does it make sense to blame ourselves for past shortcomings, lack of knowledge, or addictive behavior? Of course not.

The line between healthy and unhealthy control is dangerously thin; riding it is an art that takes practice. You can begin by learning to distinguish between the two. A woman who tends to exercise unhealthy control is often called a control freak, a term that is accurate if somewhat pejorative. Implicitly or explicitly, she believes in the potential for absolute control, and she suffers the consequences. When she's in "control-freak" mode, she is fighting a dreadful sense of helplessness she carries with her. Because she lacks underlying self-confidence, she feels she must direct every action and actor in her world, or else none of her hopes and desires will ever be realized. If she could recognize why she works so hard to manipulate her environment and other people, she might have more compassion for herself, and for others. She would be less likely to be thrown by unpredictable circumstances, such as the death of a loved one, the breakup of a relationship, the diagnosis of an illness. She would find more constructive ways to overcome feelings of helplessness.

By contrast, the woman with healthy control has a deep-seated belief in her own ability to change stressful circumstances, or at least her reactions to them. She therefore has confidence that she can improve the conditions of her life and health. She does not believe she is responsible for everyone else's problems, for the behavior of loved ones, or for causing a terrible disease in herself. Indeed, she does not believe that she has absolute control over most outcomes, because she accepts that certain factors are, alas, out of her control.

Above all, the woman with healthy control has a balanced view of her own power. She searches diligently for realistic leverage in any situation and takes action whenever appropriate. At the same time, she can identify situations where she has minimal influence (e.g., a family member's addiction) or where exerting influence would be a bad idea (e.g., trying to control her husband's every move). That's when she gracefully bows out, avoiding traps of codependence and terminal frustration. Her balanced sense of control is internal (she knows she can influence but not commandeer her bodily functions) and external (she knows she can change many stressful situations but she can't run other people's lives).

We can readily remind ourselves of the difference between healthy and unhealthy control. It's summed up by the famous prayer of theologian Reinhold Niebuhr, used today in twelve-step groups: "God grant me the serenity to accept the things I cannot change, the courage to change the things I can, and the wisdom to know the difference."

Whatever your spiritual beliefs, the serenity, courage, and wisdom referred to in the prayer are attainable. What's required of you is a choice: to actively find serenity within; to exercise courage in your relationships, work, and creative pursuits; and to practice wise discernment, so that you know when to act and when to let go. Mind-body methods support your development of serenity, courage, and wisdom.

Coping Skills:
The Toolbox of Mind-Body Medicine

I've heard one comment repeatedly from my patients, regardless of their condition. "Now, when I'm stressed and I start to feel helpless, I always have the skills I have learned. They're like a set of tools I can use to make myself feel better—more in control, more at peace—when my life and health seem to be spinning out of control."

When we can no longer cope with the stress in our lives, we end up feeling anxious, terrified, angry, helpless, or depressed. As we've seen, these emotional states have physical correlates. Ongoing states of helplessness and depression have been linked to diseases of immune dysfunction, including cancer. We can't simply stop ourselves, by force of will, from feeling these negative feelings. We can, however, develop better ways of coping with stress, ways that relieve our distress.

Each chapter that follows in this section details one particular coping skill you can learn and adopt. Each skill is psychophysical, having a mental and physical component. However, some skills are more body-oriented; others are mind-oriented. The body-oriented coping skills include relaxation practices, nutrition, and exercise. When stress takes its toll on our bodies and we become physically tense, fatigued, or overstimulated, relaxation, a healthy diet, and exercise are practical, effective ways to make ourselves less tense or exhausted. The mind-oriented coping skills (chapters 5–8) enable you to transform your relentlessly negative beliefs; establish healthy and health-promoting relationships; express anger, sadness, and joy; and treat yourself with the utmost care and kindness. But the array of tools that mind-body medicine provides for handling life's difficult patches does not offer a bunch of quick and easy fixes. Developing each skill requires commitment and the courage to confront our thorniest problems.

A patient's newfound coping skills can help her in miraculous ways. A good illustration is the case of Georgia, whose condition was infertility but whose story is similar in many respects to those of my patients with other medical conditions. She and her husband, Bill, first went to a specialist after being unable to conceive for two years. Then diagnostic tests revealed the likely culprit: Georgia had extensive endometriosis, a condition where endometrial tissue grows outside the uterus. Surgery removed 70 percent of the endometriosis, and their doctor informed them that they would be able to conceive in a matter of months.

But she did not get pregnant, even after several courses of fertility treatment. A year later, she and Bill began to feel hopeless. Georgia blamed herself, because Bill's sperm counts were fine. They seemed ready to adopt, but were continually haunted by the question, Why can't we have a child? Bill's mother read a magazine article about our Mind-Body Program for infertility, and she convinced Georgia to give it a try.

Within a few sessions, Georgia's whole mind-set started to shift. She listened regularly to our relaxation tapes, one of which provides instruction on guided imagery, a form of mental visualization to achieve inner tranquility. Georgia transported herself on an almost daily basis to a deserted beach. She also reached out to the other group members, sharing her sadness and disappointment with them. She regularly practiced the yoga she learned in the program, which revitalized her tired body. And she later added a self-styled dimension to her guided imagery practice: she would see herself holding her newborn baby in her arms, feeling the touch and smelling the smell of the baby's skin.

These efforts helped enormously, but Georgia was still hounded by the thought that she was to blame for the couple's infertility. Her self-blame had begun the day after a surgeon's laparoscope diagnosed her problem. Bill, who picked her up at the hospital, imparted the news he'd gotten by phone from the doctor: she had endometriosis. Bill interpreted the news positively: We know what the problem is, and the solution is surgery. But Georgia saw only one reality: *It's all my problem.* Bill argued, "No, it will never be your problem. It will always be *our* problem." But his words didn't sink in.

In our program, Georgia learned cognitive restructuring, a technique that would transform her entire point of view. She recognized how deeply she blamed herself for their infertility. It was the reason she'd been ready to give up all hopes of a biological baby. She couldn't withstand another failure, because it would be *her* failure. Georgia learned to restructure her self-blaming beliefs, and she was able to absolve herself of guilt by pouring her feelings out on paper. As a result, she came to embrace Bill's simple, elegant truth: *We* have a problem. And together, *we* will try to solve it.

Not only did Georgia get blame off her back, she also saw that other women in the group had been through many more cycles of high-tech treatment. With renewed strength, self-esteem, and hope, she and Bill decided to try again. After a third cycle of intrauterine insemination, she called her answering machine and picked up a message from a nurse at the fertility clinic: her recent pregnancy test was positive. "I replayed that message five times," she said. Georgia's son, Marty, is now approaching his first birthday.

Georgia's new coping skills had given her an entirely new perspective on her situation, easing her distress and preparing her for a difficult but rewarding struggle. We don't know if mind-body methods helped her get pregnant by changing her physiology, but that possibility can't be ruled out. I'll explore this controversial question in chapter 11.

The tools of mind-body medicine are mere instruments for self-development. Draw one from the box and you strengthen connections among mind, body, and emotions. Draw another and you find more courage to communicate honestly in your relationships. Draw yet another and you gain a firmer sense of mastery over your life, your health, your fate. Draw many at once and your quality of life improves on almost every level.

Swimming in the Medical Mainstream

Your gynecologist says your pap smear is positive. She instructs you to come back for a cervical biopsy. Might it be cancer?

You experience searing pelvic pain due to endometriosis, even after laparoscopic surgery and hormone treatments. Your doctor says that the only surefire cure is a hysterectomy. But you're only thirty-five, and you want to start a family.

Your surgeon tells you that your early breast cancer can be cured by a mastectomy. The thought of losing your breast is hard to bear.

Your physician recommends estrogen replacement, because hot flashes are robbing you of sleep and sanity. But you have a family history of breast cancer, and you know that estrogen might increase your risk. Should you save your sanity but possibly risk getting breast cancer?

Reading these scenarios, can't you imagine your fight-or-flight response in full throttle?

That's what can happen to us when we swim in the medical mainstream.

We're faced with scary diagnoses, conflicting opinions, agonizing choices. We rarely get all the information we need. And the stages on which these dramas are enacted are forbidding places—antiseptic offices, institutional corridors, cold examining rooms. If a playwright wanted to evoke in her audience the feeling of losing control, she'd only have to place her story in a hospital and get herself a good set designer.

Having an illness is stressful enough. Unintentionally, the medical world tends to make it worse. Even the most caring doctors and nurses cannot completely negate institutional insensitivities. Rarely can they afford the time to explain every crucial decision in full detail or provide sufficient insight into the medical literature. Physicians don't receive enough training on how to offer psychological support or teach self-help skills. Many hospitals have psychiatrists and psychologists on staff, but they are not utilized enough.

So you're cast out into the medical mainstream, to sink or swim. Here, mind-body medicine can not only keep you afloat, it can help you develop a steady stroke against a pretty strong current.

When we're faced with a painful diagnosis and difficult decisions, most of us feel three things: scared, alone, and confused. When we're scared, we can't think straight. That simple truth underscores the need for anxious medical patients to develop a committed practice of relaxation. Given the painful diagnosis and tough decisions, we *must* think straight. Take the case of an early breast cancer patient whose surgeon recommends a mastectomy. She's so frightened that she asks no questions, and has her breast removed. If she practiced relaxation, the fear in her heart might not direct all her actions; her head would enter the process, too. She'd ask hard questions, and discover that a simple removal of the lump with subsequent radiation would almost certainly be as likely to cure her cancer. Then she could make an informed choice. She still might choose mastectomy, but at least she'd have been able to consider a breast-saving option.

By some estimates, 70 percent of all hysterectomies are unnecessary. That is a tragically high figure. The percentage would plummet if most women were armed with coping skills. Indeed, the number of mistaken or unwise procedures for *any* condition will drop as women take greater charge of their medical care. Women with coping skills—especially assertiveness—ask tough questions and insist upon answers from specialists. They create a partnership with their physicians. They reach out for support from friends and family. They run every sensible option by every knowledgeable ear they can find.

In a Tufts University study of people with ulcers, diabetes, or hypertension, internist Sheldon Greenfield, M.D., and psychologist Sherrie Kaplan taught patients assertiveness skills to use with their doctors. Trained aides sat with each patient, reviewed their medical records with them, developed a set of questions they wanted to ask their doctors, and rehearsed ways they could be assertive without feeling too anxious or embarrassed.

These patients, and another group who didn't get the training, were followed and observed as they interacted with physicians. Those coached in assertiveness actually directed the conversations with their doctors. They interrupted when necessary, and obtained much more information than their noncoached counterparts. Four months later, the coached patients reported fewer symptoms, had missed less work, and rated their health as significantly better than those who'd simply followed doctor's orders.

In our culture, it can be very difficult for women to assert themselves with physicians, many of whom are male. Our fears of being disrespected or dismissed by powerful doctors are deeply ingrained. It takes enormous courage to be assertive when we walk into our doctors' offices feeling twice vulnerable—first because of their venerated status, second because our medical problems can be so distressing.

My advice goes beyond telling you to be courageous. In chapter 8, I offer encouragement and a set of skills you can apply in any interaction with health-care providers. These skills enable you to stand up for yourself in a clear, articulate way—to be assertive, not aggressive. You'll be less likely to alienate your doctor, and thus you'll have less to fear. The other key is getting your family and friends on board. When you have loved ones in your corner, your capacity to assert your needs and rights is greatly strengthened. Learning and applying these skills brings forth your native courage.

Whenever we're faced with severe illness and hospitalization, we are likely, at times, to feel uncertain and alone. Among my patients with breast, ovarian, or cervical cancer, the greatest causes of distress are fear and loneliness. Regardless of her age, a woman who undergoes a hysterectomy may feel sad about the loss of reproductive organs, and apprehensive about the surgery. Women with infertility often feel there's something terribly wrong with them, as friends and relatives blithely conceive and have children. There is no more potent medicine for all of these women than a sense of connectedness—preferably with others who've been through the same trials.

Sometimes, when facing a difficult medical decision, all the knowledge in the world isn't enough. This occurs when mainstream medicine has not reached final consensus on an issue. The examples are legion. Should an early breast cancer patient have a lumpectomy or a mastectomy? Should a woman with uterine bleeding have a hysterectomy, when one expert says yes and another says no? Should someone with pain from endometriosis take drugs with side effects, or have surgery?

As medical research and treatments for women's health conditions become ever more sophisticated, we face many of these tough calls. I tell patients in such circumstances to do all the research, get all the expert advice, consider all the options. If no definitive answer emerges, I counsel them to turn within. They can use relaxation methods both to calm down and to tap their intuition: What do *I* believe? What feels right for *me*?

So often, in the onrush of medical events, we overlook these basic questions. But they cut to the heart of the issue. Am I going to be a part of the medical solution to my own condition? Am I an equal member of a healing partnership? Aren't my body, my health, and my life ultimately on the line? If so, my deepest intuitions about myself must be part of the decision-making process, especially during tough calls. We must listen carefully to our head; we must also listen to our gut. The relaxation response helps us to do both.

For women caught between the proverbial rock and a hard place, mind-body medicine can offer practical alternatives. One of my endometriosis patients, Marcy, faced the prospect of a hysterectomy, because other treatments had failed and she was still in pain. Before taking this radical step, she developed a daily practice of relaxation and guided imagery. Within weeks, her pain subsided so significantly that she was able to avoid surgery. In instances of chronic pain, when surgery is not a matter of life and death, time can be taken to experiment with mind-body approaches. Marcy was not the only one of my patients who was spared major, body-altering surgery.

The relaxation response also reduces the pain and anxiety associated with surgery and various medical tests. When I first came to work with Dr. Benson at Harvard's Division of Behavioral Medicine, I carried out research that verified the effectiveness of relaxation techniques in reducing anxiety and pain among patients undergoing surgery.

Carol Lynn Mandle, Ph.D., and I, along with colleagues at Boston's Deaconess and Brigham & Women's Hospitals, collaborated on a study of patients receiving femoral angiography, a diagnostic procedure in which a catheter is inserted in the femoral artery, near the groin. The injection of the dye causes an excruciating sensation of burning, and the amount of medication it would take to completely stop the pain would also unfortunately stop the patient's breathing. Maximum amounts of anti-anxiety drugs and narcotic painkillers are given, but they're just not enough.

My colleagues and I included in our study forty-five patients about to undergo a femoral angiogram. We gave each one a portable audiotape player with a tape already inserted, and we put the headphones on them as they were being wheeled in for the procedures. The patients had been randomly assigned to three groups. The first group had a relaxation tape inserted, the second got low-key instrumental music, and the third got a blank tape.

The patients given the tape with instructions for eliciting the relaxation response experienced significantly less anxiety and pain. The radiologists and nurses taking care of them, who had no idea who got which tapes, confirmed that this group of patients showed fewer signs of anxiety and pain. Moreover, the relaxation group required only one third of the anti-anxiety and narcotic medications needed by the other groups. (Surprisingly, the patients listening to music experienced no less pain and anxiety than those who merely got blank tapes. At least in this instance, music was not what it's been cracked up to be as a physical relaxant.)

You can use relaxation techniques to ease the anxious anticipation, and the actual physical pain, associated with every imaginable medical test or procedure, including these:

- Mammogram
- Pelvic exam
- Pap smear
- Cervical biopsy
- Breast biopsy
- Laparoscopy for diagnosis or treatment
- Surgery for an ovarian cyst or fibroid
- Hysterectomy
- Mastectomy

You can elicit the relaxation response to calm your fears before, during, or after any of these tests or operations. In the next two chapters, I provide commonsense guidelines for the use of relaxation during medical procedures.

When you find yourself in the thick of a medical problem or crisis, remember that mind–body methods can help you in three areas: confronting difficult decisions, dealing with doctors and specialists, and undergoing medical tests and procedures. You can accomplish difficult passages through the choppiest waters, and you may be surprised to find yourself swimming rather gracefully in the medical mainstream.

The Chinese Buffet

*H*ave you ever had Chinese food at a buffet? If you have, perhaps you follow the same ritual as I do. You first select tiny portions of many dishes. Once you taste them all, you return for generous helpings of the dishes you find most delicious. I recommend such a "Chinese buffet" approach as you work your way through this book. The next chapter offers a myriad of methods for eliciting the relaxation response, and subsequent chapters offer a panoply of mind-body methods. Sample the methods detailed in each chapter, and see which ones work for you. Then develop a regular routine in which you practice methods that have proven effective to reduce your distress, improve your quality of life, and lessen your physical symptoms. Listen to your own insights and intuitions as you design daily rituals of mind-body practice.

Our tastes regarding psychological self-care are as individual as our tastes for gourmet delights. Could anyone predict precisely what you're going to like or dislike at a buffet? Even your closest family members might not know what dishes you'd select. Why should anyone dictate what methods you use to heal mind and body?

Mind-body medicine treats women as whole beings, with regard for their unique physiology and psychology. It cannot be a one-size-fits-all approach. As mind-body clinicians, we address your thoughts and feelings, family relationships, dietary patterns, physical activities, and spiritual lives. Our treatments support your personal growth and well-being, which can only be defined by you. Any technique that does not resonate with your singular history, core beliefs, and individual traits will not work.

As you create your own mind-body program, exercise freedom and autonomy. Bring with you a sense of your needs on bodily, emotional, and spiritual levels. Respect your idiosyncrasies; account for your own history. Play liberally with various approaches until you settle into a fulfilling routine. Delight in the possibilities. Listen to the call of your own mind and heart, and your efforts will bear fruit.

Peace of Mind: A Parable

A colleague of mine who used to work at Harvard Medical School's Division of Behavioral Medicine, Steve Maurer, M.A., once told me a mythic story that has stayed with me ever since.

Sometime in antiquity, a devoutly religious man who prayed every day seemed to have a pipeline to the Almighty: the man's prayers were invariably answered. But as time went on and the population grew, God got pretty busy. An overworked God came to the man and said, "You are a very loyal follower, but I just don't have time anymore to answer your prayers every day. What I'm about to offer you should compensate. I am going to grant you three wishes."

The man went home and told his wife about his three wishes. She went berserk. She demanded a new home, a new boat, new clothes. She harassed her husband day and night until one day, out of utter desperation, the man blurted out, "I wish you'd disappear." His first wish was granted—the wife died suddenly. During the funeral, the man was filled with regret. His wife did get on his nerves occasionally, but he truly loved her. As her casket was being lowered into the ground, he said, "I wish my dear wife was back with me." In a flash, there she was, back by his side. Now he'd used up two of his three wishes.

With only one wish left, the man gathered all his friends together to help him answer the question, What should I do with one wish?

One friend told him to wish for money. With money, the friend said, you can buy anything. The man disagreed. Money can't guarantee health, or a happy marriage, or a good family life. It can't guarantee anything that the eye can't see.

This led another friend to counsel the man to wish for good health. Good health is wonderful, replied the man, but it doesn't put food on the table. Good health doesn't guarantee anything except good health.

Other friends had other suggestions, but the man shot down each one with the same brand of logic. Finally, the man went to God and asked him straight out, "I only have one wish left. What should I wish for?"

God replied, very simply, "Wish for peace of mind. You can be rich or poor, in good health or bad. But if you have peace of mind, you have everything." The man wisely took God's advice.

Steve's story is a fine parable for mind-body health. My patients love the story because it suggests that peace of mind is possible even as they struggle with vexing medical conditions. (They also know that the parable applies to smart women as well as to loose-lipped guys who wish death upon their stereotypically bitchy wives!)

Each mind-body method is a way to cultivate peace of mind. Each is a pathway to a spacious inner ground where seeds of well-being can be planted, germinate, and grow. Once we inhabit this ground, we can still be hurt but we can't be spiritually destroyed by illness or infirmity. Whether you come to this book with a wish for recovery or a wish for continued good health, I hope it will also guide you toward peace of mind.

Three

♦ ♦ ♦

ROADS TO RELAXATION

*V*ivian's new life seemed to be in place. She moved with her husband, Peter, from Arizona to Boston, ready to attend graduate school and start a family. She would work toward a master's in social work, hopefully while pregnant, and take six months off from school after the baby was born. The move was stressful, but Vivian's dream kept her spirits and her energy humming.

A few years earlier, Vivian had an unplanned pregnancy that miscarried. Her doctor told her it was nothing to worry about. There was nothing physically wrong with her, and she should be able to have children when ready. Her doctor was wrong. Once Vivian and Peter started trying in earnest, she began having miscarriages—one after another. Vivian was devastated.

Her sense of devastation increased with each new unexplained miscarriage. After the third, Vivian lost her bearings. "I was in the middle of a graduate school course when I had that miscarriage," she recalled. "I was so upset that I couldn't function. We were new to Boston, I had no close friends nearby, my family was far away. I got depressed and anxious and no one seemed to care."

Vivian's dream was turning into a nightmare. They'd moved into a new neighborhood where she felt isolated. Her distress made it difficult for her to concentrate on schoolwork. After her fourth miscarriage, her sister-in-law called from England to say that she was pregnant. Needless to say, Vivian had a hard time pretending to be wildly enthusiastic. Her heart was sinking.

Why was she having all these miscarriages? Vivian didn't feel she was getting answers from her doctors. "I felt so out of control," she said, "and I felt that medicine had all the control."

The worst was yet to come. When Vivian got pregnant again, she and Peter went to a fertility specialist. After blood tests, he informed the couple that Vivian's immune system was rejecting the developing fetus—a common biological reason for multiple miscarriages. Treatments were available for future pregnancies, but the results were uncertain. One thing was certain— her current pregnancy would not come to term. But Vivian and Peter had already planned a trip to Maine for their wedding anniversary. With a sense of inevitable dread, they kept their plans. Vivian miscarried in the car on the way to Maine.

After that experience, Vivian's depression deepened. "I couldn't be a mom. I couldn't be a social worker. I couldn't be anything. It was awful. I started drinking martinis every day at four o'clock in the afternoon."

A friend had told Vivian about my Mind–Body Program for Infertility, and she thought about joining. When Peter realized what was happening to his wife, he strongly urged her to sign up. She did, but her first day was inauspicious. "On the first day of class, I was drunk," recalled Vivian. "I came home and started drinking some more. I just wanted to go to sleep and wake up when I was ready to live my life. My husband came home, and put me in a cold shower. He made me drink coffee and insisted that I go back to the program."

Vivian did return to our program. For a while, she sulked quietly during our sessions. As she admitted, she continued to drink. She doubted the program, and doubted she could regain her balance in the face of so much grief and uncertainty. After a few sessions, however, something clicked with Vivian. She began using the audiotapes that include my instructions for eliciting the relaxation response. One specific afternoon proved to be the turning point.

"The day after one of the early sessions, I returned home from graduate school," recalled Vivian. "It was four in the afternoon, and I poured my usual martini. I sat in my chair and picked up the relaxation tape I'd gotten from the program. Suddenly I realized I have a choice. I paid good money for this program and I just made myself a martini. A voice inside me said something about my responsibility to myself. So I started listening to the tape.

"The tape began leading me gently through the relaxation process. As I listened, I started to cry. I literally sat there sobbing. Then the sadness gave way to a sense of relief. I felt that this tape was playing in a part of my brain where infertility and miscarriage could not get me. I had found refuge inside myself.

"Afterward, I got up and poured the martini down the sink. An hour later, Peter called. I said hello. He said, 'What have you done?' He could tell from my voice that something was different. I said, 'Come home. I'll explain.'

"When Peter got home, he asked again, 'What happened?' I held up the tape and said, 'This happened.' The tape, and the program, had changed my life."

I disagree with Vivian. The tape and program had not changed her life. The tape and program brightly illuminated a part of her own being that was capable of change. Once that happened, there was no turning back. She became an active participant in every phase of our Mind-Body Program.

The results were dramatic. The martini Vivian poured down the sink turned out to be her last. When she first entered our program, I observed her carefully because she was so seriously depressed. I was ready to refer her to a psychiatrist and an alcohol treatment program. As it happened, neither was necessary. Vivian's participation enabled her to overcome chronic anxiety and depression, as well as alcohol abuse.

Still wanting to become a biological mother, Vivian continued to try to get pregnant. All told, she had ten miscarriages. Today, Vivian has stopped trying to have a child. But she and Peter are genuinely at peace with their decision. They do not currently plan to adopt, but have left the door open to future adoption. In the past two years, her quality of life has only gotten better, despite her traumatic history of miscarriages. She's flourishing in graduate school. She has developed a staunchly supportive network of friends and family. She and Peter moved into a lovely new home. Their marriage, which had teetered on the edge of destruction, is now stronger than before.

Vivian is one of the many courageous women I have met in my mind-body practice. The fact that her turning point occurred as she practiced the relaxation response does not surprise me. As she said so eloquently, it is possible to access an inner refuge from even the most traumatic events. Eliciting the relaxation response offers that port in the storm. It is not an escape, however. Nor is it a panacea. It is a respite and a profound reminder that we have the strength and serenity to handle the most painful and challenging circumstances. "Meditation is not an evasion," says Zen Master Thich Nhat Hanh. "It is a serene encounter with reality."

Vivian's relaxation practice gave her that strength and serenity. It calmed her anxieties and melted many of her physical tensions. It allowed her to think straight and helped her to feel her feelings rather than drown them in alcohol.

In this chapter, I offer you a variety of methods for eliciting the relaxation response. As mentioned in the last chapter, Dr. Herbert Benson discovered and defined the relaxation response as an inborn mechanism that offsets the negative effects of our fight-or-flight stress response. Dr. Benson's achievement opened doors of opportunity for the prevention and treatment of stress-related conditions. In a sense, the relaxation response is to stress-related illness what aspirin is to everyday aches and pains—a reliable source of relief. Why is relaxation so versatile? Because stress plays a role in so many chronic diseases that are so difficult to treat, including many women's conditions.

I've been asked whether the actual techniques for eliciting the relaxation response differ for men and women. The answer is probably not, but the application and selection of techniques do differ. Certain methods tend to work best for specific women's conditions, as I will explain shortly. Also, I've found that men tend to gravitate toward directive techniques with clear-cut instructions, such as progressive muscle relaxation. Women are more drawn to visualization, which depends upon the free exercise of one's imagination. But there is no hard and fast division, just as there is no hard and fast division within ourselves between so-called masculine and feminine qualities. Both genders have the need, and the ability, to exercise their logical and intuitive sides.

A major difference between men and women stems from the everyday situations that call upon the need for relaxation. Most men will cite work-associated pressures as their main source of stress, while women more frequently cite relationships. In the area of health, women have their own utterly unique stressors. Consider the woman in the middle of a high-risk pregnancy who finds herself packing a roll of white toilet paper in her pocketbook. What in God's name is she doing with white toilet paper? She wonders about that herself, because she can't believe she's doing it. But she's worried that she'll end up at the house or office of someone who has only pink toilet paper—a color that might obscure the light splotch of blood that would signal an end to her pregnancy. I've worked with more than one woman who's carried around rolls of white toilet paper, and each one lived in a state of abject fear.

Consider also the fifty-year-old postmenopausal woman who worries incessantly about social events in rooms that are too warm or crowded.

What if she has a hot flash? Will sweat start pouring down her face? Will it noticeably stain her shirt? Will the sensation of warmth become so intense that she can no longer carry on a normal conversation? Will her physical appearance during a hot flash be the equivalent of a neon sign that says to everyone, MENOPAUSE! MENOPAUSE!

And what about the otherwise healthy working woman whose latest project—a massive writing job—is due on the day after her daughter's music recital? How is she going to manage her time so she can make it to the recital and meet her project deadline, without collapsing from exhaustion or illness?

These are women who, perhaps like yourself, can use all the stress-reducing help they can get. If you practice relaxation when the going gets rough, the short-term benefits will see you through. Beyond that, you'll experience long-term benefits that will change your physiology and your outlook.

I recommend that you practice some form of relaxation for about twenty minutes every day. Beyond that, I have no rules and regulations to lay down, other than that you follow your instincts. Let your commitment be driven by your deep sense of your own needs, rather than by guilt or obligation. Experiment with various approaches. Weave several of them together, if you so desire. Develop a ritual that is both meaningful and effective for you.

The Benefits of Relaxation, Today and Tomorrow

As you consider the following choices to elicit the relaxation response, bear in mind that your practice will indeed yield both short- and long-term benefits. After your twenty-minute practice, you will generally feel refreshed and becalmed. You'll be better able to face a stressful situation at work or at home.

Let's say that your in-laws, with whom you have a tense relationship, are coming to dinner at your house. You've cleaned the house and prepared the food well in advance of their appointed arrival at 7:00. Normally, you'd spend the last hour panicking about details, even if everything was well in order. Instead, at 6:15 you go into a quiet room to elicit the relaxation response. As a result, when you greet your in-laws you are not only composed, you're actually pleased to see them. You may find that you even enjoy their visit.

A perfect example of short-term yield occurs when you practice relaxation soon before a medical test, a visit to your doctor or dentist, or a surgical procedure. You will likely experience less pain and fear. These immediate effects can last for hours. Countless women I've trained in relaxation report back to me that their breast biopsies, IVF procedures, pelvic exams, or laparoscopic surgeries—to name a few—were far less frightening and uncomfortable. (In the next chapter, I will tell you how to do "mini-relaxations," rapid exercises to calm yourself down when you don't have the time or opportunity to sit quietly for at least fifteen minutes.) These short-term results are ongoing; continue to practice relaxation, and the benefits keep on coming. But just as important are the long-term benefits. At the Division of Behavioral Medicine, we have shown that people who consistently elicit the relaxation response get a "carryover" effect. Rather than simply feeling better for minutes or hours after their practice, patients begin to feel better twenty-four hours a day. Women report that their PMS episodes or hot flashes begin to diminish, and our formal studies bear this out.

Informally, I've found that women's menstrual cramps become markedly less severe. Their anxiety levels plummet. Patients who come for one problem discover that other problems suddenly dissolve. I can no longer count the number of infertility patients who have reported that, after weeks of practicing relaxation, their back pain has completely disappeared.

These long-term benefits usually occur after patients have consistently elicited the relaxation response for two to six weeks. Almost everyone who remains committed to their practice finds improvements in their moods and symptoms. One of my patients with PMS, Martha, had begun to feel irritable all the time. The aftereffects of her weeklong PMS episodes were rippling throughout the month. After only three weeks of meditating, Martha's friends at work began making comments like, "What's up with you? You seem so centered." After hearing this repeatedly, Martha recognized that she *was* more centered. Over time, her entire outlook and state of mind changed for the better.

In the following sections, I present nine different approaches to eliciting the relaxation response. There are many other methods I have not included, simply because I have had no experience teaching them. But these are nine tried-and-true ways to become calmer in mind and body, to reap the short- and long-term benefits of the relaxation response. In each section, I explain the method, how it is practiced, and which individuals and conditions it tends to work best for. Use the guidelines in each section to learn the practice, but also consider using audiotapes to guide your practice. Refer to

Appendix B for a complete list of relaxation tapes you can order from our institute.

Before you start, here are a few basic guidelines worth following:

- Find a quiet place in your home to elicit the relaxation response. If you have a special room you can use, with a chair, bed, or pillows that provide the most comfort, all the better. Some people like to have beautiful paintings, plants, or sacred artifacts nearby—objects that have meaning or carry a message of peace. Others simply require a reasonably comfortable chair.
- Make certain that you won't be disturbed by family members, by the telephone, or even by pets. (Animals are attracted to people who are relaxed. You may love your cat or dog dearly, but a pet's presence in your lap or its licks at your face will disturb your concentration.) This is your time for inner peace, time you need and deserve.
- If you have small children, arrange ahead of time for them to be taken care of or otherwise occupied. You can schedule your relaxation practice at a time when your husband, partner, or someone else is available for caretaking. Or, if they're old enough, you can encourage them to read or watch TV for those twenty minutes, with the proviso that they interrupt you only for something very important.
- Find a regular time of day to elicit the relaxation response. For many women, first thing in the morning is best. Early morning relaxation can set a tone, nourishing the strength and serenity you need throughout the day. Others prefer to elicit the relaxation response before lunch, before dinner, or before sleep. What's preferable is that you find a particular time of day and do your best to stick with it. The sense of ritual is most important, since ritual reinforces commitment. But don't let guilt derail your commitment. If you miss your morning ritual on a hectic day, find time later—even if it's just before bedtime—to practice relaxation.
- You can elicit the relaxation response in any comfortable position. However, sitting is generally preferred, primarily because you are less likely to drift off into sleep than if you are lying down. Many people choose to sit in a straight-backed chair with a cushion or pillow that provides comfort and support. Others sit or kneel on the floor. If you much prefer to lie down on a mattress or mat, feel free to do so, but monitor any tendencies to fall asleep. (Naps don't qualify as relaxation techniques!) Most people elicit the relaxation response with their eyes closed. However, if you prefer, you may keep your eyes open.

- A single session for eliciting the relaxation response generally lasts between fifteen and twenty-five minutes. I have, however, had patients who experience the essential mental and physical changes in as little as ten minutes and others who sit for forty-five. But most patients sit, on average, for twenty minutes once a day. If you are particularly stressed out or simply want to deepen your practice, you can certainly benefit by eliciting the relaxation response twice a day.

Breath Focus

*W*hat happens when we stifle our true anger during a confrontation with a family member? We may not realize it, but we hold our breath. What happens when we hold back tears in front of an authority figure, be it a parent, a boss, or a doctor? We hold our breath. What happens when we dial the phone for results of a Pap smear, mammogram, or pregnancy test? We hold our breath. What happens when we suddenly notice that our stomach sticks out in a sexy, tight new dress? We hold our breath.

In our culture, we learn from an early age to stifle strong emotions and impulses. From a biological standpoint, there is one reliable way of doing so: holding our breath. We can essentially lock up emotions in the walls of our chests. Women are also indoctrinated to believe that a full stomach is unattractive, that the only beautiful body is one with an abdomen as flat as an ironing board. So what do we do? We rigidly hold in our stomachs, which causes us to restrict our breathing. After a while, holding our stomach and our breath becomes second nature and we forget we're doing it. That is when normal breathing becomes seriously impaired. We become shallow "chest breathers," rather than deep "abdominal breathers."

What is the distinction between chest and abdominal breathing, and why does it matter? The answer involves the diaphragm, that sheath of muscle separating the chest cavity, which houses the heart and lungs, from the abdominal cavity. As you inhale, this muscle contracts and drops down, pushing gently on the abdominal organs, making ample room for the lungs to fully expand. As you exhale, the diaphragm relaxes and moves upward as the lungs expel air out your nose and mouth. When we engage in shallow chest breathing, the diaphragm is practically frozen in place. It doesn't fully move down, and our lungs don't fully expand with air and its life-giving oxygen. The lower portion of our lungs, the location of most of the small blood vessels that carry oxygen to our cells, is robbed. Our heart rate and blood pressure may increase, as if to compensate for inadequate oxygenation.

When we engage in healthy abdominal breathing, we get superb oxygen exchange—taking in generous amounts of oxygen as we inhale, completely expelling carbon dioxide as we exhale. Our hearts don't have to work overtime, and our blood pressure tends to remain stable.

Given these physiologic changes, one way to elicit the relaxation response is to make this shift from shallow chest breathing to deep abdominal breathing for an extended period of at least fifteen minutes. This relaxation practice is known as breath focus; it is also a way to let go of mental and physical tensions. Breath focus is perhaps the simplest approach to relaxation. The only individuals who may wish to sidestep breath focus are those with a history of asthma or ongoing bouts with colds or the flu. If you have such a history, or you currently have a bad cold, you may become anxious trying to overcome your physical impediments to deep breathing.

How to Practice Breath Focus

Begin by taking a normal breath. Don't change any aspect of how you breathe; simply take note of your breathing.

Now take a deep, slow breath. Let the air come through your nose and move deeply into your lower belly. Take note of how your belly expands when you take such a deep breath; make no effort to limit this expansion. Then breathe out through your mouth. (Inhaling through your nose and exhaling through your mouth is a suggestion, not a rigid rule. Allow yourself to breathe in whatever way is most comfortable for you.)

Now do one normal breath, then one slow, deep, abdominal breath. Alternate normal and deep breaths several times. As you do so, let yourself become aware of how you feel on each inhalation and each exhalation. Compare and contrast the sensations associated with your normal breathing and your conscious deep breathing. Do you begin to notice that your normal breathing is constricted? Does the deep breathing foster sensations of relaxation?

Once you've noted the differences, take time to practice deep breathing. Let the inhalations expand your belly. Now, on long, slow exhalations, allow yourself to sigh. Repeat this process for several minutes.

For the last ten minutes of breath focus, add another layer to your practice. On the inhalation, imagine that the air traveling in through your nose carries with it a sense of peace and calm. On the exhalation, imagine that the air traveling out of your lungs and mouth is removing tension and anxiety. You may even wish to say these words to yourself on the inhalation: "Breathing in peace and calm." And, on the exhalation: "Breathing out tension and anxiety."

Continue to focus on your deep breathing, letting in peace and calm, letting go of tension and anxiety. You may complete this entire process in about twenty minutes.

The Uses of Breath Focus

Breath focus may be the most universally applicable way to elicit the relaxation response. Regardless of your cultural background, religious beliefs, or current health status, you probably won't have any trouble practicing and appreciating the benefits of breath focus relaxation.

Using the breath as an anchor for mental and physical relaxation is central to many secular and spiritual traditions. Like the ebb and flow of the oceans, breathing represents the heart of our natural biological rhythms. When our breathing is constricted, our being is constricted. After completing a course of mind-body treatment, countless patients have said to me, "I finally learned how to breathe."

Breath focus is particularly useful for women with eating disorders. As you will see, several relaxation methods, such as body scan and progressive muscle relaxation, rely heavily on awareness of the body. Whether the problem is overeating, anorexia, or bulimia, women with eating disorders may become anxious when focusing on the very source of their distress—their bodies.

Women with eating disorders are also generally obsessed with body image, and they restrict their breathing to hold in their stomachs. This often unconscious tactic increases their tension and anxiety, leaving them more vulnerable to stress-related illness. For these women, breath focus can help to overturn one contributor to their suffering—their inability to take a deep breath. Breath focus can jump-start a process of emotional healing.

For some women, breath focus can loosen the strictures they have on their emotions. Ursula, who felt riddled by anxiety, was one such patient. As soon as she began practicing breath focus, everything "began to slow down, like a forty-five-rpm record going down to thirty-three." As her sense of relaxation became deeper, her eyes would fill with tears. "I would almost always have teary eyes," said Ursula, "even though I couldn't always connect the tears to a specific emotion." Over time, however, Ursula did find herself more aware of sadness, anger, and joy. She also experienced tensions in her face, which she would relax with other techniques, such as the body scan. As Ursula became more aware of her underlying emotions, she became considerably less tense and anxious.

Body Scan

We hold tension in every conceivable part of our bodies. Why we store anxieties in certain muscular bundles and not others remains something of a mystery, but each of us has our own special repositories.

After a tough day at work, do your shoulders seize up? Do knots of tension grip the back of your neck and head? Does your forehead feel squeezed by taut bands of muscle? Do you hold anger in your jaw? Anxiety in tight stomach muscles? Grief in a taut little ball in your throat? During an emotionally painful period, does your chest ache? Do you feel a ring of tension around your waist, as if you're wearing an invisible girdle? Is there a constant achiness in your pelvic region?

Though we all carry tension differently, most of us *do* carry tension. Often, we've carried that tension for so long we are barely conscious of its locations in our body. Pauline, a patient in one of my mind-body groups, began to recognize her own bodily tensions only after practicing the body scan relaxation exercise.

"I only did the exercise a few times before I became considerably more relaxed," said Pauline. "It was relatively easy to do and the results were obvious. But what struck me was just how stressed I was. There was so much tension in my body that I wasn't even aware of. As I did the body scan, I became fully aware of that tension, and how much better I felt once I was able to let go."

During the body scan relaxation, you use your mind's eye to scan your body, becoming aware of bodily tension. You also use your breath to focus on these tensions, and to gradually, gently let go of them.

How to Practice Body Scan Relaxation

- Pay attention to your breathing. Allow your stomach to rise as you inhale, and to slowly fall back down as you exhale. Take some time to breathe deeply before you begin the body scan.
- Now concentrate on your forehead. As you breathe in, note the muscles of your forehead. Let yourself become aware of any muscle tension in your forehead. Now, as you breathe out, let go of any muscle

tension you may have in your forehead. Continue this practice—awareness of forehead tension on the in-breath, letting go of forehead tension on the out-breath—for several slow, deep breaths. Now, move down to your eyes and repeat this process. As you breathe in, become aware of any muscle tension around your eyes. As you breathe out, let go of that tension around your eyes. Continue this practice for several slow, deep breaths.

- For the remainder of the body scan exercise, repeat this process: concentrate on any muscle tension in a particular body area as you inhale; let go of that tension as you exhale. Again, make certain to take nice, slow, deep breaths, perhaps noticing how your stomach rises as you inhale and falls as you exhale.

Now move down gradually and repeat the process in these bodily areas:

- Scan your mouth and jaw. You may notice that your jaw drops a bit as you exhale, letting go of tension in that area.
- Scan your neck.
- Scan your back, all the way from the top of your spine down to your tailbone.
- Scan your shoulders.
- Scan your upper arms, from where they meet your shoulders down to the elbows.
- Scan your lower arms, from the elbows down and including your hands and fingers.
- Scan your chest.
- Scan your stomach.
- Pause for a moment to do a quick mental check on the upper half of your body, from your forehead down to your waist. If you notice any area of muscle tension, concentrate on that area as you breathe in; let go of that tension as you breathe out.

Now move on to the following:

- Scan your pelvis and buttocks.
- Scan your upper legs.
- Scan your lower legs, ankles, and feet.
- As your body scan relaxation comes to a close, do a mental check on your entire body, from your head down to your toes. If you notice

remaining areas of muscular tension, let yourself become aware of them as you breathe in. Let go of these muscle tensions as you breathe out.

The Uses of Body Scan Relaxation

As you can see, body scan is a method for eliciting the relaxation response that offers fairly specific instructions. Others, such as meditation, simply give your mind a "one-pointed" focus—a single word or meaningful phrase. If you have a naturally wandering mind, meditation may be difficult. That doesn't mean you should never attempt to meditate; just that meditation may not be right for you at all times. When particularly anxious, the wandering mind wants guidelines. Body scan offers those guidelines. It is not as directive as some other methods (namely autogenic training and progressive muscle relaxation) but it gives your mind a clear purpose: scanning your body and releasing areas of tension with the help of deep breathing.

Thus, body scan relaxation is a fine choice when the daily grind leaves you physically tense and mentally agitated. Body scan also makes sense if you are someone, by dint of personality or temperament, who has a great deal of trouble keeping your mind focused.

One of my patients, Lorrie, a forty-year-old career counselor, struggled with irritable bowel syndrome (IBS), anxiety, and depression. She had grown up in a dysfunctional family, with both parents in the medical profession. Her father, a psychiatrist, had repeatedly hypnotized her as a child. "They treated me more like a patient than a daughter," she said.

Lorrie's gastrointestinal pains were so intense that she could not tolerate any medication for her mental distress, including Prozac. She went to several psychiatrists but felt they had little empathy. After she finally found a caring psychiatrist who enabled her to make progress with her psychological issues, he moved his practice to another state. She developed toxic hepatitis from one of her IBS medications and eventually required gallbladder surgery. For several years, Lorrie was continually being hospitalized. After so much suffering, Lorrie became suicidal.

Then Lorrie's gastroenterologist told her about our mind-body group. She learned several relaxation methods, including body scan, which released tensions in her lower abdomen. "After a few weeks, I was able to get relief from the IBS," said Lorrie. "I actually had a period of time when I had no pain, no nausea," she said. "My internist thinks the results I've gotten from this group are a miracle."

Much of Lorrie's emotional distress stemmed from her body's betrayal—

the constant pain, uncontrollable symptoms, and rejection of medicines that offered the prospect of relief. Once she learned a method for controlling her physical symptoms, her anxiety and depression began to lift. She found another psychiatrist who could help her, and medication for her depression that she could finally tolerate. Her mood gradually improved. So have her relationships, her zest for living, and her religious faith.

Now, Lorrie says, using the body scan to relieve gastrointestinal pain "is like turning on a switch." She has not had to be hospitalized once over the past three years. The pain still comes in occasional waves, but she can manage it effectively.

"Wednesday morning I woke up at three A.M. feeling like I had an elephant on my chest," she said recently. "The nausea and pain probably stemmed from something I ate that I shouldn't have. I stayed home from work, and I used the body scan tape. I returned to work the next day, just a bit sore. This may be the best I've ever done after an attack. I was able to manage it without medication."

Body scan meditation may not be helpful to women who become anxious when focusing on their bodies. Women with anorexia, bulimia, and other eating disorders might not choose body scan. A woman who has recently had a mastectomy for breast cancer might not wish to concentrate on her chest, if doing so will interfere with her effort to let go of tension. This may also apply to a woman who's undergone a hysterectomy. You may wish to wait until your physical and emotional scars have healed sufficiently to allow you to scan your body with a gentle exploratory spirit, rather than anxious preoccupation.

Many women participating in the Mind-Body Program for Infertility have benefited from body scan relaxation. One of them, Katherine, believes that body scan actually facilitated her medical treatment. Katherine had been trying to conceive a child for three years. She had had several intrauterine inseminations (IUIs), in which her husband's sperm was chemically "washed" and inserted with a small catheter into her womb during ovulation. On these occasions, the infertility specialist performing the procedures had trouble placing the catheter properly. "My cervix was like a closed fist," said Katherine. "He just couldn't get the catheter in there."

After Katherine joined our program, she practiced body scan on a regular basis. She was convinced that relaxing every part of her body, including her pelvis, helped to relax her cervix as well. The next time she had an IUI procedure, she brought her body scan audiotape along with her. This time, the specialist had no trouble placing the catheter. "I'm convinced it was because of the relaxation," commented Katherine. Eventually, with the help of hormone treatments, Katherine was able to conceive a child.

Body scan may be useful for any woman who feels that muscular tension contributes to a health problem, whether that problem is migraines, TMJ, fibromyalgia, gastrointestinal disorders, menopausal hot flashes, pelvic pain, or PMS. Some women with acute or even chronic pain won't wish to focus on their bodies at all; others find that the body scan relaxation relieves their pain. The solution for some is to use body scan when their pain is relatively quiescent.

Progressive Muscle Relaxation (PMR)

*P*rogressive muscle relaxation takes the body scan to another level of concreteness. It is practiced in a similar fashion, but instead of simply noticing tension in particular bodily areas, you actually *increase* the degree of muscular tension before you relax and let go. While this exercise enhances awareness of tension, it also enhances your sensation of release.

PMR, as it is commonly called, was developed by University of Chicago researcher Edmund Jacobson. According to Jacobson, the typical stressed person "does not know what muscles are tense . . . does not clearly realize that he should relax and does not know how. These capacities must be cultivated or acquired anew." Jacobson authored a famous book about his PMR method with the ironic title *You Must Relax*.

Women with acute or chronic pain (e.g., endometriosis, fibromyalgia, migraines, severe backaches) might not wish to practice PMR, since it involves tensing of muscles and could either cause more discomfort in the affected area or call more attention to the source of pain. If you have a condition of acute or chronic pain, yet PMR appeals to you, try tensing and releasing muscles in every part of your body except the area in pain. As with the body scan, women with eating disorders might not wish to utilize such a body-oriented method of relaxation.

How to Practice PMR

- Close your eyes; pay attention to your breathing. (If you'd rather not close your eyes, keep them open and focus on the floor or an object.) Allow your stomach to rise as you inhale, and to fall back down as you exhale. Take some time to breathe deeply before you begin PMR.

- Now concentrate on your forehead. Consciously tighten the muscles of your forehead while counting slowly from one to five. Hold your forehead muscles as tight as you can for the duration of this count. Then let go of your tense forehead muscles while taking a nice, slow, deep breath. Notice your stomach rise as you inhale, and fall back down as you exhale. Now do this again: tighten your forehead muscles for a count of five; release those muscles as you take a slow, deep breath.
- Now, move down to your eyes, and repeat this process. Tighten the muscles around your eyes while counting slowly from one to five. Then let go of these tense muscles while taking a slow, deep breath. Now do this again.
- For the remainder of the PMR exercise, repeat this process twice for each bodily area: tighten the muscles in a particular body area for a count of one to five; release that tension as you take a slow, deep breath.

Now move gradually from one region to another as you practice PMR in these body areas:

- Tighten and release your jaw, letting go of any tension.
- Tighten and release your neck.
- Tighten and release your back, all the way from the top of your spine down to your tailbone.
- Tighten your right shoulder, bringing it upward as high as you can. Let go of the tension.
- Tighten your right upper arm, from the shoulder to the elbow. Then let go of the tension.
- Tighten your right forearm; let go of the tension.
- Tighten your right hand into a fist; let go of the tension.
- Take a moment to notice if your right and left arms feel different now. Is your right arm more relaxed?
- Repeat this process on your left side, tightening and releasing your left shoulder, upper arm, forearm, and hand in the same manner you did on your right side.
- Tighten and release your chest.
- Tighten and release your abdomen.
- Tighten and release your pelvis and buttocks.
- Tighten and release your right upper leg muscles.

- Tighten and release your right lower leg.
- Tighten your right foot by pointing your toes upward; let go of the tension.
- Take a moment to notice if your right and left legs and feet feel differently now. Are your right leg and foot more relaxed?
- Tighten and release your left upper leg muscles.
- Tighten and release your left lower leg.
- Tighten your left foot by pointing your toes upward; let go of the tension.
- As progressive muscle relaxation comes to a close, do a mental check on your entire body, from your head down to your toes. If you notice remaining areas of tension, tense those muscles for a count of one to five; then let go of those muscles as you take slow, deep breaths.

The Uses of PMR

PMR is among the best relaxation practices for people with hyperactive minds. It is especially effective for women who are acutely stressed, whose jobs, families, and social lives have them whirling with activity. If you pictured what went on in their minds, it might look something like a computer running Windows, the program that allows you to open little boxes onto the screen with lists of choices. They have these multiple lists in their heads, constantly floating in and out of awareness. Their bodies are left in the dust by their brains, which speed ahead at a hundred miles an hour, no matter how exhausted their limbs.

Such women often have trouble with less directive methods for eliciting the relaxation response, such as meditation. Progressive muscle relaxation occupies their minds with concrete instructions; there is little opportunity in PMR for women to get lost in repetitive thoughts and laundry lists of things they haven't done that day. At the same time, the active tensing and releasing of tight muscles gently coaxes them to become aware of their neglected bodies.

I know about these hyperactive minds firsthand, because I have one. I love to quietly meditate, a process I will shortly describe. But all too often, my mind is too active to wind down to a single focus, even in a twenty-minute exercise. That's when I find PMR to be a most effective choice for eliciting the relaxation response.

Jeanine came to me troubled by her monthly bouts of PMS. Her mood swings were wild, and she experienced headaches, breast pain, and insomnia. She was a high-powered lawyer with three children, and her mind was constantly racing with details of recent cases, her kids' schedules, social plans, household items to be bought, and chores to be done. Trying to quiet her own mind was a herculean task. Once Jeanine learned PMR, however, she was able to complete a powerful relaxation exercise without getting lost in the endless corridors of mundane thinking. She invariably felt refreshed and more aware that a body was attached to her frenetic head. Over time, her PMS symptoms became far more manageable.

Another patient, Theresa, was undergoing gynecologic tests to determine the cause of her pelvic pain when a large mass was discovered on one of her ovaries. Before she had the mass surgically removed and biopsied, Theresa was in a state of silent panic. Fear raced around her mind in the form of catastrophic thoughts: "I have terminal ovarian cancer." "I'll never have children." During this waiting period, Theresa was able to use progressive muscle relaxation. It gave her mind a simple activity, and it allowed her to release some of the physical tensions caused by so much anxiety. Fortunately, her mass turned out to be a benign cyst.

Many women who have trouble with other techniques, for whatever reasons, respond well to progressive muscle relaxation. You don't have to have a hyperactive mind to benefit; most women, with the previously noted exceptions such as eating disorders, can enjoy PMR. I suggest you turn to this exceptionally helpful method when other approaches are not proving effective.

Meditation

To some, the idea of meditation is fraught with odd images: burning incense, gurus with stringy hair sitting on oversized pillows, pot-smoking devotees of 1960s counterculture. The images are unfortunate, since meditation has a vaunted history, going back at least 2,500 years, as a spiritual practice with no links whatsoever to sex, drugs, or rock 'n' roll.

Many Eastern and Western spiritual traditions have some form of meditative practice, from Buddhism to Hinduism to Judaism. Although each tradition has its own unique philosophic and practical approach to meditation, certain essential features span these traditions. Herbert Benson, M.D., has found that meditation can elicit the relaxation response when it has these basic elements: you turn your attention inward, and focus repetitively on your breathing and a simple word, phrase, or prayer. You also adopt a nonjudgmental attitude toward any thoughts or feelings that float through your consciousness.

When practiced regularly, meditation is a discipline that can yield a profound sense of mental and physical calm. It can clear the mind of cognitive and emotional "clutter." Committed meditators experience an increasing sense of inner peace, and for some, a spiritual connectedness. Spirituality does not need to be the focus of your meditation, though it can be. If you choose a focus word or phrase, it can be entirely secular (e.g., "Peace," "Let It Be") or religious (e.g., "Hail Mary" for Christians, "Shalom" for Jews). Your choice of a focus word or phrase is important; it should have personal meaning for you, or at least foster feelings of tranquility.

For the purposes of the following simple instruction, I offer the old Sanskrit mantra, *Ham Sah*. (*Ham* means "I am"; *Sah* means "that.") Many patients use it because the sounds comfortably reflect the sensations of breathing and letting go. Feel free to substitute other words or phrases.

As mentioned, meditation may be difficult if you have a wandering or racing mind. Some women with racing minds do eventually master and enjoy the practice; it is one discipline that allows them to shift out of mental high gear. Others try so hard to keep out intrusive thoughts that they never relax while meditating.

If you find yourself continuously frustrated, don't bang your head against the wall, as it were. Move on to another technique, or meditate when your mind is not so active. Remember, you should never come to view relaxation as the mental equivalent of vacuuming or defrosting the freezer. Don't use meditation if it feels like a chore.

How to Practice Meditation

Find a comfortable place to sit and either close your eyes or, if you'd rather, keep them open. Plan to sit for about twenty minutes. Starting with the number ten, count down to zero, one number for each breath you take. Notice that your breathing may get slower as you count down.

As you breathe in, begin to concentrate on the word *Ham* (pronounced "Haam") in your mind. Let the sound reverberate, like the Hmmm feeling you get when you sink into a hot bath. As you exhale, concentrate on the word *Sah* (pronounced "Saah") in your mind, like a sigh. Do this for several moments. (Inhale through your nose and exhale through your mouth, if that is most comfortable.)

If your attention wanders, gently bring it back to *Ham* as you inhale, and *Sah* as you exhale.

Continue to note your breathing. As you inhale, pause for a few seconds. As you exhale, pause for a few seconds. Let your breathing slow as you think *Ham* while you inhale, *Sah* when you exhale.

If your mind starts to wander, gently return to *Ham Sah*. Stay as focused as you can on your breathing and these words.

Don't judge yourself as you meditate. If thoughts or feelings intrude on your practice, don't encourage them or push them away. Just gently return to your breathing and *Ham Sah*.

As your time for meditation comes to a close, continue to be aware of your breathing, but start to be aware of where you are, the sounds around you, where you are sitting. When you feel ready, slowly open your eyes, look down for a few moments, and get up gradually.

The Forms and Uses of Meditation

It is normal for meditation to be a circular rhythm, in which you "go off" into thought, then repeatedly come home to your breath and your word or phrase. Over time, you will become more focused and more relaxed. You will especially be able to tune out the negative tape loops in your head—the critical voices, anxious concerns, endless lists of things undone. Liberated from those mind traps, you may achieve a genuinely tranquil state of mind and body.

How do you choose a focus word or phrase? Try out ones that feel right or have meaning, and stick with the one that works best. One of my infertility patients, Yolanda, had been trying to get pregnant for four years. After several high-stakes, high-tech treatments had failed, Yolanda was drained. She was fast losing hope and patience. Yolanda chose the focus phrase *calm perseverance*. In her mind she'd say *calm* as she inhaled, *perseverance* as she exhaled. This practice helped her to continue treatment, with renewed energy and hope.

Iris, a patient who'd suffered multiple miscarriages, used *we will/get there*. Frances, a young woman with breast cancer, selected a focus phrase that many patients with varying conditions have chosen: *calm* on the in-breath, *peace* on the out-breath.

Some patients like a single word or very short phrase on both the in-breath and out-breath. Examples include One, Let Go, Relax, Ocean, Oh Well, Let It Be, My Time, and Love. Repetitive prayer is essentially meditation with the use of phrases that have religious or spiritual significance. I will discuss prayer in the following section.

As mentioned, body-oriented relaxations may not always be suitable for women with eating disorders. By contrast, meditation can be a fine option for these women. Betsy, a slender, fashionable career woman with two children, had developed bulimia, the binge-and-purge syndrome. She had

had an intrusive mother who insisted that she always conform to modelesque proportions. A few years before I met her, work and family pressures had become overwhelming. That's when Betsy felt compelled to binge, but she couldn't accept the idea of any additional poundage. So she began her binge-purge habit.

Betsy's addiction was tenacious, and her treatment was not proceeding as I had hoped. So I made a contract with her: when she got the urge to binge and purge, she would choose instead to listen to an audiotape that guided her through meditation practice. If, after practicing meditation, Betsy still wanted to binge and purge, she could do so. I actually wrote up this agreement, and we both signed on the dotted line.

Though it wasn't easy, Betsy held up her end of our bargain. The fact that our contract had not been compulsory—one more dictate for her to follow—was clearly helpful. So was the meditation practice itself. On almost every occasion, meditating released Betsy from the tensions that drove her to binge and purge. Over a period of months, her bulimia ceased entirely. It's been four years since Betsy has had a bulimic episode.

Prayer

As physician Larry Dossey showed in his book *Healing Words*, the idea that prayer can aid physical healing is more than spiritual fancy. A variety of studies suggest that prayer and spiritual belief can strengthen our own healing capabilities. Jeffrey S. Levin, Ph.D., Associate Professor of Family and Community Medicine at Eastern Virginia Medical School, has turned up "over 250 published empirical studies" in the medical literature that show statistical relationships between spiritual practices and positive health outcomes.

Does prayer work by reducing our psychological anxieties? Does it work by connecting us more deeply to our families and communities? Does it work by invoking a healing energy or higher power? As scientists, we don't have answers. As individuals, we can only turn within to find our own perspectives, ones that acknowledge and honor our most personal beliefs.

Any woman with any medical condition can benefit from prayer, as long as her practice stems from her core beliefs. Individuals who have no ongoing religious or spiritual commitment may choose not to pray, or they can experiment to discover whether the practice is either relaxing or meaningful, or both. Some women may rekindle the flame of early religious experiences or spiritual feelings.

Prayer, of course, comes in many forms. Practice prayer in any way that is comfortable and meaningful for you, given your religious history and spiritual proclivities. Dr. Benson believes that prayer can specifically be used to elicit the relaxation response when practiced in a fashion similar to meditation, with a repetitive word or phrase. The only practical difference is that your phrase or word has a personal, spiritual meaning to you.

The Practice of Prayer

You can practice prayer exactly as you would meditation. (See the script on pages 56–57 for guidance.) However, choose a focus word or phrase that has a personal religious or spiritual meaning for you. The following is a list of focus words and phrases from the major religious and spiritual traditions. (The list is from *The Wellness Book,* by Herbert Benson, M.D., and Eileen M. Stuart, R.N., M.S., published by Birch Lane Press, New York, 1992.) Don't feel constrained by this list; find the focus word or phrase that speaks to you.

Common Focus Words or Phrases for Prayer

Christian

Come, Lord
Lord, have mercy
Our Father
Our Father, who art in heaven

Lord Jesus, have mercy on me
Hail Mary
The Lord is my shepherd

Jewish

Sh'ma Yisroel ("Hear, O Israel")
Echod ("One")
Shalom ("Peace")
Hashem ("The Name")

Eastern

Om (the universal sound)
Shantih ("Peace")

Aramaic

Marantha ("Come, Lord")
Abba ("Father")

Islamic

Allah

The Uses of Prayer

Prayer is especially helpful for patients with life-threatening conditions, including breast and gynecologic cancers. I have also found it useful for women at menopause, who may be coming into or discovering a mature spirituality. For many of these women, prayer offers a dimension of inner peace that cannot be achieved in any other way.

Consider the case of Sophia, who at sixty was struggling with some painful passages. After losing her first husband to illness and her second to divorce, she had settled into her third marriage with a man she loved. But strains appeared in the relationship since she started working for him in his law office. She'd raised her four daughters largely as a single parent, and all of them were now out on their own. Separation anxieties caused difficulties between Sophia and several of her daughters. At the same time, Sophia suffered with aggravating menopausal hot flashes, even after she had started taking estrogen.

Sophia had to work through many psychological issues in order to handle her losses, strengthen her family relations, and find her own path. But most helpful was her practice of prayer. Having been raised Catholic, Sophia returned to her roots in parochial school to find the perfect focus phrase: "Hail Mary Full of Grace."

"I drew on something that was part of my history," explained Sophia. "I repeated 'Hail Mary Full of Grace' as I meditated. It made me feel supported whenever I felt most anxious and alone." Over time, not only did Sophia's hot flashes abate, so did her sense of disconnection and loneliness.

Mindfulness

Based on ancient principles of Tibetan Buddhism, mindfulness is a philosophy as well as a meditation practice that can be summed up in one phrase: being in the moment.

Without realizing it, many of us spend our days so preoccupied with the past or the future that we literally lose touch with the present. Our minds cling to memories or regrets or they hang feverishly on fears and hopes about future events. When this occurs, the here and now starts to slip away, until we go through our daily routines with little awareness. When this form of "mindlessness" takes hold, we cannot be fully present for small pleasures and events, or even for the significant ones.

Mind*ful*ness is the antidote to mind*less*ness. In his wonderful book *Wherever You Go, There You Are*, Jon Kabat-Zinn, Ph.D., founder and director of the Stress Reduction Clinic at the University of Massachusetts Medical Center, referred to mindfulness as "the direct opposite of taking life for granted." Mindfulness is a daily practice that nourishes our capacity for being in the present, which naturally results in a greater appreciation of everything life has to offer, as experienced through our senses, intellects, and emotions.

Mindfulness can be developed by practicing a particular form of meditation, for which I will shortly provide guidelines. But mindfulness is also developed by taking time, each day, to allow ourselves to become fully absorbed and engaged in an activity, whether that activity is a creative work project, washing the dishes, making love, eating a meal, playing with children, or taking a shower.

I recommend a daily practice of mindfulness during some activity, and a patient in one of my groups, Zelda, chose one that she particularly dislikes: making a salad. For her, salad-making was akin to vacuuming—a drawn-out process devoid of pleasure. But when Zelda began taking time to appreciate the process of making a salad, moment by moment, with her senses fully engaged, the experience was transformed.

For the first time, Zelda saw the brightness and vibrancy of the orange carrots and red peppers, and she heard the crunch and snap as she cut vegetables. She recognized the visual splendor of the salad as she tossed in each new ingredient: the mixtures of greens, reds, yellows, and oranges; the design and texture of cut cucumbers and the long spine of each romaine lettuce leaf. From that time on, making a salad was no longer a chore for Zelda. It was an opportunity to be in the present, to find pleasure in ordinary experience.

Mindfulness, as both a daily practice and a meditation, can also help us to manage stress. How so? The feeling of being stressed-out can melt away when we anchor ourselves in the here and now, experiencing an object, engaging in an activity, or just being fully present as we sit quietly.

Several years ago, I was buying my first house and was about to be married. The house closing and wedding plans coincided to create an inordinately stressful period for me. Although the events were happy ones, the massive changes in my lifestyle, and the seemingly endless list of responsibilities and chores, set me on edge. During this time, I was having some trouble eliciting the relaxation response.

Then I began taking a pottery course every Thursday night. I would invariably come to the class in a state of overload from house- and wedding-related problems. I was learning how to use the electric wheel to throw pots. When you make pots at the wheel, absolute concentration is required; one slip and your pot is ruined. I would sit at the wheel with total focus for two hours, and I would leave the class every Thursday in a state of bliss. The house, the wedding, and the people I felt I had to keep happy—it all fell away at the altar of the whirring pottery wheel.

In other words, my stressful preoccupations about the future evaporated as soon as I found an anchor in the present. You can find a similar anchor, and it matters not what activity you choose, but rather the quality of attention you bring to that activity. As Kabat-Zinn writes, "Mindfulness means paying attention in a particular way: on purpose, in the present moment, and nonjudgmentally. This kind of attention nurtures greater awareness, clarity, and acceptance of present-moment reality." By gently putting aside our mental attachments to the past and future, this kind of mindful attention opens up the here and now, the only realm in which we are capable of joy and fulfillment.

Remember that mindfulness can be applied to everyday activities, but it is also cultivated through a specific meditation practice. (I recommend Kabat-Zinn's first book, *Full Catastrophe Living*, for a complete discussion of mindfulness practices.) Here, I offer you an exercise in mindful activity as well as a mindfulness meditation, and I suggest that you try both.

The Practice of Mindfulness

Use the following exercise to give yourself an opportunity to become mindful during the simplest imaginable activity: eating a Hershey's Kiss.

MINDFUL ACTIVITY: Go get yourself a Hershey's Kiss and eat it mindfully. By that I mean, eat it with full awareness of every movement, bite, and sensation from moment to moment. First, peel off the foil wrapper. Notice the little white tag that twirls inside the kiss. Crunch up the foil and notice how this sounds and feels. Look at the chocolate kiss. Observe its shape and texture. As you take your first bite, attend to every sensation on your lips, tongue, the roof of your mouth. Eat slowly, savoring each bite and fully receiving every taste sensation.

Take as much time as you need to complete this exercise. You may also peel and eat an orange, or eat a raisin, as Jon Kabat-Zinn recommends. Remember that the purpose is the gradual cultivation of awareness in the present, anchored by your senses and a deliberate effort to savor each moment as it unfolds. When in doubt, eat more slowly. The slower your practice, the more likely it is that you will experience the state of being in the moment.

MINDFULNESS MEDITATION: Mindfulness meditation is simply another way to cultivate experience in the present, although it is a more disciplined approach. Begin as you would with meditation, becoming aware of and focusing on your breathing. You may wish to use a focus word or phrase, but for mindfulness meditation this is not necessary. Use one if it feels comfortable to do so. If you don't use a focus word or phrase, simply concentrate on the sensations of your breathing—your belly as it rises and falls, the air as it enters your nostrils and leaves your mouth.

You may notice that thoughts are continuously arising, perhaps in the form of worries, anxieties, fears, hopes, or fantasies. This is a natural process of the mind. So as you sit in stillness, your body in a state of quiet and relaxation, watch each thought as it comes and goes. Be mindful toward the process of thinking. Notice how the thoughts are always subtly shifting, moving, dissolving.

When you notice that you've been carried away in a stream of associations, in a stream of thoughts, just observe that this has happened. Without judgment, without being hard on yourself, gently return to awareness of your breath, being aware of the breath in the foreground, while the thoughts may continue in the background. The breath is the most natural way to center ourselves and be anchored in the present moment.

For the remaining time, keep your breathing in the foreground of your awareness. To the best of your ability, keep whatever else may arise—sensations in the body, thoughts in the mind, sounds in the environment—in the background. If they intrude, don't struggle with them. Rather, be aware of them and simply return to your breathing.

As you complete this mindfulness meditation, know that the benefits can expand, enabling you to bring full attention to whatever you do during the rest of the day. Now, at your own pace, bring your awareness back to your surroundings.

The Uses of Mindfulness

Jon Kabat-Zinn reminds us of a basic truth, one worth remembering as we practice mindfulness: "If you have a mind, it is going to wander." A key to mindfulness meditation is your ability to accept rather than judge this wandering tendency.

Let go of anxiety about how you're doing. Intrusive thoughts and emotions can't be avoided; they are not a sign that you're a failure at mindfulness or any other meditation. Neither cling to these thoughts nor push them forcefully out of your awareness. Mark them in your mind, as you might an interesting dream that has drifted in and out of your sleep. Observe and acknowledge them; then gently bring your awareness back to your breathing.

If you try mindfulness meditation, let the experience seep into your everyday life. Bring your newfound ability to be in the moment along with you as you conduct business, take care of your home, enjoy your environment, exercise, eat, make love, relate to your friends and family. No matter how stressed you are by ongoing events, you will still appreciate small moments if you remain mindful. You can enjoy the scent of soap or shampoo as you shower; the crunch of your breakfast bagel; the smell of fresh air when you first step outside on a lovely spring morning. The notion of stopping to smell the roses may seem a cliché, but it certainly applies to overburdened women.

Many of my patients with emotionally devastating conditions turn to mindfulness practice to find peace and stillness within. Rediscovering the capacity to enjoy the smallest of pleasures becomes an authentic priority. On occasion, these patients are too anxious to sit quietly and meditate, mindfully or otherwise. I recommend to them that they take a mindful walk.

Mindful walking is among the most useful and pleasurable ways to become relaxed, to reorient yourself in the present. Take the most pleasant route you can think of, then let your senses be the guide. Walk slowly, fully experiencing the sensations of walking, one step at a time. Smell the aroma of grass, trees, the city, whatever odors waft into your space. Notice the sights—houses, buildings, your neighbors and their activities. Really listen to the sounds of birds chirping, dogs barking, flies buzzing, cars honking. If anxious, negative, or repetitive thoughts intrude on your awareness, gently return to your focus on the sensations of walking and the sights, sounds, and smells around you. When thoughts intrude, don't judge them. Just nudge yourself gracefully back into the present moment.

Andrea was thirty-two years old when she was diagnosed with vaginal cancer. The diagnosis came immediately after the birth of her second child. A vital woman with enormous energy and heart, Andrea was overwhelmed by her prognosis, which was extremely poor. Like so many other cancer patients, she began to live by the philosophy of *carpe diem*—seize the moment. In tune with that philosophy, she found it most useful to take mindful walks, especially when it was too hard to sit quietly and meditate.

Andrea had lived near a lovely ocean beach most of her life. During the worst times after her diagnosis, she would take mindful walks on that beach. "I had strolled that stretch of beach a million times before," she told me. "It wasn't until I did so mindfully that I really saw and felt the beauty of that beach."

But you certainly do not have to have a life-threatening illness to live in the moment, because every facet of your quality of life improves when you become mindful. Lydia, a young woman who struggled with infertility for three years, had been through countless medical procedures and hormone shots with no success. When her older sister conceived within a few months of trying, Lydia was unable to experience any emotion other than stark envy. Her unhappiness kept her at a distance from her family and it colored every experience, most especially the birth of her niece.

But the assignment that week in the Mind-Body Program for Infertility was to do something mindfully. Lydia decided to visit her sister and her new baby in the hospital. She was miserable on the way over, but she entered her sister's room with the intention of tuning out the past.

"I decided to be in the moment," recalled Lydia. "And when I got there, I saw my grandmother, who was ninety years old, holding my niece. I really took in that image—my niece, barely a day old, in the arms of my ninety-year-old grandmother. Then I held the baby in my arms, and I let myself enjoy that completely, in the moment. While I was there, everything my husband and I had been through seemed to fall away."

Allowing herself to be in the present with her sister, her niece, and her grandmother had a healing effect on Lydia, and on her relationships with her family members.

Guided Imagery

You can elicit the relaxation response by imagining mental pictures of scenes, places, or experiences that evoke a sense of inner calm. This process, known as guided imagery, is a mind-body approach with a vast variety of forms and uses.

Guided imagery was first popularized as a treatment for cancer patients. In the late 1970s, two teams of practitioners—Jeanne Achterberg, Ph.D., and Frank Lawliss, Ph.D., and O. Carl Simonton, M.D., and Stephanie Simonton, Ph.D.—developed a method by which cancer patients would visualize their white blood cells, or their chemotherapy drugs, destroying their cancer cells. The white cells or drugs would be viewed as saviors on white horses, heroic soldiers, snapping Pac-Men—any image that conjured strength and ruthless efficiency for a good cause. The cancer cells would be viewed as confused or weak—spineless jellyfish, for example. In the mind's scenario, the heroic cells or drugs were seen attacking and overwhelming the less powerful cancer cells.

These research teams produced data suggesting that cancer patients who used guided imagery, along with psychotherapy and other supportive treatments, could outlive their doctors' expectations for their survival. But some of the researchers' scientific methods have been questioned, and the notion that guided imagery can be used to fight cancer directly remains a complex and controversial one.

What has been shown, beyond a shadow of a doubt, is that guided imagery can lessen the side effects of chemotherapy and reduce pain in cancer patients. Guided imagery has also been proven as an effective approach to stress management, relaxation, and psychological well-being.

Since I cannot shed any new light on whether guided imagery helps people overcome cancer or any other disease, I recommend to my patients that they use this approach, first and foremost, as a method for relaxation, self-awareness, pain reduction, and the management of side effects and symptoms. Should they receive additional benefits in the form of disease remission, all the better. But the most effective psychological approach—the one least complicated by uncertain or unproven expectations—is to use imagery to improve your quality of life.

For this purpose, guided imagery is among the most powerful methods available. Rachel Naomi Remen, M.D., has described imagery as the "language of the unconscious." Indeed, we can rediscover lost parts of ourselves—including the part capable of deep tranquility—through the use of guided imagery.

You can elicit the relaxation response by conjuring images that others have developed for this purpose. I use a number of specific imagery exercises that my patients find helpful. In one, you see yourself taking a walk on a deserted beach; another has you strolling a path toward a mountain stream; yet another has you slowly entering a luxurious hot bath. The easiest way to introduce yourself to guided imagery is to use an audiotape. You can order these specific tapes, and other relaxation tapes, by writing to our institute at the address listed in Appendix B. But I also suggest that women develop their own imagery exercises, ones that speak to their own unique past and present experiences, memory stores, and dreams.

The Practice of Guided Imagery

Find a quiet place where you can sit in a comfortable position. Take several slow, deep, cleansing breaths.

Now go in your mind to a special place that you love, a place where you have felt relaxed or know you would feel relaxed. It can be a favorite vacation spot; your parents' or grandparents' backyard; a place you have seen in the movies. It does not matter what environment you choose, as long as it makes you feel at peace.

Now spend time in this place, seeing yourself sitting or standing in one spot, if that is most peaceful; or moving along, if that is most peaceful. Take in the sounds, smells, and views all around you.

Focus on colors and shapes. If you are out of doors, note the color of the sky, the shape of the clouds. See the whole expanse of sky, or sand, or grass, or forest, or stream. If you're in your grandmother's backyard, see the scene in its entirety.

Focus on smells. If you're on a beach, smell the ocean smells or the suntan lotion. If you're in your grandmother's backyard, recall the smells there and conjure them up. Savor the fresh-air smells deep in the forest, by your favorite brook.

Focus on sounds. Listen to the ocean waves breaking; the sound of your grandmother's voice; the gurgling of water across rocks in the brook.

Focus on movement. See the movement of clouds, or water, or seagulls, or cars. If you wish, see yourself moving—walking on the sand inspecting seashells; traipsing through high grass in the backyard; bounding from rock to rock in the brook.

Focus on sensations. Feel the salty ocean air on your skin; the grass tickling your naked feet; the slippery surfaces of the rocks as you step along in that brook.

Allow yourself to become totally absorbed in the sensual aspects of these images, all in a place where you feel comfortable, at home, at peace. If your sense of peace is interrupted by anxious or disturbing thoughts or images, observe them. Then gently return to the specific sights, smells, and sensations that surround you.

The Uses of Guided Imagery

One key reason that it's useful to create your own images relates to the deeply personal aspect of visualization. Put simply, one woman's beautiful beach scene may be another woman's nightmare. Indeed, some practitioners of guided imagery will have all their clients imagine a beach scene as a way to relax. But what about the red–haired, fair–skinned woman who was constantly burned by the sun as a young child? For her, visualizing the beach might not be the least bit relaxing. As with any relaxation method, there is no one–size–fits–all approach, because each of us brings our own singular history to the practice.

When I was first taught guided imagery, I was led to visualize a scene where I would stroll in the middle of a sprawling field full of budding flowers during midsummer. Sound relaxing? It wasn't for me, and it didn't take long to figure out why. I have a potentially fatal allergic reaction to bee stings. A sprawling field of budding flowers is not a place I want to be!

Hannah, a thirty–five–year–old participant in one of my mind–body groups, was led in a guided imagery of walking along the banks of a river. Suddenly, she burst into sobs. As it happened, as a young child Hannah had been walking along a river when she came upon a dead body. She had completely repressed this memory until the imagery exercise.

If you are looking to unearth repressed memories, then visualizing disturbing scenes or places might actually be useful. But if you are trying to experience inner peace, you must conjure images that are peaceful to you and you alone. You must honor your own history.

One breast cancer patient, Marla, was struggling with the side effects from her chemotherapy. Nothing seemed to allay the terrible nausea and vomiting. It had gotten to the point where she was becoming nauseous long before her next treatment—what is known to oncologists as "anticipatory nausea." Finally, Marla hit upon the relaxation technique that effectively relieved her anticipatory nausea and reduced her vomiting. She remembered how calm and happy she felt as a child lying in a hammock in her grandparents' backyard. Before, during, and after her chemotherapy treatments, Marla would breathe deeply and take herself back to that hammock, where she would see and hear the same sights and sounds she did as a child, when she felt so safe, serene, and loved.

Some women have difficulty transporting themselves to an imaginary place. If you find visualization difficult, don't judge yourself; not everyone sees pictures clearly in her mind's eye. But I have found a method that helps some women who have difficulty transporting themselves to imaginary scenes. Taught to me by Irene Goodale, the technique is relatively simple: first imagine yourself on a magic carpet, then have the carpet take you to that special place of beauty and serenity.

The magic carpet ride isn't for every woman, either. But it can evoke that magical childhood belief in limitless possibilities. Whether you have trouble visualizing or not, you might try this exercise. Renée, a woman who said she felt hounded by daily stressors, loved the magic carpet imagery because it produced some ecstatic sensations. "More than flying, I had a sense of floating and weightlessness," recalled Renée. "It was wonderful and incredibly relaxing." Renée would then be transported to mountaintops, meadows, ocean beaches. But the carpet ride was often the most joyful part of her imaginary trips. "One time I got my husband to come along for the ride," she said. "I gave him a real guided tour."

Autogenic Training

*A*utogenic training uses verbal suggestions to help you achieve a state of profound relaxation. It was developed by the German doctor Johannes Schultz as a form of progressive relaxation for the body. The verbal suggestions, called orientations, are a subtle form of self-hypnosis. When you use autogenic training, you are essentially bypassing your conscious mind in order to instruct your body to relax. There's a sound logic to this process: since our minds so often obstruct our body's effort to calm down, we can set up more direct lines of communication with the body. That's what happens during autogenic training.

For women who have trouble doing breath focus or meditation, autogenic training is a sensible choice. It gives your mind a clear focus, so intrusive thoughts are less likely to derail your practice. Autogenic training also works well for women who get mentally waylaid during body scan, or who don't respond to the muscular activity of PMR.

The Practice of Autogenic Training
Get comfortable and have someone slowly read you these instructions (adapted from Herbert Benson, M.D., "The Relaxation Response," in *Mind-Body Medicine,* edited by Daniel Goleman and Joel Gurin, published by Consumer Reports Books, New York, 1993), or make a tape recording to use until you get the hang of it.

Focus on the sensations of breathing. Imagine your breath rolling in and out like ocean waves. Think quietly to yourself, "My breath is calm and effortless . . . calm and effortless. . . ." Repeat the phrase to yourself as you imagine waves of relaxation flowing through your body: through your chest and shoulders, into your arms and back, into your hips and legs. Feel a sense of tranquility moving through your entire body. Continue for several minutes.

Now focus on your arms and hands. Think to yourself, "My arms are heavy and warm. Warmth is flowing through my arms into my wrists, hands, and fingers. My arms and hands are heavy and warm." Stay with these thoughts and the feelings in your arms and hands for several minutes.

Now bring your focus to your legs for a few minutes. Imagine warmth and heaviness flowing from your arms down into your legs. Think to yourself: "My legs are becoming heavy and warm. Warmth is flowing through my feet . . . down into my toes. My legs and feet are heavy and warm."

Now scan your body for any points of tension, and if you find some, let them go limp, your muscles relaxed. Notice how heavy, warm, and limp your body has become. Think to yourself: "All my muscles are letting go. I'm getting more and more relaxed."

Finally, take a deep breath, feeling the air fill your lungs and move down into your abdomen. As you breathe out, think, "I am calm . . . I am calm. . . ." Do this for a few minutes, feeling the peacefulness throughout your body.

Then, as your practice session ends, count to three, taking a deep breath and exhaling with each number. Open your eyes and get up slowly. Stretch before going back to everyday activities.

The Uses of Autogenic Training

Women with breast or gynecologic cancers, as well as women struggling with infertility or multiple miscarriages, often respond well to autogenic training. Their ongoing stressors are so intense that they require a directive practice that guides them into a state of relaxation. They can "give themselves up" to the gentle suggestions, and their bodies follow suit.

Autogenic training also provides relief for many patients with chronic pain. For women whose pain or anxiety keeps them up at night, autogenic training is a superb treatment for insomnia. The sensations of warmth and heaviness often put them to sleep within minutes.

Although autogenic training is effective for some women at menopause, others who experience hot flashes might not respond well, since several suggestions require them to generate sensations of warmth. Women with eating disorders may not wish to focus on their bodies so much. Those struggling with obesity, anorexia, or bulimia don't necessarily want to experience parts of their bodies as being heavy.

Yoga

Yoga is a three-thousand-year-old practice, based on Indian philosophical teachings, that involves physical postures, meditation, and deep breathing. Although many people associate yoga with the famous lotus posture, this extraordinary discipline is much more than sitting with legs folded in the shape of a pretzel. Yoga is undoubtedly the earliest known mind-body system designed to heighten awareness and promote healing.

There are many different yogic systems, but certain basic elements are shared by them all, including *pranayamas,* or breathing purifications; *asanas,* which are stretching postures; and various meditation practices. Pranayama practices are exercises in directing breath within the body, which helps to improve oxygenation and revitalize our energy. (According to the ancient traditions, *prana* is our vital force or life energy; pranayama practices assimilate that vital force into the body.) Asana postures, which also involve rhythmic breathing, help to increase body awareness and flexibility while releasing muscular tensions. Yogic meditations involve centering and the development of inner tranquility.

Hatha-yoga is one yogic system that includes a variety of asanas, or physical postures. Margaret Flood Ennis, M.A., Director of Training and Relaxation Therapies at our Division of Behavioral Medicine, teaches hatha-yoga to our patients, including the women who attend my mind-body groups. The hatha-yoga exercises she teaches are practiced while seated in a chair or on the floor, or standing. These exercises combine breathing with slow, gentle physical postures and movements.

Many of my patients with widely varying women's conditions find yoga to be an enormously valuable and effective way to relax, release tensions, reconnect with their bodies, and relieve symptoms. Margaret Caudill, M.D., Ph.D., who directs the mind-body groups for chronic pain patients in our division, points out that yoga is helpful to anyone with pain because the exercises are slow, nonstrenuous, and coordinated with breathing.

The Practice of Yoga

Yogic exercises are not like aerobics or calisthenics; they represent a gentle, noncompetitive system of stretching, moving, and breathing in coordinated ways that relax, balance, and revivify our mind-body systems. These exercises should also be calibrated carefully to individuals, which is why I would rather not offer a laundry list of poses. Margaret Ennis strongly suggests that women who wish to practice yoga for health, stress reduction, and relief from specific symptoms should "shop around" for a yoga teacher whose instruction and techniques meet their needs. Because there are so many different systems, it makes sense to try a few different teachers before settling on one who inspires your commitment. A good yoga teacher will provide advice on postures and adjustments that are specific for you.

Ms. Ennis believes that teachers are better than books for learning how to do yoga, but you can get a flavor, as well as some guidance, from a few books she recommends, including *Yoga for Women,* by Paddy O'Brien, and *Complete Stretching,* by Maxine Tobias. I also recommend Ennis's chapter in *The Wellness Book* by Herbert Benson, M.D., and Eileen M. Stuart, R.N., M.S. In this chapter, entitled "Tuning In to Your Body, Tuning Up Your Mind," Ennis offers a variety of yogic exercises with clear directions. She instructs anyone who does yoga to bring to their practice two essential elements, which actually apply to any method for eliciting the relaxation response: focused awareness and a nonjudgmental attitude.

In her clinical experience, Ennis has found certain postures to be particularly useful for women with conditions affecting their reproductive organs. "I often teach women the forward-bending postures, as well as other postures that essentially massage the female organs by moving them in gentle ways." According to Ennis, exercises such as "knee to chest," in which the person lies on her back and draws the knees in toward the belly, can massage these organs, enhancing blood circulation and releasing tensions. Other postures with similar effects are the "child pose," and the "cat pose," which are detailed in "Tuning In to Your Body, Tuning Up Your Mind." (The child pose has repeatedly been observed to alleviate panic attacks.)

Yoga is about tranquility and mind-body unity, and, like mindfulness, should not be practiced in feverish pursuit of some goal, be it weight loss, muscle-building, fertility, or a cancer cure. The purpose, as Ennis so rightly points out, is not to "tie our body up in knots," but rather to take better care of our bodies, with gentleness, kindness, and a fine-tuned awareness.

The Uses of Yoga

Yoga can be a godsend to women with racing minds. Whether healthy or ill, women who can't sit still to elicit the relaxation response, because their heads are filled with lists and anxious thoughts, can tune right into their bodies through yoga. Margaret Ennis points out that yoga, by releasing muscular tensions, helps to quiet the mind. (Many mind-body practitioners hold the view that we carry mental tensions in muscular bundles; relieving these tensions—whether through yoga, t'ai chi, or physical exercise—relaxes not only the body but also the mind.)

Many of my most stressed-out female patients love yoga, and the long-term benefit is better overall health and the reduction of specific symptoms. For instance, the forward-bending postures recommended by Margaret Ennis may help relieve PMS and menstrual cramping. In *The Endometriosis Answer Book,* Neils H. Lauersen, M.D., a leading obstetrician/gynecologist, recommends similar poses to increase pelvic circulation and relieve menstrual cramps.

In *The Menopause Self-Help Book*, Susan Lark, M.D., recommends certain yoga postures as helpful for relieving the hot flashes, vaginal changes, and insomnia so common among menopausal women. Poses such as "the locust," "the wide angle," and "the pump" are suggested for women with these symptoms, and I recommend Dr. Lark's book for a complete description and guidelines.

Yoga may also carry psychological and spiritual benefits for women suffering emotionally from medical conditions. Women who have had mastectomies or hysterectomies, or who struggle with infertility or miscarriage, may not feel whole and complete. Margaret Ennis explains the value of yoga for these women:

> Many women believe that they are not complete because they have lost a breast or cannot have a child—whatever the reason. The experience of relaxation they get from Hatha yoga includes a sense of completeness, of fullness, of being enough, of being okay. And that is really their basic state. Before, they were saddled with stories imposed by our culture, which led them to thoughts such as: "I'm not good enough." "I'm not accomplished enough." "I'm not a whole woman." Yoga and relaxation enable them to experience themselves as whole and complete. It has the power to change thought structures, because it takes them to an expanded yet firmly grounded experience of themselves. With this understanding, they can create their lives anew.

Developing Your Own Relaxation Ritual

Cultures other than our own carve out much more time for relaxation. Many European countries break their workdays in two, allowing for relaxation at midday. The Spanish siesta is a perfect example, where people stop work and return home for a sumptuous feast and hours of relaxation. Our nonstop culture keeps us going from early morning to early evening, and sometimes longer, with only minimal time for breaks and lunch. As we whiz through life, we often forget our profound needs for mental respite and bodily rest.

Women often forget these needs so completely that they feel they don't *deserve* mental respite and bodily rest. Before you begin to develop a relaxation ritual, you must accept—on a deep level—that you deserve to take twenty minutes out of your day for mental and physiologic relaxation. It is a need, a right, and a health prescription you ought to take.

Other people, including your mate, may interfere with your relaxation ritual. Certainly, many of us have mates who will be thrilled by and supportive of our efforts, but some mates won't be. I've observed cases where husbands wittingly or unwittingly sabotaged their wives' efforts to elicit the relaxation response. Why would they? The reasons are many, but I've seen instances where husbands were threatened by their wives' increasing sense of control as they became less anxious. These husbands seemed to depend upon their wives' being needy and uncertain. Other husbands were jealous of their wives for the time they took to relax, time they would not allow themselves.

You may therefore have to assert your need and right to twenty minutes per day to practice relaxation. One woman with chronic pain delivered this sermon to her family: "I am taking my time now to practice relaxation. I want to be left alone. I want to be protected from the phone and any other outside interference. Only interrupt me if someone is hemorrhaging."

Lauren was a recently divorced single parent of three preteens; she also had a difficult part-time job and a load of monthly bills. Given the enormous stress of her work and financial situation, Lauren was often overwhelmed by the demands of her energetic kids. How could she ever steal away time for relaxation? At one point, she began taking her audiotape player with her into the bathroom. She'd sit on the toilet, stick on her headphones, and lock the door.

As I have emphasized, use only those relaxation methods that you learn from experience are effective. But don't feel you must stick with only one method. Your personality changes, your moods change; let your relaxation practice change with them. Use what works when it works; move on when it doesn't. Cultivate a commitment to your relaxation practice, but never let it become an obligatory drag. If you miss a day, return to your practice the next day. My hope is that you will become motivated to elicit the relaxation response because it is so pleasurable, and because the short- and long-term benefits are so welcome.

Eliciting the relaxation response is the best first step in any program of mind–body transformation. Dr. Benson hits upon the reason, I believe, when he speaks and writes about the way relaxation opens the mind and heart. "Immediately after you elicit the relaxation response, you become calmer, less anxious, and you learn better," he explains. "If you are anxious, you can't learn. It's like dropping seeds on concrete. With a quiet mind, people take things in."

Regardless of their state of health or illness, women who regularly elicit the relaxation response are better able to "take things in." They are more open to changing their negative thoughts, sharing their feelings, seeking help, asserting their needs, taking time out to enjoy life. In short, they are more able to grow. Seeds of awareness take root, and in time, they sprout into full flower.

Four

• • •

MINI-RELAXATIONS:
THE PERFECT PORTABLE
STRESS MANAGERS

*T*he young mother is having a bad day. Her infant son has been crying for twenty minutes, and she can't figure out what's wrong. He doesn't seem interested in the breast, so he must not be hungry. He clearly doesn't need a diaper change. Is she holding him too much? Not enough? She's not sure. He keeps on crying, and now his frustration has rubbed off on his three-year-old sister, who starts flinging pieces of a puzzle to different corners of the living room. The mother picks up each piece and puts it back in the puzzle box. Her baby's cries get louder, so she moves back toward him. With mother's back turned, daughter dumps the puzzle pieces back onto the floor, and begins tossing them all over again.

The mother has had it. "How can I handle this on my own?" she asks herself, and she has no answer. All she wants to do is crawl under the covers. She can feel her insides churning. Then she remembers her fallback strategy. In the middle of the living room, she stops for a moment, standing between one screaming infant and one angry toddler, and simply breathes. She slowly takes a deep breath. As she takes in air, she says in her head, "One, two, three, four." Then she pauses. As she lets out air, she says, "Four, three, two, one." She does this a few more times, then turns her attention back to the living room chaos.

The mother feels saner now. Her body isn't as tight, and her mind is clearer. Without anger, she firmly instructs her daughter to put the pieces back in the box herself. Her daughter, taken aback, complies, while the mother goes over to her son still crying in his crib. She picks him up, this time bouncing him around in the air. His crying slowly subsides. She guesses that her son needed that kind of stimulation. The mother goes back about her business in a world that no longer seems unmanageable.

This young mother, one of my patients, turned around her day with the help of a "mini-relaxation" exercise. Mini-relaxations, or "minis" for short, are among the most useful tools of the mind-body medicine I practice with women. The primary purpose and focus of mini-relaxations is to shift from shallow chest breathing to deep abdominal breathing. You may wonder, "Can such a quick breathing exercise really enhance my ability to cope in a meaningful way?" Based on my clinical experience, the unequivocal answer is yes.

Most of the women I work with, regardless of their condition and whether they are currently sick or currently well, use mini-relaxations to handle havoc in their inner and outer environments. I have had patients who use minis over a hundred times in a single day. These women report that minis are among the most important skills they have learned, because they can rely on them to provide a physical and psychological lift anywhere, anytime, in any circumstance. Within moments, they say, minis take the edge off their anxiety, quiet their racing physiology, and revive their sense of control.

The Breath That Makes a Difference

*W*hat explains such swift and salutary effects? How could such a brief exercise in deep breathing make such a profound difference? The answers lie in our normal tendency toward inadequate breathing, with serious negative consequences for our mental and physical well-being.

As I discussed in the "Breath Focus" section of the previous chapter, when we're anxious or upset, we restrict our breathing. Very few of us are immune to this effect; when tense, we unknowingly engage in shallow chest breathing rather than abdominal breathing.

Unless we consciously change this state of affairs, the mind-body connection starts to work against us. How so? When we don't get sufficient oxygen exchange, alarms are sounded in our brains and bodies. The fight-or-flight response increases, even if stress in our environment is stable or recedes. A vicious cycle ensues: Fight-or-flight and its attendant stress hormones keep us anxious and sustain the shallow breathing. Our diaphragms remain stuck, and so does our state of agitation. We often can't think straight, and we experience a variety of emotional and physical symptoms. We lose oxygen, energy, and we no longer recall what it feels like to be calm.

Have you ever watched a baby breathe? Take note: babies are abdominal breathers. It takes years of this cycle of anxiety, along with cultural conditioning, before we become habitual shallow breathers.

Over time, shallow breathing results in emotional distress and physical exhaustion. Some medical reports, dating back to the 1940s, implicate shallow breathing in chest pain and heart disease. Breathing disorders have also been noted in vast numbers of people who suffer with fibromyalgia, irritable bowel syndrome, TMJ, insomnia, chronic dizziness, and imbalanced immunity. Shallow breathing has been observed in people who are fatigued, and in people with full-blown chronic fatigue syndrome. This link should not be hard to understand: every one of our billions of bodily cells requires oxygen as a source of energy.

"We have become a nation of shallow, thoracic—chest—breathers," writes researcher and clinician Sheldon Saul Hendler, Ph.D. "Most of us do not use the diaphragm the way it was intended to be used; many of us scarcely use it at all. Rapid, shallow breathing, often punctuated by frequent sighing, yawning, and erratic breathing rates characterize this epidemic of oxygen starvation. Futile breathing results in serious disturbances in blood chemistry, altering proper acid-alkaline balance."

To make matters worse, women have special difficulty with deep breathing. It has nothing to do with genetic differences between men and women, or the fact that men have wider chest cavities. Our difficulty is strictly societal: we've been taught to hold in our stomachs because the hallmark of beauty is thinness. In *The Beauty Myth*, author Naomi Wolf points out that few women are immune to the emotional effects of our rigid cultural definitions of beauty. She's right, but the effects are also physical; holding in our stomachs prevents us from taking a single healthy breath. And women with eating disorders are often further hampered by the inability to take full natural breaths, which only exacerbates the stress cycle that causes them to either overeat, undereat, or binge-purge in the first place.

To understand the effects of chest breathing, try this exercise. Sit or lie down and contract your abdominal muscles with all your might. As you do, take note of your breathing. Only your chest will rise as you inhale. Notice that your diaphragm is stuck in place, and that air fills only the uppermost portions of your lungs. Now relax your stomach muscles and breathe into your abdomen. Notice how your diaphragm moves downward, and the lower portions of your lungs fill up. While you're at it, take note of differences in how you feel, in mind and body, as you engage in chest versus abdominal breathing.

After doing this exercise, you may recognize that how you breathed when you held in your stomach is a mere exaggeration of how you normally breathe. And sensations associated with shallow breathing—constriction, light-headedness, mild anxiety—may be modest exaggerations of how you often feel, especially when stressed out. That's what happens when we chronically hold in our stomachs. We may be robbed of the rich oxygenation we need to run every cell in our bodies.

After years of holding in our bellies, the process becomes unconscious, automatic. Often we don't know we're tensing our abdomens, and the muscular tensions become chronic. We therefore must make a conscious effort to relax those tensions, to restore normal function to our diaphragms, and to take deep, natural, abdominal breaths once again. That's where minis come in. Practiced regularly, the mini-relaxation exercise can change our bad breathing habits. By doing so, minis can instantaneously help to break the vicious cycle of tension and anxiety.

By shifting our breathing patterns, minis perform a function similar to the longer breath focus relaxation. But they don't last long enough to elicit the relaxation response and therefore do not carry the same long-term benefits. Yet minis *do* bring about the beneficial psychological and physiological changes I've described here within minutes or even seconds. Thus, you can do a mini in the midst of almost any event that taxes your patience, energy, or capacity to cope. I recommend that you practice minis *and* regularly elicit the relaxation response, since the former can pull you through tight situations, and the latter can, over the long haul, bring about a deeper enhancement of mind-body health.

How to Do Minis

In the last chapter, I described techniques for eliciting the relaxation response. Each one requires you to take at least fifteen or twenty minutes, alone in a place where you won't be disturbed, to gradually enter a state of emotional and physical tranquility. By contrast, you can practice mini-relaxations anywhere, anytime. You can do them with your eyes open or closed. You can do a mini whenever you are feeling anxious, or even when you anticipate feeling anxious. You can do them in the presence of others, and more often than not, they won't even know you are practicing a mind-body technique.

I teach four different methods of mini-relaxation, although other approaches can be used. Based on my own experience and my patients' reports, these four are the easiest and most reliable methods. The first version helps you to learn the basic approach for switching from chest to abdominal breathing. It can be practiced in any position, but it is useful initially to lie down, a position that makes you more aware of your breathing patterns. Otherwise, you can practice minis sitting, standing, lying down, or hanging by your feet from a chandelier—any position you find yourself in when you're stressed out!

Mini Version 1
Sit down or, preferably, lie down in a comfortable position. Take a deep, slow breath. Notice any movement in your chest, and any movement of your abdomen. Place a hand on your abdomen, just on top of your belly button. Allow your abdomen to rise about an inch as you inhale. As you exhale, notice that your abdomen will fall about an inch. Also notice that your chest will rise slightly at the same time that your abdomen rises. (Abdominal breathing does not mean that you don't take air into your upper chest; you do. But now you are also bringing air down into the lower portion of your lungs by using your diaphragm to expand the entire chest cavity.)

Become aware of your diaphragm moving down as you inhale, back up as you exhale. Remember that it is impossible to breathe abdominally if your diaphragm does not move down. And it is impossible to let your diaphragm move down if your stomach muscles are tight. So, relax your stomach muscles! If you are having trouble, try breathing in through your nose and out through your mouth. Enjoy the sensations of abdominal breathing for several breaths, or for as long as you desire.

Mini Version 2
Make the shift from chest breathing to deep abdominal breathing. Count down from ten to zero, taking one complete breath—one inhalation, one exhalation—with each number. Thus, with your first abdominal breath, you say "ten" to yourself, with the next breath you say "nine," and so on. If you start to feel light-headed or dizzy, slow down your counting. When you get to zero, see how you are feeling. If you are feeling better, great! If not, try doing it again.

Mini Version 3

Make the shift from chest breathing to deep abdominal breathing. As you inhale, count very slowly from one to four. As you exhale, count slowly back down, from four to one. Thus, as you inhale, you say silently to yourself, "One, two, three, four." As you exhale, you say silently to yourself, "Four, three, two, one." Do this for several breaths, or for as long as you wish.

Mini Version 4

Make the shift from chest breathing to deep abdominal breathing. Use any of the other three methods as you breathe: simply breathe as you feel your stomach rise, add a ten-to-zero count with each breath, or add a one-to-four/four-to-one count as you inhale and exhale. But this time, regardless of what method you use, pause for a few seconds after each in-breath. Pause again for a few seconds after each out-breath. Do this for several breaths, or for as long as you wish.

Minis in Everyday Life

*W*hat do rosary beads, Valium pills, amulets, teddy bears, and talismans have in common? They are things people carry around to ease their anxieties in circumstances that threaten to overwhelm. Yet they have something else in common. They are things people can forget to take with them.

But we can't forget our lungs, no matter where we go. And our lungs can be an immediate source of relaxation, comfort, and control—if we use them properly. When we practice minis, we use our lungs to restore balance to our breathing, and balance to our perspective about events swirling around us.

As many of my patients do, you can use minis while driving in heavy traffic. You can use them during a family argument. You can use them in any pressure-filled job situation. You can use them during a bout of acute or chronic pain. You can use them as you anticipate or undergo stressful medical procedures. You can use minis any time you are upset, anxious, fearful, or in pain. Here are a few everyday instances that would call for a mini:

- You are already running late for an important meeting or appointment, and traffic is bumper to bumper.
- You are the mother of several young children, with a husband at work. You're trying to cook dinner while keeping watch over the kids, who

roam about the house making noises that suggest breakage of household items.

- You feel awkward as you attend a party with many interesting, attractive people, none of whom you know.
- Your husband has a group of friends over to watch a sporting event, and they don't clean up their own mess, expecting you to do it.
- Your teenage daughter is two hours late coming home from a Saturday night date.
- A friend who is going through a period of depression calls for the umpteenth time, and you don't know if you can listen anymore.
- After a shopping spree, the credit card bills arrive. You know that you have to sit down with your partner that evening to figure out how you are going to pay these bills.

I've already mentioned the physiologic effects of minis—improved oxygen exchange, lower heart rate and blood pressure. The psychological effects are also pronounced. First, minis are a distraction. They momentarily take your mind off fear or pain, especially during stressful or unpleasant medical procedures. Second, minis enhance your perception of control. When you know you can count on minis to make you feel physically and emotionally better, you regain that sense of control. Third, minis can be psychological touchstones—little reminders that you can find your center, even when events or other people seem utterly out of control.

Sena was always being undone by daily irritations: heavy traffic, the minor mischief she'd come to expect from a teenage son, the silly demands of customers at the clothing store where she worked as a salesperson. Minis returned Sena to an awareness of her body and they immediately gave her a balanced perspective.

"I'll do minis five or six times a day," she said. "It's become a conditioned response, almost subconscious. Now when I get cut off in traffic, I do a mini and wave to the people who cut me off. I almost got shot one day by a guy who assumed that my wave was really a call to arms. Minis enable me to stop myself long enough to ask, 'How important is this anger?' The answer is almost always, 'Not very.' They help me not to sweat the small stuff. And it's all small stuff."

Minis can also help people get through some of the big stuff. Harriet, a middle-aged woman, came to our mind-body group one evening and told a harrowing story of a car accident. She'd been sideswiped by another car going through an intersection. Her car was nearly totaled. Had the other driver been going any faster, Harriet might have suffered life-threatening injuries. As it was, she suffered a minor case of whiplash. But the immediate impact was, of course, frightening beyond words. Within seconds of impact, what came to Harriet's mind was not a replay of her life's best and worst moments. "Before I even stepped out of the car, I told myself to do a mini," she told the group. "My panic subsided, and it helped me to handle the whole trauma."

That such a simple method can be so beneficial causes it to stay in women's minds. Recently, a patient I had not seen in six years called me requesting some information. I had to go into my desk drawer to retrieve it, and in my haste to return to the phone I closed the drawer on my hand. I let out a little yelp, which my patient obviously heard. Her immediate comment was, "Do a mini." She had remembered minis over the span of six years because she continued to do them on a regular basis.

Minis are especially helpful in situations that evoke panic, an emotion that can wreak havoc on both our emotional well-being and our physiology. The renowned Harvard cardiologist Bernard Lown, M.D., has long studied the negative effects of panic on the cardiovascular system, and he has developed a clinical cardiology practice that emphasizes psychological support to help reduce the abject fear experienced by his heart patients. That panic, he believes, can worsen their condition, and perhaps even hasten the outcome they dread the most. Over time, panic can also have destructive effects on other biological systems, including the endocrine and immune systems. People subject to feelings of panic, whether heart patients or not, can use a variety of psychological skills to calm themselves down, and minis are among the most applicable.

Several years ago, my husband and I were returning from a vacation on a flight that included a group of people with whom we'd become acquainted at our hotel. We were about to land at Logan Airport in Boston when the plane, which had been steadily descending, suddenly shot back up into the air. As we headed back out over the ocean, the pilot announced that he didn't want to scare us (hah!) but that a warning light indicated that the plane's landing gear would not lock into place.

As we began to fly in circles over the sea, the passengers could not contain their panic. Some were anxiously murmuring, others were audibly praying. I turned to my husband and commented, "We must be circling because they're preparing at Logan for a crash landing." It was obviously the wrong comment at the wrong time.

I should say that my husband had not been inclined to learn the many relaxation methods I teach to my patients. He had always supported me in every aspect of my work, but his native skepticism led him to demur politely when it came to practicing mind-body techniques, including minis. However, after my ill-timed remark, my husband surprised me with his reaction. Of all the comments he might have made under these dire circumstances, he turned to me and said, "Maybe now is a good time for me to learn minis."

When the other passengers who knew us, and who knew something of my work, heard me teaching my husband how to practice minis, they clustered around and asked me to teach them, too. What ensued, as we circled above the Atlantic with no idea whether we would ever land safely, was a rather hurried seminar in mini-relaxation techniques. Several rows of passengers, including my husband and me, began abdominal breathing as we counted "ten, nine, eight," and so on.

Our collective practice of minis continued for what seemed like an eternity but was probably closer to forty-five minutes. It was pitch dark when we finally made our approach, and we could see lights from fire engines and ambulances that had gathered on the runway. As we got closer, we could also see rescue workers dressed in silver suits. We didn't know the status of the landing gear until we actually landed safely. We were later told that the problem had been not with the landing gear but with the warning systems.

Needless to say, all of us felt our panic subside, at least to some extent, as we began to practice minis. In this laboratory of fear, we discovered that minis can be useful under extreme circumstances. They served as a distraction; they gave us a sense of control when our world seemed completely out of control; and they acted as touchstones—reminders that we could find a few moments of peace even when confronted with the possibility of imminent death.

The plane experience was instructive, but minis are clearly most useful in the grip of the daily grind, particularly for women who are doing too many things at once. Tania, the woman I described in chapter 1, was coping with an undermining boss, two troubled adult children who'd returned home for her support, and continuing flare-ups of rheumatoid arthritis. When the going got rough, Tania also suffered from insomnia. She was able to use minis throughout the day, whether in the midst of difficulties with her boss or her children, episodes of arthritis pain, or simply while waiting out a traffic light. She also used minis before going to sleep, and whenever she awoke in a state of anxiety. Shifting to abdominal breathing enabled Tania to prevent those frequent bouts of insomnia.

The time to do a mini is any time you tune into mind and body and discover that you are tense, anxious, or upset. But you may also prevent emotional and even physical symptoms by practicing minis *before* a stressful event, one you know is likely to make you tense, anxious, or upset. For instance, you are at work and you've received a message from a supervisor with whom you have an ongoing conflict. You know it's going to be a difficult conversation, so you do a mini-relaxation before picking up the phone. Or you find yourself at a family dinner with an uncle who pushes your buttons, so you practice a mini before you even enter the house. Or you're on the cusp of a potentially destructive fight with your spouse or partner, so you do a mini to keep yourself from completely losing your composure. You may also do minis before any stressful medical test, procedure, or office visit, a subject I will return to shortly.

Women dealing with medical conditions can use minis to calm their fears, and in some cases to quell their symptoms. Minis are particularly useful and effective for women who suffer with PMS or menopausal hot flashes. Their symptoms often strike without warning, smack in the middle of their day- or nighttime activities, with no regard for their social environment. A woman whose PMS makes her irritable to the point of exploding can't just leave work and go home to ride out her emotional swings in solitude. Neither can a woman whose hot flashes cause so much discomfort and potential embarrassment. Minis are often a solution for these women, both because they can be readily practiced in these circumstances, and because they so frequently reduce emotional and physical distress within minutes.

Minis can also be anxiety-blockers for women with breast or gynecologic cancers, who frequently feel overwhelmed by their medical treatments, side effects, and the sheer emotional impact of their diagnoses. The same holds true for women with infertility problems or multiple miscarriages who are faced daily with painful reminders of their plight: friends or relatives with babies, friends or relatives who are pregnant, friends or relatives who make unknowingly insensitive comments, spanning the spectrum from, "Oh, of course you'll come to term," to "Maybe it's time for you to let go." My patients do minis the moment these unpleasantries occur, and they are spared much unnecessary distress.

Miriam was a fifty-six-year-old nurse whose hot flashes had no regard for her work schedule; they came on when she was treating patients, huddling with doctors, trying to get a good night's sleep. She found that minis helped to quickly reduce the intensity of her flashes. "It's been a long time since I learned how to do minis in our group," said Miriam. "But I continue to use them. They remind me that I have some control over my body, rather than my body having control over me."

Minis in the Medical Mainstream

*I*n 1987, I was walking across the street when I was hit by a car. The impact, and the spill I took, left me with significant injuries to my knee and elbow. My treatment took place at the hospital where I work. I had to undergo an arthrogram on my elbow, a radiologic procedure in which air is injected into the joints so the doctors can view the damage with an X ray. I was not aware of how painful this procedure would be until I was told by the radiologist in no uncertain terms: "Feel free to scream."

I thought to myself, "I can either scream and embarrass myself in the hospital where I work, or I can actually do what I tell my patients to do." I opted to do what I tell my patients to do in such circumstances, which is to use minis. Throughout the procedure, I did every version of minis that I teach. When I ran out of versions, I made up new ones. I kept on doing minis throughout the procedure, and I experienced next to no pain.

I was surprised by how effective the minis were in reducing my own discomfort. So surprised, in fact, that I began to doubt whether the minis had indeed been responsible for protecting me from such excruciating pain. I must simply have a much higher threshold of pain than most people, I thought.

A month later, I returned to the hospital for an arthrogram on my knee. Because I had come to believe that my prior experience was due to my high pain threshold, I neglected to do any mini-relaxations. As the radiologist began to inject air into the joint, the pain was searing. Although I did not scream, I felt about as much pain as I believe I can endure.

Never since have I doubted the potential efficacy of minis as an effective tool for managing pain. I eventually underwent two operations on my knee, and used mini-relaxations consistently—during blood tests, insertion of IV needles, injections, and preparation for surgery.

Minis reduce the anxiety we experience as we anticipate painful medical procedures, and they distract us from the pain itself as the procedure is being conducted. For women, certain procedures are associated with particular anxieties. Pelvic exams may not only be uncomfortable, they can be emotionally difficult or distressing. Certainly any woman who has reason to be concerned about a particular condition—be it a fibroid, cervical dysplasia, ovarian cyst, or any type of gynecologic cancer—will be especially tense during the examination. I have counseled teenagers undergoing their first pelvic exams, who are often embarrassed and afraid that the exams will be terribly painful. Minis put the focus on themselves and their breathing to such an extent that they lose awareness of what the gynecologist is doing.

In addition to during pelvic exams, consider doing mini-relaxations at these times:

- Prior to and during any blood test
- Prior to and during any injection
- Before and during insertion of an IV needle prior to surgery
- During any stressful phase of preparation for surgery
- During a mammogram
- Before and during every phase of chemotherapy for cancer: as you anticipate treatment, during insertion of IV needles, immediately afterward, and later, when nausea may occur
- Before and during radiation therapy for cancer
- During any ultrasound test, including those used at various phases of treatment for infertility and those used during pregnancy
- Before calling the doctor's office for test results
- When you are awaiting a call from your doctor
- When you are put on hold by your doctor's office

As I will detail in Part II, every condition carries its own unique stressors. Women dealing with infertility interface with the medical system constantly, going to their doctors' offices for blood tests, ultrasounds, and hormone injections on a regular basis. As they await test results to determine whether they can get pregnant, or whether they are pregnant, such women experience ragged emotional dips and sways. Women with high-risk pregnancies are constantly on a fearful lookout for signs of miscarriage; often their doctors consign them to long periods of bed rest. Women with cancer typically cope with distressing examinations, tests, surgeries, and treatment protocols. All of these circumstances call for the use of minis.

♦ ♦ ♦

Why are minis the perfect portable stress managers? Because they can calm and center us in daily life, when symptoms arise, or when we have stressful encounters with doctors or hospitals. But the reason for their utility is another matter. Minis do not help us to achieve some extraordinary state of consciousness. Rather, they help restore a fundamental physiologic reflex—breathing—to its natural state. When we breathe deeply, easily, and naturally, the effects on both mind and body may *seem* extraordinary, but we have only relearned the most ordinary of biological functions. However, proper breathing can quiet our stress responses, distract us from pain, enhance our energy, and sharpen our awareness. As Karlfried Durckheim wrote, "In breathing we partake unconsciously in the Greater Life."

Five

· · ·

CATCHING THE NASTY MIND:
COGNITIVE RESTRUCTURING

If I spoke to any of my friends or my family the way I spoke to myself, then I would truly be alone in the world."

So said Amanda, a woman in her forties who was just discovering the harshness of her own inner voices. Periodic bouts of depression, coupled with a string of chronic physical ailments, had led Amanda to one of my mind-body groups. She learned that all of us are vulnerable to negative thought patterns, and that like the proverbial tape loop, they play over and over in our heads. She also learned that women are subject to particular negative thoughts, most of them bequeathed by our culture and our families. One of Amanda's recurring thoughts was "I'll never amount to anything." It took some intense one-on-one discussions, but Amanda eventually came to realize that this belief was both cruel and inaccurate. Once she was able to supplant "I'll never amount to anything" with a kinder, more realistic assessment of her own potential, Amanda's depression, and many of her physical symptoms, began to lift.

Amanda had undergone a process called cognitive restructuring. It is a technique based on principles of cognitive therapy, which was largely developed by Aaron T. Beck, M.D., and popularized by David D. Burns, M.D. Cognitive restructuring has become a mainstay of mind-body groups, because our thoughts can determine our emotional states, which in turn can influence our physical health. Put simply, if I constantly think that I am a worthless know-nothing who will never succeed in my career or relationships, I am likely to become seriously depressed, and anxious to boot. If these thoughts continue unabated, and my depression and anxiety become chronic, I also become vulnerable to a host of physical ailments.

Cognitive restructuring is a tried-and-true method that helps us to identify our negative thoughts, question their veracity and validity, and replace them with new thoughts that are kinder to ourselves and more accurate. As with Amanda, once we "restructure" these negative thought patterns, we rid ourselves of a major cause of our emotional and physical distress. We can overthrow tyrannical ideas that, without our consent and barely with our knowledge, have seized control of our consciousness.

I use cognitive restructuring for women who are anxious or depressed, whether or not they are physically healthy. This method has special applications for women, because women have many specific, socially conditioned negative thought patterns. For instance, we are often beset by negative thoughts about our bodies and self-worth. (So are men, but the prevalence of such thoughts among woman in our society is clearly greater.) "I'm fat" is a veritable mantra for countless women, one often murmured by those who aren't even overweight. Another broken record is Amanda's "I'll never amount to anything." Among the most pernicious is "If I'm not perfect, I'm no good at all." I have helped women to restructure these dysfunctional thoughts, a process with profoundly positive effects on mind, body, and spirit.

Cognitive restructuring also has special applications for women with specific health conditions, each of which carries with it a particular set of common negative thoughts. Many of these thoughts are merciless self-judgments and social stigmas that must be restructured if women are to free themselves from undue suffering.

The Negative Tapes Within

*A*s my former colleague Steven Maurer always emphasized, all of us have certain tape loops in our heads—recurring thoughts or phrases we say to ourselves repeatedly. In my experience, for most women about 90 percent of these tapes are negative. Few of us wake up in the morning, look in the mirror, and say to ourselves, "You look maaahvelous!" to borrow Billy Crystal's time-honored line as Fernando on *Saturday Night Live*. Instead, most of us say things like: "My God, look at my hair!" "What am I going to do about these thighs?" "I'll never get rid of those wrinkles." "I'm going to blow that big project at work." "My finances are completely out of control."

We carry these and other negative tape loops with us throughout our days and nights. Some of them are relatively benign. But many of them haunt us, and others gradually beat us down with their harshness. After years of replaying, these tapes—whose messages are not only unfair but usually false—take on a life of their own. Our inner response to almost any situation becomes unconscious and automatic: a button gets pushed and one of our greatest (i.e., nastiest) hits is played for the umpteenth time.

I once helped lead a conference for health professionals in which all the participants had either M.D.s, Ph.D.s, or M.S.W.s (master's of social work). Many were leaders in their respective fields. In a discussion of cognitive therapy, the group leader with whom I was working said to the participants, "Quickly, without thinking about it too long, tell me the most common tape loops running in your heads." I was astonished by the answers given. Without exception, they were ruthless self-defamations such as, "I'm lazy," "I'm stupid," "I'm fat," "I'm a slob," "I'll never really make it in this field."

Cognitive restructuring offers a way to erase such tapes, and to "re-record" new tapes that are both more fair and more truthful. The first step is to fully acknowledge these thoughts, which are usually so automatic that we either don't know what they are, or we have no sense of their impact. An often revelatory aspect of acknowledging negative tapes is our discovery of their origins. Typically the tapes are eerie echoes of someone else's voice. That someone may be a person from early life—a parent, sibling, or teacher whose judgments mattered because we were dependent upon him or her. Or the tapes may mimic a person in the present, one who has power over us or one we've granted too much power—an insensitive doctor, a disapproving spouse, or a competitive friend.

Lorretta Laroche is a wonderful humorist from Plymouth, Massachusetts, who uses humor to teach stress management. An adjunct member of the faculty of the Mind/Body Medical Institute, Lorretta tells patients (and anyone else who will listen) to think of their minds as being like a bus. Her inevitable follow-up question is, "So who's driving *your* bus?" Is it your boss? Your mother-in-law? Your mother? Your father? A guy who broke up with you years ago? For people beset by negative tapes, the usual answer is anyone but themselves.

In some instances, the negative tapes do not originate with someone else, but are internal representations of our own worst fears. We allow the voice of rational assessment to get drowned out by the far louder voices of fear and trepidation.

Whether the tapes originate in the past, in the present, or from parts of ourselves that wield too much power, they can be erased. But first we must uncover their messages, which sound and seem true until we really put them to the test of reason. Some negative tapes contain a hint of reasonable self-criticism that gets turned into a torrent of self-hatred. Other tapes carry glimmers of truth that only conceal deeper truths, ones that could free us from shame, guilt, and self-denigration.

The process of discovering the deeper truths—of recording over false and cruel messages with ones that are more truthful and compassionate—involves a series of steps that any woman can learn.

Four Questions to Catch the Nasty Mind

Cognitive restructuring should be a search for inner truths. While such truths can certainly be painful on occasion, they are rarely more painful than the suffering we inflict on ourselves with the lies and half-truths we tell ourselves every day of our lives. The deeper truths my patients discover when they utilize cognitive restructuring liberate them from the punishing voices in their heads.

The method of cognitive restructuring I teach is quite simple, although the process itself isn't always easy. It begins with four basic questions, which I have adapted from the work of leading practitioners of cognitive therapy.

First, identify one common negative thought pattern, one tape loop that plays repeatedly in your head. Now, ask yourself these four questions about this negative thought:

1. Does this thought contribute to my stress?
2. Where did I learn this thought?
3. Is this thought logical?
4. Is this thought true?

Before you can restructure an automatic negative thought, you must first honestly confront that thought, discover its origins and effects, and put it to the test of logic. That is the purpose of the four questions.

One patient, Carol, was constantly feeling burned out by the stress in her life. Her most common negative thought was "I'm a terrible slob." I asked her the four questions as probes for her to explore this thought and its effect on her life, which was profound. Yes, the nonstop thought that she was a slob contributed to her stress by making her feel worthless. "There were times when I literally did not want to go home," said Carol. "I didn't want to enter my own house because it reminded me of my inadequacy."

Where did Carol learn this thought? It did not take long for her to identify the main source. Carol's mother-in-law was always on her case about the state of her home. Earlier in her life, Carol hadn't thought of herself as a slob. And clearly, she cared about how her mother-in-law viewed her and was therefore vulnerable to her judgments.

Was Carol's thought logical? Carol had some trouble with this question. "What do you mean?" she asked. I clarified my question in the plainest way I knew how: "Well, is your house really gross?"

"It is pretty cluttered," she replied. "I sometimes let the newspapers and magazines pile up, and there are often shirts on the backs of chairs and shoes under the coffee table."

"Okay, but is your house disgustingly filthy?" I asked, moving the inquiry along.

"Of course not!" said Carol, with a hint of indignation. "It's not really *dirty*, it's just cluttered."

I moved on to the fourth and pivotal question. "So is the thought that you are a slob actually true?"

In response to this question, Carol did what one is supposed to do when answering the four questions: she took her time and searched for an honest answer rather than a quick emotional retort.

"Well, no," she replied. "My house is often cluttered but it is always clean." Carol went on to describe her home in more detail, and it became clear that her house was actually *quite* clean. Moreover, the clutter was the often unavoidable result of Carol's hectic lifestyle. Her husband worked long hours, and she held down a part-time job as a waitress while bearing most of the responsibility for raising their two children. Yet her mother-in-law's criticisms had gotten to Carol, and they added to her burden by making her feel so inadequate.

By identifying and restructuring her negative thought, Carol was relieved of that burden. She no longer harbored constant feelings of worthlessness, because she was able to transform "I'm a slob" into "My house is cluttered but clean." Indeed, from that point on, whenever she entered her home and saw clutter, she responded in an entirely new way. Instead of viewing the clutter as evidence of her inadequacy, she viewed the clutter as evidence of her demanding life. What's more, she'd been doing her best to manage it all—her job, marriage, kids, and home.

One key to cognitive restructuring is to take time with your answers.

Apply your intelligence and self-awareness with laserlike precision, and you will discover surprising truths about your automatic thoughts and their influence on your state of mind and health. In my mind-body groups, participants ask these four questions in small groupings of four or five, and share their answers with other members. I frequently hear gasps of self-recognition rising from each small group. Women often burst into tears as they come to grips with negative tapes that have hounded them for years, sometimes decades. Uncovering the lie at the heart of these long-accepted beliefs may be experienced as a release from a kind of mental prison.

A patient in one of my groups, Jennifer, had had five miscarriages in her attempts to bear her first child. Jennifer's most painful negative thought was "God does not want me to have a child because I'm going to be a bad mother."

I and the other group members were surprised by Jennifer's tape, because she appeared to be such a warm, caring figure—someone who would be a wonderful mother. Where had she learned this thought? After much soul-searching, Jennifer uncovered a long-forgotten memory. She was the oldest of four children, and her parents had often put her in charge of her younger siblings. When she was about ten years old, one of the siblings had gotten into some mischief. Jennifer's mother held her responsible. "You're going to grow up to be a terrible mother!" her mother raged at her.

There it was, plain as day. Jennifer had not known that the tape she heard in her head every day, in the midst of her suffering over multiple miscarriages, was first recorded in a scene with her mother some twenty-five years earlier. It never left her because it had been so damningly painful, and every new miscarriage seemed to confirm her mother's stinging words. Of course she could not come to term, she thought, because she did not deserve to be a mother.

This breakthrough enabled Jennifer to explore deeper truths. Yes, she'd made a few mistakes with her younger siblings. But she was herself a child, and she'd been given far too much responsibility by her parents. The group also let Jennifer know that they experienced her as a warm, loving person. Having identified the source of her false and heartless mind tape as a voice from the past, Jennifer could finally see herself clearly in the present. At one point in our group process, in a voice rising with passion, she blurted out, "You know what? I'm going to be a damn good mother!"

Within months of completing our group, Jennifer not only became pregnant again, she finally came to term. She recently celebrated her daughter's first birthday. Neither Jennifer nor I can possibly know whether her cognitive restructuring played any role in her ability to have a biological child. But there is no question that she was emotionally ready to be a mother by the time she did give birth.

You may not be able to clearly identify one person in your past or present as having laid down your negative tape. Take the case of Judy, a highly regarded college professor. Between her lectures to students and her talks to professional societies, Judy spoke in public regularly. She came to me because she was suffering from severe panic attacks about her public speaking. Every time she got up to speak—which was almost every day—she became terrified, experiencing shakes, sweats, and other physical as well as psychological symptoms. When we practiced cognitive restructuring, Judy suddenly realized that her panic attacks were associated with one dreadful thought: "I am a terrible public speaker." That thought had been so automatic, and so overshadowed by her symptoms, that she hadn't realized that it was causing her panic attacks.

Judy did not know why she thought of herself as a terrible public speaker; she couldn't think of anyone who'd implanted this idea in her head. But it was enough for her to recognize that the thought was rooted in fear rather than reason. As we discussed her work, she made it clear to me, and to herself, that her students loved her lectures. So did her fellow faculty members, who always complimented her. During one session, she restructured her thought: "Actually, I'm an excellent public speaker!"

Afterward, when Judy began to lecture, her panic attack would begin, accompanied again by the thought that she was a lousy lecturer. At that very moment, she'd challenge the old tape with, "Wait a minute, I'm a terrific lecturer." Within seconds, her panic attack would subside.

Knowing the source of a negative tape can yield profound insights, but it is most important to restructure that thought, source or no source. Perhaps Judy's fear came from a deeply ingrained cultural message that women are not supposed to place themselves front and center as powerful leaders and teachers. We cannot know, but what Judy needed most was to jettison the lie so she could relieve her panic, which allowed her to move forward with confidence as a powerful leader and teacher.

Thought Restructuring:
Kinder, Gentler, Truer

*T*he process of thought restructuring can be simple or it can be complex. It's simple when we clearly see the falsity and cruelty of a particular negative thought. It's complex when the thought is a mixture of truth and falsehood, or when the thought is a "true-sounding lie." In the latter cases, we must tease fiction from truth, a process that can be as delicate as microsurgery. But you don't have to be a genius or expert to do it, as I will demonstrate shortly. However, you may need the help of a close friend, supportive group, or therapist.

Most of the time, our automatic negative thoughts are shot through with lies, and no teasing apart is needed. Sally, a participant in one of our mind-body groups, was a "Type A" woman who constantly strived for higher levels of corporate success. The side effect was stress burnout; she was always on the verge of physical and emotional exhaustion. Like Amanda, whose story began this chapter, Sally's negative thought was "I'll never amount to anything."

Sally never before realized that this tape loop was fueling her struggle. She constantly tried to prove to herself and others that she would amount to something, because she was tormented by the inner message that she never would.

The discrepancy between her thought and her reality could not have been more dramatic. Sally was already a phenomenally accomplished executive who'd not only scaled the corporate ladder, but had a lifestyle that reflected her financial success. Though they were completely sympathetic, the other group members had a bit of trouble understanding how someone so comfortable and successful could think and feel the way Sally thought and felt.

A breakthrough came when Sally answered the second question, "Where did I learn this thought?" She remembered several incidents as a child when her father specifically told her, "You'll never amount to anything." Her negative thought had been her father's voice in her head, reverberating until this day.

Once Sally discovered the thought's origin, she recognized that it did not reflect her current reality. "I'll never amount to anything" was nothing more than an old tape, but it was a powerful one, because it carried all the hurt she experienced when her father expressed so little regard for his young daughter.

Having brushed away the cobwebs in her mind, Sally began to think clearly. Her restructuring was simple: "I already *have* amounted to something!" She could step back and appreciate her remarkable successes and her comfortable lifestyle. When others in her group complimented her, she was able to take in their regard. Sally continued to work toward higher levels of accomplishment, but she no longer did so with the desperate edge of someone whose entire sense of self was on the line with every new project or potential promotion.

Sally's story illustrates the usefulness of all four steps in cognitive restructuring. If she had never identified the source of her negative tape, she might never have accepted, on a gut level, the fact that she was a smashing success. Although cognitive restructuring focuses on thought processes, it works best when we experience truths on a deep emotional level.

Sally's story also shows how social messages can get inside our heads and cause tremendous trouble. Her father's ruthless assessment probably had something to do with the fact that she was female. Women who hear such voices at an impressionable young age grow up to discover that society does in fact make it harder for them to amount to anything. This double whammy saddles them with all kinds of negative tapes: "You'll never make it." "You're not smart enough." "You're not tough enough." Cognitive restructuring is needed to subvert these nasty messages.

Though Sally's restructuring took work, the falsity of her tape was quite apparent. Other negative tapes are much trickier. For instance, the first negative tape reported by many women is simply, "I'm fat." In cases where a woman is clearly obese (as opposed to being a few pounds overweight), this tape cannot be branded a lie. Though it may be true, it is also a cover-up. I say to such women, "The phrase 'I'm fat' describes a physical state; it's not the crux of a negative thought. What is the underlying thought or feeling you associate with 'I'm fat'?" After some contemplation, the answer is usually something like: "I'm disgusting." "I hate myself." "I'm not worthy of looking good." "I'm scared of attention."

These thoughts can be restructured. If a person is overweight, it does no good to deny this reality in the name of cognitive restructuring. But it is very useful—indeed, it can be healing—to pry apart this reality from the merciless thoughts and feelings that get "stuck" to it. The fact that a woman is overweight does not mean she is disgusting, worthy of hatred, or unworthy of love. She must reject any voice—from society or family, past or present, without or within—that equates being overweight with worthlessness. Then she can restructure thoughts such as "I'm disgusting" and "I'm hateful" by focusing on physical features and inner qualities she feels good about.

I practice cognitive restructuring as a search for truth, not a newfangled form of denial. If we have a negative thought that contains a hint of painful truth, there's no point "restructuring" that reality to make us feel good. We're better off confronting that truth, as long as it is not a cover for self-hatred.

Consider the woman who has long stifled her creativity because her husband insisted that she remain housebound with chores and children. Her negative thought is "I have not lived up to my potential." She's right, and she can only benefit by exploring that thought rather than prematurely restructuring it. On the other hand, if she beats herself with this thought, the truth will get lost. She'll blame herself with other negative thoughts like "I obviously have no talent." Thus, she ignores the true reasons she has not lived up to her potential, reasons that have nothing to do with lack of talent. She ends up punishing herself in ways that only keep her stuck.

As you can see, cognitive restructuring is not brainless optimism, in which we plaster a smile on our faces no matter the circumstances. At its best, cognitive restructuring fosters a *realistic* optimism, in which we grapple with hard realities at the same time that we cultivate kindness toward ourselves.

Take the case of Elaine, who was despairing when she joined one of my mind-body groups. She was forty years old and recently had had a mastectomy after a diagnosis of breast cancer. The surgery had a profound impact on her self-esteem and sexual identity.

When we came to the part of our program for cognitive restructuring, Elaine identified her main negative tape: "I'll never be a complete woman." This repetitive thought had been the cause of her self-doubts, creating a rift between her and her husband, Jim. Despite his reassurances, Elaine could not shake her belief that she was "damaged goods."

Working with me and the group, Elaine struggled to restructure her own hurtful thought patterns. After much work and many tears, she did come to believe that "I'll never be a complete woman" was basically illogical and untrue.

It had been difficult for Elaine because there was a hint of painful truth in "I'll never be a complete woman," although the phrase was unduly harsh and unnecessarily global. She had lost a part of her female anatomy, and she needed to grieve that loss. But she did not have to accept *any* indictment of her femininity or her humanity. Suddenly, Elaine was able to restructure her thought: "You know, I may not be a complete woman," she told the group, "but I am a complete person."

Elaine's restructuring did not anesthetize the sadness associated with her mastectomy. But it completely healed the gratuitous pain inflicted by her own mind. Her self-esteem was restored, and she and Jim were able to retrieve their capacity for sexual pleasure and loving communication.

Most cognitive restructuring is less complex than in Elaine's case. When we ask the four questions about our automatic negative thoughts, we'll discover that the majority are clearly illogical and false. But I tell Elaine's story to illustrate how negative thoughts can contain bits of truth. In such instances, it is our job to separate truth from fiction. Then we must accept the realities, reject the lies, and come up with new thought structures that reflect our new understanding. Invariably, these new thoughts are kinder, gentler, and more truthful.

I also tell Elaine's story because so many women are confronted with similar circumstances. If you are coping with infertility or menopause, or you've had either a mastectomy or a hysterectomy, you may feel that you are no longer a "complete" woman. Elaine's restructuring may apply to you. Yes, you've lost one biological aspect of being female, but you have not lost the wholeness of your femininity or your humanity.

Other negative thought patterns that are commonly associated with particular women's conditions include "I'll never be as attractive, energetic, and creative as I once was" (menopause); "I have no control over my mind or body" (PMS); "My body will never be slim enough to make me feel attractive" (eating disorders).

I provide many possible restructurings for these negative thoughts in the appropriate chapters in Part II, but in every case, the messages are true-sounding lies, and they can be transformed. But you must be on the lookout for your own mental trickery, and leave no stone unturned in your search for inner truth.

What happens if you work hard at this process, and you still can't tell whether a negative thought is truly dysfunctional? You may be helped by the list on the next page—developed by Dr. David D. Burns—of so-called cognitive distortions, or disordered thoughts, "Definitions of Cognitive Distortions." Ask yourself whether your negative tape falls into any one of these ten categories. If so, use the guidance in this chapter to challenge and restructure this thought to the best of your ability.

Definitions of Cognitive Distortions

1. *All-or-nothing thinking*. You see things in black-and-white categories. If your performance falls short of perfect, you see yourself as a total failure.

2. *Overgeneralization*. You see a single negative event as part of a never-ending pattern of defeat.

3. *Mental filter*. You pick out a single negative detail and dwell on it exclusively, so that your vision of all reality becomes darkened, like an entire beaker of water discolored by a single drop of ink.

4. *Disqualifying the positive*. You reject positive experiences by insisting that they "don't count" for some reason or other. This way, you can maintain a negative belief, even if it would tend to be contradicted by your everyday experiences.

5. *Jumping to conclusions*. You make a negative interpretation even though there are no definite facts to prove your conclusion. For example, you may automatically conclude that someone is reacting negatively to you, without bothering to ask that person.

6. *Magnification or minimization*. You exaggerate the importance of things that make you feel bad (such as your own mistakes or someone else's achievement) or minimize positive things (your own desirable qualities or the other person's imperfections).

7. *Emotional reasoning*. You assume that your negative emotions reflect the way things really are: "I feel it, therefore it must be true."

8. *"Should" statements*. You try to motivate yourself with shoulds and shouldn'ts, as if you had to be whipped and punished before you could be expected to do anything, and you feel guilty if you don't do what you think you should.

9. *Labeling and mislabeling*. Instead of describing your error, you attach a negative label to yourself: "I'm a loser." When someone else's behavior rubs you the wrong way, you attach an emotional label to that person: "He's a damn louse."

10. *Personalization*. You see yourself as the cause of some negative external event that, in fact, you were not primarily responsible for.

(Adapted from David D. Burns, *Feeling Good: The New Mood Therapy*. New York: New American Library, 1981.)

Goose in the Bottle:
A Riddle for Our Times

*I*magine that you have in front of you a large glass bottle that contains a large, healthy, and happy goose. How can you get that goose out of the bottle, without either breaking the bottle or harming the goose?

Are you stuck? Here's a hint. You are approaching the problem too concretely.

Are you still stuck? Another hint: Ask yourself how the goose got in the bottle in the first place.

Still stuck? Here's a final hint. Where is the problem? Where is the goose in the bottle located?

The answer to this question, which you may have spent several minutes pondering, can be found in my initial posing of the riddle. Since I only asked you to *imagine* the goose in the bottle, all you need to do is remove the goose in your *imagination*. Imagine the goose in; imagine the goose out.

This riddle makes a point that I drive home to my patients: many of our everyday worries are as illusory as that goose in the bottle. We imagine inescapable traps that are nothing more than figments of our worst fantasies. The goose-in-the-bottle exercise illustrates that many of our problems can be solved when we realize that our minds are creating them—and our minds can undo them.

After completing my mind-body programs, patients often stop in the middle of an anxiety attack, saying to themselves "Now *that's* a goose in a bottle." They suddenly realize that the cause of their upset is all in the mind. It doesn't matter whether they were worried about unwashed dishes, unsatisfied kids, or unfinished work projects.

Goose-in-the-bottle is really a shorthand version of cognitive restructuring. It's an image that reminds us how we conjure up negative notions that make us anxious, notions that have little basis in reality. One way to break the cycle of anxious thoughts and feelings is to stop and ask ourselves: "Is this a goose in a bottle?" So often, our daily worries have no more substance than the web-footed bird we imagine in our heads when we first ponder the riddle.

Goose-in-the-bottle is an especially useful response to those small but aggravating worries that afflict so many women. My patients use this mental image to defeat the little anxieties and angers that would otherwise snowball into mountainous fears and rages. One of my patients, Naomi, told a perfectly illustrative story. Before heading off to work, Naomi asked her husband to defrost the chicken she'd cook for dinner. On her way home, she thought, "I bet he forgot to defrost the chicken." With that seemingly innocuous thought, Naomi began packing together her snowball. With increasing anger, the progression went like this:

"He always forgets to do stuff like that."

"I'm sick of this. He expects me to work full-time, do all the shopping and cooking, and he can't even defrost the bloody chicken."

"We're going to fight about this. And I know how we fight. It's going to get ugly."

"I'm going to have to move out of our apartment."

"I can see us getting a divorce."

Naomi arrived home fully prepared to do battle. She stepped into the kitchen where, of course, the chicken was plopped on a plate on the countertop, dripping wet.

Had Naomi stopped her racing mind for just a moment and asked, "Is this a goose in a bottle?" (or, "Is this a bird in the freezer?") she'd have saved herself a lot of emotional and even physiologic distress, as her fight-or-flight response took off with each increasingly rageful thought. Even if he hadn't defrosted the bloody chicken, why make that a test case for the whole marriage?

Here are some similar circumstances, and the domino effect of negative thoughts that followed, based largely upon stories I've heard from my patients. Each of these could potentially be defused by the goose-in-the-bottle question:

- I made a faux pas with a client today. I'm not going to get the sale. I'm going to have a bad year. I'm going to lose my job, and my house.
- My ten-year-old child got one D on his report card. Clearly, he'll never get into college.
- I suddenly realized that the recipe I'm making for dinner could include an ingredient that my father-in-law is allergic to. He's going to get terribly sick. Imagine if he died right in my dining room.
- I've been dating a lovely man for three months. We're going away together for the weekend, and I'm sure that when he sees my thighs for the first time he's going to head for the hills. I'll be alone forever.
- My daughter has been asked to the prom by a guy she's always had a

major crush on. She's really worried that he won't show up. If he doesn't, she'll be utterly humiliated. What if she gets so upset that she drops out of school? God knows, she may even join a cult.

- My doctors tell me that my breast biopsy came back negative from two different labs. My cancer must be so advanced that they're afraid to tell me the truth.

Goose-in-the-bottle represents a swift challenge to thoughts such as these, which are pretty transparent. But it is an important practice, because women can eventually be toppled by the irritating little thoughts that peck away at their strength and self-confidence on a daily basis.

In a sense, goose-in-the-bottle is to cognitive restructuring what minis are to the relaxation response. In other words, the image is a quick but often effective version of cognitive restructuring that can work in lieu of a more extended process. Like minis, goose-in-the-bottle can and should be used in the course of daily living, when dysfunctional thoughts add to our stress. For instance, our employer makes one mildly cutting remark and we worry that we're getting fired. By contrast, "big issue" thoughts such as "I'll never amount to anything" and "I'll never be a mother" require the deeper inquiry of cognitive restructuring.

In our efforts to gain peace of mind, we benefit by using both minis and the longer techniques to elicit the relaxation response. By the same token, we benefit by using goose-in-the-bottle for everyday worries, and cognitive restructuring for big-ticket problems and issues that cause us to suffer day in and day out.

Perfectionism Is a Pathogen

Society "infects" women with certain negative thought structures. We usually pick them up in our families when young, and have them reinforced by social learning and media indoctrination. Among the most prevalent socially conditioned negative thoughts are those linked to shame about our bodies. But a related negative thought structure, and a rather all-encompassing one, is rigid perfectionism.

Many of us have come to believe that our bodies, our behavior, our creative output, our parenting, our conduct in relationships, and our capacity to stitch every patch of our lives into a lovely quilt must all achieve perfection. Anything less, and our self-assessment is brutal: we just don't make it.

Many women are haunted by voices that belittle them for not performing brilliantly at every turn. This crazy brand of perfectionism makes them feel helpless when they can't achieve their goals, many of which were unreachable to begin with (i.e., many women set themselves up with unrealistic ambitions). And extreme perfectionism robs the lifeblood from women who feel they can never do enough. That is why perfectionism is a pathogen—it makes women sick.

Cognitive restructuring reveals the distorted thinking that underlies perfectionism. Indeed, perfectionism can be so dysfunctional that it entails most of Dr. Burns's ten cognitive distortions: all-or-nothing thinking, overgeneralization, mental filter, disqualifying the positive, minimization, emotional reasoning, "should" statements, and mislabeling. Using the techniques of cognitive restructuring, we can finally recognize what we do to ourselves in the name of perfectionism. By so doing, we can reject the tyranny of impossibly high standards.

Frances, a forty-year-old woman who was constantly fatigued, was married and had two young children, and she worked part-time as a word processor. Here was a typical scene from Frances's life: She was already tired from a full day of work and chores, and she had just made dinner for her family. She gave her four-year-old son the orange juice she bought earlier in the day, and he started to cry. He was upset because she should have known that he can't stand orange juice; it's apple juice he likes. Even though she worked all day, did the laundry, picked up the kids from day care on time, and prepared a tasty meal, she felt like a total failure.

Frances's belief that she had to be perfect led her into several of Dr. Burns's traps: all-or-nothing thinking (one shortfall and she's a failure), overgeneralization (one negative event becomes a never-ending pattern of defeat), disqualifying the positive, and minimization of all the good things she accomplished.

Another bane of the perfectionistic woman is her reliance on a mental filter: she picks out a single negative detail and dwells on it so exclusively that her vision of herself is completely darkened. Take, for instance, the female executive who meets with her male employer for a job evaluation. He tells her that she has handled her accounts superbly, she deals with clients beautifully, and she has shown great promise as a planner of new projects. In the coming year, he would like to see her pursue new accounts more aggressively. He ends the evaluation by telling her that a promotion is in the offing.

But our female executive spends the next several days with only one thought in mind: I've done a lousy job pursuing new accounts. She can't stop obsessing about her boss's comment, and she assumes that his overall assessment of her is poor, even though he praised her many strengths without reservation! She doesn't even take in his comment that she is likely to be promoted. She loses all perspective until she actually starts expecting a pink slip.

Of course men may be subject to the same dysfunctional thinking. Workplace pressures are extremely hard on men, who often succumb to mental traps similar to those of our female executive. But society has placed peculiar demands on women to do it all, and do it all spectacularly. According to the most rigid social conventions, we're expected to be perfectly sexy yet perfectly motherly; perfectly dutiful at home yet perfectly tough on the job; perfectly available to our mates yet perfectly engaged in every aspect of social planning. It is no wonder that some of us view one slip as a sign of total collapse. And the new expectations of '90s women have not *replaced* the old; they've simply been added on, like so many weights pushed onto the ends of a barbell.

Working women today have a hard time fending off extreme expectations, because society often puts them in a tough spot: if they're not perfect, their world may indeed come tumbling down. Consider the single woman who supports two school-age children by holding down a job as a receptionist. She has already taken all her sick days due to several bouts of the flu. Moreover, she has an unsympathetic boss who's already expressed displeasure about the missed days. Now, one of her daughters has the lead in a school play and desperately wants her mother to be there. Does she ask her boss's permission, and risk losing a day's salary? What if her finances are so tight that she can't even afford that loss? And what if her boss is so miffed that he threatens her with an even worse sanction? Finally, how will she and her daughter feel if she misses the performance?

Some women's lives are pitched at a delicate balance, and one minor conflict or mistake can throw everything off. These women need cognitive restructuring to restore their sense of balance and perspective. The working woman with the prickly boss won't find the perfect solution to her and her daughter's dilemma. But whatever road she takes, she can do so with compassion for herself—understanding that her peculiar pressures just won't let her be perfect.

I have had many perfectionistic patients who can't sleep at night because they lie awake thinking about a presentation at work the next day. They wake up at 2:00 A.M., and the chain reaction of negative thoughts begins. The perfectionist's snowball thinking goes like this:

> "I can't fall back to sleep."
> "I'm going to be exhausted tomorrow."
> "My exhaustion will leave me totally ineffective during my presentation."
> "We're going to lose the new account."
> "I'm going to lose my job."
> "I'll be miserable for the rest of my life."

What begins as a twinge of anxiety becomes a tremor of despair. Perfectionism and its relentless cognitive distortions leave no room for the slightest human error. While the insomniac is not likely to get fired no matter how tired she is the next day, her spiral of anxious thoughts certainly worsens her insomnia. If you find yourself in such a spot, do a mini and remind yourself that such thoughts are late-night geese in variously shaped bottles. If that doesn't work, put your thoughts to the four-question reality check.

For many women, their extreme perfectionism has less to do with current pressures than with voices from the past. Jody, a sixty-four-year-old party planner, was experiencing constant migraines that she attributed to stress. She had moved from city to city three times over the previous five years, as her husband, a store owner, kept needing to relocate. The most recent move was indeed most stressful: the couple left behind a lovely home, a reasonably profitable business, and the proximity of their oldest son. No doubt these stresses did contribute to Jody's emotional and physical distress. But when I probed her state of mind, it became clear that she was having trouble adjusting to the social scene. Here she was, once again in a new city, and it was very important to Jody to attract a new group of friends. Her migraines were most severe when she had company to their new home.

"I know I'm a perfectionist," said Jody. "When I would entertain, everything had to be just so. If it wasn't, and it never was, I began to get those migraines again. I kept wondering, 'What are they thinking about the house? The food? The decorating?' "

Here was a woman who was a *professional* party planner, who excelled at creating elegant events for crowds of people. Yet she worried obsessively that she would be judged poorly for what was arguably her greatest talent.

I worked with Jody to cognitively restructure her negative thoughts about her social events. It did not take long for her to recognize that she was a superb party planner, whether the parties she planned were at other people's places or her own. But the pivotal question was, "Where did you learn these thoughts?"

"It finally occurred to me that I never had any positive feedback as a child," said Jody. "I know my parents loved me, but they did not know how to show it. That's why I may know that I am loved or appreciated, but I often don't feel it. That's when the pain manifests itself in my head. I need words that prove it to me."

Once Jody realized where her self-judgments came from, she was able to restructure her thinking. She also had to nurture herself and explore and express her emotions, factors I will focus on in the following three chapters. But her transformation began when she discovered that her perfectionism had originated in childhood, and it had caused her to judge unfairly her talents and her worth to other people. Over time, her migraines also began to abate.

Perfectionism can be brutal to women with medical conditions. For instance, many women with breast and gynecologic cancers blame themselves for their condition. They didn't have perfect diets or perfect emotional lives and are now worried that they are paying the price with a life-threatening condition. Others believe they waited too long to check out a lump or other symptom and blame themselves when the prognosis is not favorable.

For such women, there may or may not be a bit of truth in their beliefs. But they use that bit to punish themselves with self-blame. How can any woman be expected to sustain a perfect diet and a perfect emotional life? (The role of emotions in cancer is controversial. But if psychological factors do contribute to cancer, they are only one contributor among many. And no woman can be held responsible for emotional states or traits she did not know were unhealthy, and could not control because they were unconscious.) Moreover, many women delay going to doctors either because they do not recognize a sign of trouble, or because they are downright scared. While such delay is never a good idea, it is often understandable when it happens.

One of my patients with breast cancer, Cindy, was told by her physician that her breast lump was benign. "But I'll keep an eye on it," he said. He did, and kept insisting that it was benign. After several months, during which time the lump grew larger, Cindy went for a second opinion. When it turned out to be breast cancer, Cindy blamed herself. "I should have known, I should have seen another doctor sooner." It took several sessions before I could convince her that she was not to blame. I reminded Cindy that she'd been frightened and vulnerable, a state of mind that makes it hard to aggressively pursue second opinions, new specialists, and so on. I also asked her if she had had any reason to doubt her physician. The answer was no—he had always treated her skillfully in the past. It made sense for her to trust him.

Many of my patients with infertility or multiple miscarriages blame themselves, citing some behavioral imperfection as the cause of their childlessness. The negative thoughts range from "I can't do anything right" to "I'm going to be a bad mother" to "I should have tried sooner." Frequently, multiple-miscarriage patients will blame the tiniest slip for their loss of a pregnancy. One woman who took a car trip before a miscarriage blamed herself: "I should never have traveled at all." These negative thoughts are demonstrably false. But women who are so tyrannized can be liberated only by putting such thoughts to the most rigorous reality check.

Whether we are sick or well, perfectionism takes its toll by robbing us of self-esteem and the capacity to experience ease and tranquility in daily life. Of course, I am not referring to rational perfectionism, which might be defined as the healthy drive for excellence. I am referring only to rigid perfectionism, which leaves no room for error, exhaustion, or even experimentation. To the best of your ability, use the skills of cognitive restructuring to banish irrational perfectionism from your heart and mind, and your body will thank you.

Cognitive Restructuring in Action

I practice cognitive restructuring with my patients on an individual basis, but, as mentioned earlier, I also practice it in my groups. I have found that it is easier for women to challenge and transform their negative thoughts with the help of others. Think about it: most of us have had painfully critical tapes playing in our solitary heads for as long as twenty, thirty, or forty years. Changing them isn't easy. We can be assisted by a caring, supportive environment, even if it involves only one other person. Not only does it help to have emotional support, it's useful to have another set of eyes and ears, someone with a more objective view when we cannot seem to escape our nasty minds.

Some negative tapes are so painful that they cause long-lasting depression and/or anxiety. In these instances I recommend that you find a therapist who can assist you in cognitive restructuring, which may be combined with other forms of psychotherapy as well as medication. Even if you aren't clinically depressed, a therapist who specializes in cognitive therapy can offer extraordinary assistance as you work to free yourself from tyrannical tapes.

You can also sit down with a friend or loved one and ask each other the four questions about your most brutal negative thoughts. As you speak, your friend or loved one can write down your answers. You can then try to restructure your own thought. If you hit a snag, you can ask for feedback, but don't expect your friend or loved one to do the work for you. (It is counterproductive and counter to the principles of good therapy to rush in with a solution to someone else's negative thought or feeling.) Then you can switch roles and listen as your partner answers the four questions about his or her own negative tape.

When you practice cognitive restructuring on your own, you may wish to write down your negative thought and your answers to the four questions. Many of my patients have found this process useful. Even just writing down the negative thought alone has therapeutic value: *There it is, the cause of so much suffering.* If you aren't sure whether a negative thought is truly dysfunctional, refer to David Burns's list of cognitive distortions and see if any of them fit.

Some of my patients keep a literal "diary of distortions," in which they write down their automatic negative thoughts every day. The records they keep are powerful testimony to how much suffering is caused by mental trickery. They also use the diaries to challenge and restructure these thoughts, writing down their new thoughts and reminding themselves to live by them.

Regardless of your state of health, I recommend that you elicit the relaxation response (see chapter 3) before attempting cognitive restructuring. I do not mean that it is necessary to practice relaxation right before you practice restructuring, rather that you begin a regular routine of relaxation before you commit yourself to cognitive change. Relaxation helps to clear the mind and body of excessive tensions that work against your effort to think and feel with clarity. Thus, the relaxation response and cognitive restructuring can work together in a synergistic fashion.

As you work to catch the nasty mind, be open to words, phrases, or ideas that suddenly shift your perspective. So many of my patients have been transformed by a spontaneous realization. I once gave a talk to participants in the Mind-Body Program for Infertility, in which I referred to a patient from an earlier group, who said, "I spent my thirties being miserable because of my infertility." One of the women in the group, Helen, was stunned by the comment. She was thirty-four and had already spent all of her thirties up to that point trying unsuccessfully to have a child. Countless high-tech treatments had failed, and the broken record in her head sang, "I'll never feel good if I can't have a biological child." She suddenly realized that she did not want to spend the rest of her thirties being miserable, a thought that spoke to her more profoundly than the broken record. Helen and her husband have since adopted a son, and she marks that moment as a turning point—the cognitive breakthrough that led her to adoption.

As you practice cognitive restructuring, remember that you don't have to be a genius to do it properly. You only have to apply common sense, and make a commitment to be as open as possible regarding your own thought processes. Remind yourself that everyone has negative tapes, and that most of them are half-truths or outright falsehoods. We all have emotional wisdom, and that's all you need to catch the nasty mind.

Six

· · ·

HEALING THROUGH
SELF-NURTURANCE

*R*ecall a time when you were head-over-heels in love. You probably saw the object of your affections as an individual of matchless intelligence, grace, and goodness. You demonstrated your devotion with a continuous stream of gifts and acts of kindness. If you happened to notice his or her minor mistakes, you saw them as signs of humanity, which only made the person *more* attractive. This early phase of a relationship exemplifies what we often call unconditional love, and it usually lasts only a few weeks or months. It's a gilded time when everything your mate does is wonderful.

When was the last time you treated *yourself* with that same unconditional love?

If you are like most of my patients, trying to recall the last time you treated yourself that kindly will be a head-scratching affair. It may come as no surprise to you to learn that you are not alone, that many women deny themselves the same compassion and care they readily shower upon others. We have too often been conditioned to caretake others, to focus our energies on the needs of spouses, family members, and even strangers. Because we are brought up to be selfless, we are too guilt-ridden to take much time for ourselves, for our pleasures, our growth, our development. Many of us lack the healthy sense of entitlement that forms a foundation for self-esteem.

This phenomenon goes by many names, some of which may be familiar—self-denial, codependence, enabling, the other-directed personality, the caretaker syndrome. It doesn't matter what name it's given; the point is, our tendency to caretake others and neglect ourselves is endemic among women, even among those who know better. I know smart, sophisticated women, many of my patients among them, who remain stuck in a pattern of self-neglect despite a high level of awareness.

The problem of selflessness and low self-esteem among women has long been recognized by sociologists, psychiatrists, and psychologists. However, in my view the problem is not strictly a psychological issue. *It is a health issue.* The ceaseless caretaking and striving of women who never give themselves a break takes its toll on their emotional *and* their physical well-being. Mind-body studies have associated self-denial of one form or another with autoimmune diseases and even with the progression of certain types of cancer.

Take, for example, the 1960s research of George F. Solomon, M.D., and his Stanford University colleague Rudolf Moos, Ph.D., who evaluated the personality characteristics of women with rheumatoid arthritis (RA), the autoimmune disease that inflames joints, causing episodes of intense pain. They described this group of patients as generally "quiet; introverted; reliable; conscientious; restricted in their expression of emotion, particularly anger; conforming; self-sacrificing; tending to allow themselves to be imposed upon; sensitive to criticism; distant; overactive and busy," among other traits. In a later study, they did not find these same traits among the subjects' sisters, women who did not have RA.

Although emotional repression, conformity, and self-sacrifice may not actually cause RA, they do appear to contribute to the disease's progression. In three decades of clinical work, Dr. Solomon has found that women with arthritis and other autoimmune diseases who begin to assert their needs and nurture themselves can bring about improvements not only in their self-worth, but in their physical condition as well. They can exert some control over bouts of inflammation and pain by finally tending to their emotional needs.

In my clinical practice, I, too, have seen evidence that women with low self-esteem who sacrifice themselves on the altar of caretaking are more prone to various physical symptoms and diseases. When these women learn to nurture themselves, their self-esteem and health improve markedly.

And women with medical conditions may enhance their recovery when they nurture themselves. My patients with infertility, multiple miscarriages, cancer, chronic pain, migraines, or autoimmune diseases need and deserve more enjoyment, because their lives have been steeped in stress. Women at menopause who take more time for themselves turn the "change of life" into a period of renewed energy and possibility.

In the last chapter, I discussed how harshly we treat ourselves in thought.

In this chapter, I focus on how harshly we treat ourselves in action. In what ways do we deny ourselves? To quote Elizabeth Barrett Browning, let me count the ways. We carve out too little time each day for pleasurable activities that have no objective other than our own enjoyment. We look to others to make ourselves feel good about our bodies, our talents, our homes, our dress, our worth as human beings. When we do take time for pleasurable activities, we often ruin the aftermath by reprimanding ourselves with self-judgments. In the guise of a diet or health program, we punish ourselves over a single indulgence in fatty or sugary foods. We often engage in romantic relationships in which we look to our partners to reinforce our sense of worth, virtually ignoring our own needs as we find new ways to struggle for that person's unconditional love.

Certainly, not all women can be described in these ways. If you recognize yourself in none of these descriptions, you need not dwell on this chapter. But many of us have chinks in our self-esteem; some of us have black holes. Our sense of deservedness does not run deep. We may *think* we deserve love, care, and compassion, but we often don't *feel* in our hearts that we do.

This gap has led to some serious misunderstandings about the problem of selflessness and low self-esteem among women. For instance, the media have frequently mocked the quest for self-esteem, as though it were nothing but an indulgent preoccupation of psychobabblers. You may have seen Stewart Smalley (played by the hilarious Al Franken), the twelve-stepping twerp on *Saturday Night Live*, who starts his cable talk show with a mirror-gazing mantra: "I'm good enough, I'm smart enough, and doggone it, people like me!" Fortunately, there is a sweetness to Franken's characterization that softens the judgment, but many people take Stewart as a huge joke on people's efforts to recover from addictions and build self-esteem. In the paperback edition of *Revolution from Within,* a serious work about women's self-esteem, Gloria Steinem documents the media's vicious attacks on the book when it was first released in hardcover. She also describes the media's dismissal of a California Task Force on Self-Esteem, which identified low self-esteem as "a primary causal factor" in major social problems such as crime, drug and alcohol abuse, teen pregnancy, welfare dependency, and child abuse. I would add women's health problems to this list. The effect of low self-esteem on mind and body is no joke.

Consider the effect of low self-esteem on Lorrie, the career counselor whose success with relaxation I described in chapter 3. Lorrie was raised by parents who did not know how to love unconditionally, and she and her siblings suffered on many levels. All four had emotional, behavioral, and learning problems. "The message I got from my parents," said Lorrie, "was that in order to have value, you must achieve great things. Now I constantly feel as though I've accomplished nothing." The only activities Lorrie and her siblings were taught to value were those oriented toward success. "To this day, all of us have a hard time doing anything that's not part of that struggle," she said. "We feel guilty just relaxing, just trying to chill out."

Though her father was not physically abusive, Lorrie clearly remembered incident after incident in which he violated her private space. "If you think of the inside of your heart and soul as being a house, then I felt like my father barged into my house and wrecked everything in sight."

Over the years, Lorrie, who is now forty, has suffered with anxiety attacks, clinical depression, and a myriad of physical symptoms. Her irritable bowel syndrome was sometimes so severe that it laid her out in bed for weeks or months at a time. She spent years in and out of the hospital for multiple surgeries and gastrointestinal symptoms. She had difficulty sustaining a romantic relationship, largely due to her low self-esteem and her anger toward men. The list of medications she had taken for her psychiatric and gastrointestinal disorders is too long to mention.

Lorrie's turnabout occurred when she entered one of our mind-body groups and began tending to her needs. In addition to taking time for relaxation, which had been very hard for her, Lorrie took time to enjoy friends, engage in church activities, and take herself out to social events. She experienced our group in the spirit I always wish for my patients: as an opportunity finally to take good care of herself. For Lorrie, this meant pursuing pleasurable activities for their own sake, enjoying the other group members, nurturing her friendships, and entering her own "private space" without feeling guilty or afraid.

Once she began tending to herself with compassion—in thought, feeling, and action—Lorrie's symptoms began to abate. She can now control her IBS attacks, and her ability to function in the world has improved markedly. Before entering our program, she was hospitalized numerous times each year for seven years; since then, she has not been hospitalized once. She'd seen many therapists before, but only recently did she find one who helped her to overcome anxiety and depression. In therapy, Lorrie allowed herself to express anger toward her parents; now, she's begun to forgive them. She finally found a job with a group of men she admires and has learned to trust. Lorrie would still like a mate, but she no longer engages, as she once did, in superficial sexual relations that only chip away further at her self-esteem. She's too busy pursuing her interests, friendships, and spirituality.

Obviously, we don't all have self-esteem problems as severe as Lorrie's. But many of us lack a deep sense of deservedness and self-worth. Our bouts of anxiety, depression, and physical illness can often be directly or indirectly related to this underlying lack. Some of us have veneers of self-confidence that we fool ourselves into believing. But the truth can only be found when we give honest answers to these questions: Do I take time out each day for my own pleasure? Does my sense of worth depend largely on other people's approval, gifts, or gratitude? Do I feel that the only way I can get my needs met is to give? Is my identity largely bound up in my abilities as a caretaker?

In this chapter, I provide practical ways that you can meet your own needs. By so doing, you can break your dependence on other people's responses in order to feel good about yourself. The key is learning to give yourself the nurturance you desire, by taking time out for pleasurable and soul-satisfying activity. Just as we must transform our self-negating thoughts into ones that are more truthful and compassionate, we must transform our self-negating actions to more self-nurturing ones. Strange as it may seem, I have come to the firm conclusion that being good to ourselves is essential to our medical self-care.

Are There Healthy Pleasures?

Does being good to ourselves really have any physical health benefits? According to psychologist Robert Ornstein, Ph.D., and David Sobel, M.D., authors of *Healthy Pleasures,* the answer is unequivocal. Ornstein and Sobel put forth the proposition that "the healthiest people seem to be pleasure-loving, pleasure-seeking, pleasure-creating individuals." Although they advocate healthy dietary and lifestyle habits, they believe that our culture has emphasized a strictly pleasure-*denying* road to health, to the point of absurdity. Moreover, they cite intriguing scientific studies that support their views. These studies demonstrate, among other things, that living the life of the senses can lead to better health, as shown by a variety of medical measures.

Positive moods and emotions tend to enhance the immune system, and, in some studies, they've been associated with disease recovery. What brings about positive moods and emotions? According to Ornstein and Sobel, the answer is social support in the form of loving friends and spouses; enjoyable activities ranging from creative hobbies to vacations; and any responsible pursuit of pleasure rooted in the senses, as long as it does not compromise health on some other level (e.g., smoking) or trample upon other people's needs. The joys of literature, painting, movies, and music are indisputably soul-satisfying; some studies suggest they are also health-promoting. Ornstein and Sobel even argue that the oft-disparaged "indulgences" of food and drink, when practiced in moderation, lift our moods without a life-threatening price tag.

Here are just a few of the studies that support the concept of healthy pleasures, organized according to the five senses:

- *Sight:* Researcher Aaron Katcher and his colleagues found that people who stared at an aquarium replete with colorful tropical fish, living plants, and rocks not only achieved a state of relaxation, their blood pressure dropped significantly. For those who already had high blood pressure, their readings often fell into the normal range. This effect was largely negated if the subjects were then asked to stare into an empty tank. Apparently, giving ourselves time to delight in visual splendor calms both mind and body.

- *Sound:* Although one study I conducted did not show music to have a positive effect on reducing the pain of a diagnostic procedure (see chapter 2), other studies have shown that music effectively reduces anxiety and pain in pre- and postoperative patients. Music has also been used successfully to treat depression; chronic pain, including headaches; the side effects of cancer treatment; and the pain experienced by accident and burn victims. In one study, music therapist and researcher Mark Rider showed that nurses who were stressed by working odd hours had reduced stress hormones after listening to tapes that combined relaxation, guided imagery, and soothing music.

- *Smell:* Though more research is needed on the physiologic effects of aromatherapy—the use of various, mostly pleasant scents to bring about positive changes in mood and health—some studies confirm its efficacy. In one experiment, people hooked up to physiologic monitors were asked stress-provoking questions. Some subjects were given a whiff of a fragrance before being questioned. The researchers discovered that the scent of spiced apple moderated the stress response in people, whose blood pressure was lower, heart and breathing rates were slower, and muscles were more relaxed.

- *Taste:* Certain foods trigger the release of neurotransmitters—brain chemicals—associated with positive moods and feelings. For instance, foods high in carbohydrates such as pastas and cereals have been shown to stimulate serotonin, a neurotransmitter that relaxes us, eases tension, and aids in sleep. Animal studies suggest that when we eat sweet foods, we experience an increase in endorphins, those pain-killing and mood-enhancing brain chemicals.

- *Touch:* Data supporting the mental and physical health benefits of touch are so extensive that it can take an entire book to document them. Ashley Montagu's *Touching: The Human Significance of the Skin* is a fine introduction, though many recent scientific investigations have confirmed and expanded upon his findings. Both animal and human studies have shown that early handling and touch have a significant, positive effect on long-term growth patterns. But can touch help protect us against disease? In one study, UCLA psychiatrist George F. Solomon, M.D., joined with colleagues to show that rats who receive early handling as infants develop stronger immune systems over time. Psychiatrist Gail Ironson, M.D., of the University of Miami showed that HIV-positive individuals who received massages had improved immune cell functions.

While I cannot support every one of Ornstein and Sobel's contentions (e.g., I feel they downplay too much the risks of fatty foods and alcohol), their overall point of view in *Healthy Pleasures* is scientifically sound. These and other studies suggest that our nervous, immune, and cardiovascular systems are as "delighted" by sensual experiences as our minds. Beautiful sights, melodious sounds, sweet smells, delectable tastes, and warm touches should not be denigrated as hedonistic thrills. They are portals of pleasure and meaning that enhance our well-being.

What do we look forward to? What soothes our souls and gives us hope and inspiration? The answers almost always involve the senses, because we receive life and love through them, whether in the form of the sights and smells of nature; the tastes of foods we need to thrive; the sounds that stir the spirit, be they from songbirds or CDs; and the touch of people in our lives whose care and support sustains us.

What does this mean for women and their health? Unfortunately, the prescription is not as easy as "Delight in the senses." Usually, women who lack for pleasurable experiences are stressed out by the dueling pressures they face every day. Often, they are self-sacrificing caretakers, or the "superwomen" trying to do too much to please their families or live up to cultural standards. Also, as I've emphasized, they may lack the underlying deservedness that would otherwise motivate them to meet their own needs. These women—and perhaps you're one of them—have come to believe that there *is* no time for relaxation, and there is certainly no time for "frivolous" activities that serve no purpose other than their own enjoyment.

Our health is bolstered when we take care of our emotional, physical, sensual, and spiritual needs. Yet we've tended to deny ourselves the time and freedom to care fully for ourselves. Our health and well-being demand that we grant ourselves that time, and that freedom.

Seize the Time

*F*or many years, Deirdre worked as a nanny for a family with three young children. When she and her husband had their own child, Deirdre had to ask for time off, and she worried that her employers would find another nanny. She was pleased when they did not, because she liked the job and genuinely cared for the three children. But afterward, when she managed to find child care for her own baby and returned to work, she began to feel stressed out by her wall-to-wall caretaking responsibilities. Though she was delighted by motherhood, she felt as though she was being stretched in every direction.

I counseled Deirdre, who was in one of my groups, to take time for herself, not just to elicit the relaxation response (which I also recommended), but to experience pleasure that did not depend on anyone else. She began doing small things, like getting herself a manicure, which was not only tending to her appearance but doing something solely for her own benefit.

Then, one day during late spring, Deirdre was inspired to go to her local plant nursery. There she did something that seemed to her and her family entirely out of character, given their tight budget and her cautious personality. She spent $350 on potted plants. Deirdre brought the plants home in the trunk of her car, then set them out on their front porch. For the rest of spring and summer, she'd often just sit and look at the splendid array of flowering plants, with their rainbow spectrum of colors.

Deirdre was a caretaker by profession, and by choice. She was clearly devoted to all her children, biological and otherwise. She enjoyed her work, and she enjoyed being a mother. But she suffered because her own needs— apart from her identity as caretaker—were not being fulfilled. Tending to those potted plants, which demanded almost nothing save a watering, was tending to herself. The porch became her space, her opportunity to experience some beauty and a sense of peacefulness whenever she found some free time in the crevices of her days.

Though a vital step of stress management is to be kind to yourself in thought, the next step is to be kind to yourself in action. That is what Deirdre was able to do, and it had a strikingly positive effect on every aspect of her life. Her relations with her family, her ability to enjoy her work, and her self-esteem all improved.

Healing through self-nurturance means seizing time for yourself. In chapter 3, I recommended that you take about twenty minutes each day to elicit the relaxation response, which is one way of taking care of yourself. Here, I recommend that you take an additional half hour (at least) each day to engage in some activity that is soul-nourishing. This is quite different from relaxation, even though the activity may be relaxing. This is time to care for your own needs, to enjoy a facet of yourself, to experience pleasure via your senses.

Start by giving yourself permission to take this time. This may be the hardest step, because many of us were not raised to do so. Frequently, our mothers, especially ones who reared us during the 1940s and '50s, took little if any time for themselves. They were too busy as housewives and caretakers, and they didn't have the same amenities—such as dishwashers and micro-waves—that we have today to compress time for household chores. Also, many of our mothers were raised by mothers who handed down strict teachings about devotion to family in the form of constant self-sacrifice.

Know that if you find it hard to give yourself permission, it is due to your own lack of a self-nurturing role model. There's no need to blame your mother for this. You may have learned this tendency from her, but she learned it from her mother, and so on down the ancestral line. Think of your effort as a midcourse correction in generational drift toward excessive self-sacrifice. Consider the probability that your mother would have been better off had she granted herself more time. And, if you have a daughter, consider the fact that she'll be better off with a maternal role model who cares for herself.

Some of my stressed-out patients feel so unentitled that I am moved to take out my mock prescription pad and write, "One half hour per day for yourself. Doctor's orders." Once they've been instructed by a health profes-sional to take time for their own enjoyment, they finally take this need seriously, recognizing that their self-esteem *and* physical health are at stake.

Recently, a clue to the healing potential of self-nurturance was uncov-ered by two leading mind-body researchers. George F. Solomon, M.D., and Lydia Temoshok, Ph.D., studied longtime survivors of AIDS—a group of individuals who had outlived their doctors' predictions. Among these unusual patients, Solomon and Temoshok discovered links between certain behaviors and stronger immune cells. One of the behaviors was assertiveness. Another one, based on an answer to one of their questionnaire items, was the willingness "to withdraw to nurture the self." Patients who took time to care for themselves had more suppressor cells, which seem to play a key role in resistance to AIDS. These cells also help us to resist autoimmune diseases. Solomon and Temoshok's research provides preliminary evidence that we take care of our immune systems when we take care of our emotional, physical, and spiritual needs.

This entire chapter is my prescription to you to take time for yourself. Over time, patients for whom I have written these prescriptions learn to refill them themselves; they no longer need me to write them out. Their own enhanced well-being and joy are motivation enough. If you follow this prescription, you will probably find that you, too, will be motivated to continue based on the many positive repercussions.

But your guilt about taking time may run deep. To reclaim your sense of entitlement, recognize that others around you—perhaps other members of your family—have no such trouble. Don't let this cause simmering resentment, which is only counterproductive to your health and well-being. Let it motivate you to action on your own behalf.

A stereotypical but undeniably common example is the husband who has no trouble taking the better part of Sunday with his male friends in the living room to watch sporting events. (Super Bowl Sunday is a prime example of such an all-day extravaganza.) It's hard to imagine many women with families taking three or more hours out of any day to do anything strictly pleasurable.

I've known women who resent their husbands' sports-drenched Sundays, and who hassle them with sarcastic remarks or requests made during the climax of some crucial game. (And we all know that every game is crucial.) Here's what I say to these women: As long as he doesn't demand that you serve him, let your husband have his time with his friends and his games in peace. He (presumably) works hard; he deserves it. Focus instead on the fact that you deserve the same. Indeed, your resentment may have stemmed from the fact, often unrecognized, that you never give yourself such opportunities. Rather than trying to rob his leisure time, seize your own. You may wish to strike a bargain with him: "Enjoy your games while I watch the kids. However, on Sunday morning (or evening) you take charge of the kids and the house while I do something for myself." You might take yourself on a morning walk in the park, or to an evening movie. Whatever you do, it will extinguish the fires of your resentment, and reinforce your healthy sense of entitlement.

If you don't seize time to take care of yourself, you're not going to take such good care of your loved ones, either. Eventually, your energy and compassion get drained, until you carry out your responsibilities as if they were drudgery. That's when you lose patience at the drop of a glass; one mishap and you fly off the handle. Though it may be a cliché, you're not doing your loved ones any good by sacrificing yourself to the hilt. As Gloria Steinem recently wrote, "It's a truism that we can't love others until we love ourselves—but truisms are also true."

The Time Pie

Another way to motivate yourself is to take an unblinking look at how you spend your time now. Ann Webster, Ph.D., my colleague in the Division of Behavioral Medicine at Deaconess Hospital, taught me a wonderful tool to help people see more clearly how they treat themselves. Try the following exercise.

Draw a circle on a piece of paper, and turn it into a pie chart that represents your typical twenty-four-hour day. If you generally sleep six hours a night, draw a slice that represents one quarter of the pie. If you generally sleep eight hours a night, draw a slice that represents one third of the pie. Then draw a slice that represents how many hours you work each day. Next, determine how much time you spend for commuting, running errands, cooking, shopping, caretaking children, exercising, having sex, showering, watching TV, and so on. In each of these "slices," write down the activity and the number of minutes or hours you expend. Be as honest with yourself and as accurate as you can. Use the sample pie (Figure 6-1) as a guide.

Put your twenty-four-hour time pie aside. On a separate piece of paper, number 1 through 20. Then, as fast as you can without too much deliberation, list twenty things that bring you joy.

Now, compare this list with your time pie. How much time is indicated on the pie for any of the twenty activities that bring you joy? I have had women who follow this exercise only to discover that they spend no time whatsoever for activities that bring them joy. Many count the time in minutes rather than hours.

The next step is to create an ideal time pie for the future. Using your current pie as a guide, draw another pie and make changes to create more time for the most important joys on your list. The key here is to be *realistic*

FIGURE 6-1

Sample Time Pie

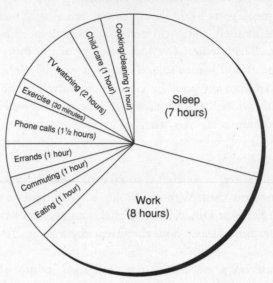

in your assessments. Perhaps you can't cut back on work or child-care hours; you probably shouldn't cut back on sleep. I don't mean for you to fantasize endless hours of leisure time, in which you have your nails done while sipping margaritas on a seaside veranda. I mean for you to consciously play with your own building blocks of time, shifting them here and there until you've created a modest block that is solely for your own enjoyment.

Many women who do this exercise discover that they waste a good deal of time. Time wasting is common among people who are anxious. I call this running in place. For instance, women who can't relax and don't take time for meaningful pleasures often spend excessive amounts of time vegging out in front of the TV or talking on the phone, which are futile attempts to relieve their tensions or their loneliness. (I have nothing against vegging out in front of the TV or talking on the phone, but we all know when we've crossed a line.) In your future time pie, borrow minutes or even hours from these time-wasting activities and redirect them into soul-nourishing activities. Instead of watching hours of sitcom reruns, take yourself to a fun or interesting new film. Rather than gabbing on the phone for hours with a disembodied friend, go with an embodied friend to a weeknight concert or play.

Use your realistic future time pie as a guide. Although I suggest that you find at least a half hour per day for your own pleasure, you might be able to find more time. You may also wish to schedule bigger slices of time for lengthier activities, alone or with friends. The point is not to create a rigid new set of expectations, but rather to be certain that you find time each day for yourself.

The Purple Outfit:
Varieties of Self-Care

*T*he varieties of self-nurturance are as limitless as our individual tastes and personalities. That's why I don't offer a list of specific things you should be doing, but rather examples that may inspire you to find your own ways to nourish soul and body.

Zelda was a patient in the Mind-Body Program for Infertility. For three years she'd been stuck on the infertility treadmill of high-tech medical treatments, with many disappointments. Her self-worth as a woman had plummeted, because she blamed herself for her childlessness, even though her infertility was unexplained. Zelda had little compassion for her own suffering. She spent almost no time on herself. She hadn't bought any new clothes in years, feeling that she'd gained weight and wasn't entitled to such a luxury.

Zelda confided her anguish to the group, and we recognized that she was depressed. But she used relaxation to gradually regain her bearings. Then, during the third session of our program, the assignment was to do something wonderful for yourself and share the experience with the group the following week. Zelda took the assignment quite seriously, because at the next group she not only described what she'd done, she provided show-and-tell.

Zelda waltzed into our meeting in a glorious, flowing purple outfit. The blouse, long skirt, and even her lovely fedora were all the same brilliant shade of purple. The group cheered as she walked in, and they listened with rapt attention as she spoke about her choice. Zelda said she realized how hard she'd been on herself. Purple was her favorite color, so she decided to deck herself out in purple. She did so with great style, and the group celebrated her for taking such flamboyant good care of herself. Zelda's mood had changed as radically as her attire; her spirit was as iridescent as her new outfit. (A mere four weeks later, the group had another reason to celebrate Zelda: she came in and announced that she was pregnant.)

What's your equivalent of Zelda's purple outfit?

A specific aspect of self-nurturance is doing nice things for yourself, as

Zelda had done. When I give my patients that assignment, their choices are as unique as their personalities. Many patients schedule regular massages, which are not only physically pleasurable but represent an hour of time devoted solely to their well-being. The same can be said for other forms of bodywork, such as shiatsu or acupressure. Others tend to their physical appearance, with manicures, pedicures, or facials. Still others buy themselves flowers, new clothes, or shoes. And it doesn't require vast sums to treat yourself well; I know women who can get blissed out over cappuccino and a fashion magazine.

Many women allow themselves to have foods that they normally would not eat, or foods they'd sometimes eat but punish themselves mercilessly for having done so. For them, an occasional ice cream cone, or whatever their guilty food pleasure happens to be, can satisfy a normal craving—*if* it's enjoyed without self-flagellation.

In a recent mind-body group, the women wrote down the good things they had started doing for themselves. Here is the list I compiled from them, a sampling of self-nurturing acts:

- Taking naps in the late afternoon
- Having a regular massage and enjoying it mindfully
- Reading trashy novels
- Having a great bottle of wine with Friday night dinners at home
- Listening to wild music in the morning
- Buying new boots I've thought about for months
- Taking long, hot baths every other night
- Enjoying extended walks on the beach
- Treating myself to a haircut with a new hairdresser
- Playing hooky once every few months from a highly stressful job
- Mindful gardening
- Not going to the in-laws' for Passover
- Going to a country bed-and-breakfast for the weekend
- Getting a regular pedicure

The key here is not to exult in luxury; few of us can afford to do that. *The key is to indulge yourself in pleasures that you would normally deny yourself, as often as you can.* For instance, if you are an addictive shopper, more shopping would not be a self-nurturing act. But if you haven't bought new shoes in years, by all means do so. If you're an addictive eater, binging is no act of self-love. You probably need to nurture yourself in areas that stimulate other senses—for instance, touch (e.g., massage) or sound (e.g., listening to soul-nourishing music). But if you never allow yourself the slightest slip from a strict dietary regime, an occasional treat may be called for.

Your choices might not be unusual. For instance, you may find it relaxing and empowering just to find more time to read. Calibrate your choices to your specific needs. If your work or creative activities are highly cerebral, give yourself a break with, for instance, a trashy novel. If you waste time on distractions, you might choose poetry, literary novels, or biographies. If you find yourself run down, you might choose music that animates the body. If you find yourself jazzed up, you might choose music that soothes the soul. If you lack for solitude, take yourself out to movies. If you lack for social contact, join a club or organization that interests you.

Self-nurturance should never feel like another obligation. Your choices should emphasize pleasure, play, and a sense of fun. Going to a museum exhibit because your erudite friend says you must, when you have no abiding interest in that type of art, is rarely self-nurturing. Although your choices should feed mind, body, and soul, I put particular emphasis on body and soul. Many of us are overloaded with intellectual stimulation and media information.

George F. Solomon, M.D., summed up my own view: "Freud talked about the need for fulfillment in love and work," said Solomon. "But he didn't mention play. Play is not goal-directed behavior, it is frivolous behavior that's enjoyable for its own sake. And some people don't know how to play. I believe that people need balance among love, work, and play in order to stay healthy."

Whose Self Is It, Anyway?

Self-nurturance affirms the healthiest messages you can deliver to your conscious and unconscious mind: "I can take care of my needs, and I can feel good about myself without anyone else's confirmation."

They don't like to admit it, but many women do feel dependent upon others to feel good about themselves. Perhaps you are one of them. The classic example is the woman in a budding romance whose self-esteem hangs on every act of her beloved. Will he call? Will he bring flowers? Will he remember her birthday? Will he ask her out for next weekend?

Allowing your self-worth to rise and fall on someone else's actions is a perilous course. By cultivating this type of relationship, you reinforce your own passivity and insecurity. The reasons you do so may run deep, with origins in your early family life. If you believe this to be so, I recommend psychotherapy to explore the roots of your insecurity. However, whether or not you do therapy, you can benefit by making a conscious shift in your behavior. Namely, don't wait for others to make you feel good about yourself; claim that power for yourself. Don't wait for your beloved to bring you flowers; buy them yourself. If your boss does not affirm your good work, ask friends at work for their support. Don't let yourself be victimized by other people's moods, whims, or limitations.

One of my patients, Gina, always had some stress-related health complaint, from colds to backaches. She also felt lonely, because at the age of thirty-five she had not found "Mr. Right." Gina fantasized about the type of man she wanted to marry, and about how the romance would unfold, from the first meeting through engagement and marriage. She specifically wished for a diamond-and-sapphire engagement ring. After several therapeutic sessions, Gina came to understand that she could be whole and happy in the present, even without Mr. Right.

While on vacation in the Caribbean, where such jewelry is relatively inexpensive, Gina saw the perfect diamond-and-sapphire ring. She wondered how long it would be before she met someone who would buy it for her. With her new mind-set, a strange thought took hold: "Why not buy it for myself? Okay, so it won't symbolize an engagement. Instead, it will symbolize my care for myself." Gina bought the ring.

Was it coincidence that Gina met the man she would marry a few months later? Probably, but I have observed, time and again, that women often get what they want when they stop clinging to an idealized goal and instead take care of their own needs. Such women have an air of self-sufficiency that is attractive; they are also more responsive to potential mates who treat them with the love and respect they deserve.

When I emphasize self-nurturance, I don't mean that women should never depend on others for help, care, and support. Women who are independent—"autonomous" may be a better term—are not disconnected islands who could, if necessary, live in isolation. As I will explore fully in the next chapter, part of self-nurturance is the ability to ask for and accept others' help, care, and support. We are all interdependent members of families and communities, and our health and well-being are sustained by our social connections. But the autonomous woman does not live and breathe for others' approval; her sense of self is sturdy. She has a strong core identity that enables her to be alone without feeling lonely. She can experience the joys of living—of nature, beauty, the life of the mind and the body—

without needing someone else to validate that experience. She can bestow worthiness upon herself.

When women who depend on others for self-worth try to change, their families and friends may respond with warmth and support. Husbands, lovers, sons, daughters, siblings, and colleagues may feel relieved of an inappropriate sense of responsibility for her emotional well-being, and happy for her positive transformation. But in some instances, family members or friends are threatened. A delicate balance can be disrupted when a woman shifts from overdependency to a capacity for self-care. These loved ones may resist her changes, because they fear no longer being needed. Or they may worry that more time for herself means less time for them.

If you find that family members and/or friends resist or resent the time you take for yourself, gently but firmly continue to assert your right to this time. Let them know that you are not trying to disconnect. On the contrary, you are living the dictum that your relationships can only be strengthened as your self-esteem is strengthened. By treating yourself with compassion and care, you become more able to give compassion and care, out of desire, rather than duty. You'll have more energy and you'll be more present, because you no longer suppress yearnings for pleasure, or meaning, or fun, or solitude.

Be careful how you communicate this need. Don't blame your husband, partner, parents, kids, colleagues, or friends for your lack of time, past or present. It wasn't their fault, and it wasn't yours. The problem arose in the crucible of a stressful existence, and now you recognize this and wish to take responsibility for changing it. Avoid statements that begin with "You haven't given me the time to . . ." or "You don't give me the opportunity to . . ." When you make such statements, you not only lay blame, which causes fights and bruised feelings, but you take the position of imprisoned victim.

I've had patients who tell their husbands, "I have to take better care of myself." The husband, mistakenly assuming that she is criticizing his ability to take care of her, reacts defensively. I've counseled these patients to state explicitly that they are not passing judgment on his caretaking; they are declaring a need that only they can fulfill. If your language is similarly misunderstood, simplify it: "I need some time to rest." "I need time to draw." "I want to take walks to get exercise and some time for myself."

If your loved ones still have difficulties, be as patient with them and yourself as possible. Know that as you nurture yourself, as you become stronger and more assertive, a process unfolds that makes it easier for you to tolerate their anxieties. It will gradually become easier for them to recognize and appreciate your newfound self-esteem. If they do not, you may need some professional help—a counselor or family therapist—to help you forge more significant changes in how you relate.

"Water" Your Self-Esteem

Sylvia worked for a talent agency for the better part of a decade, and she was beginning to experience stress burnout. Her superior was dictatorial, and he fostered bitter competition among the agents. The frequent demands of narcissistic clients only added to the pressure-cooker atmosphere on the job. The toll on Sylvia's energy and self-esteem was profound, and she was plagued by various symptoms—headaches, backaches, frequent colds.

Before taking on this job, Sylvia's self-esteem was robust. "My mother was always positive about herself," said Sylvia, "and she wanted me to feel good about myself." But the relentless job stress overwhelmed her otherwise healthy ego, striking at hidden vulnerabilities. When I first saw her, Sylvia had long since ceased taking time for herself. "After years of struggle and put-downs, you begin to feel you don't deserve any good stuff," she said. "I wouldn't even give myself a twenty-minute shower."

Once Sylvia realized how she'd been treating herself, she turned a corner. Time for herself became a top priority. "I had not gone for a facial or a massage in years," she said. "Now I go every four weeks. I golf every Sunday. I take leisurely walks. And I take long, hot showers."

For some women, a sense of deservedness can be destroyed by a dysfunctional family. But for others like Sylvia, who'd always been taught to love herself, the sense of deservedness is gradually eroded by current life circumstances. Whatever the sources of your low self-esteem, you can begin the rebuilding process as Sylvia did, with small acts of self-nourishment. By way of analogy, imagine that you have a clay pot filled with rocks, and nestled in the rocks is a bulb. The bulb will grow into full flower when watered on a daily basis. Now see that bulb as a symbolic representation of your self-esteem; if you "water" it every day with acts of self-care, it will gradually blossom. Once Sylvia's self-esteem began to bloom, she refused to get sucked into competitive madness on the job. She took more time off for pleasure, and the positive ripple effect touched every aspect of her life, including her relationships.

"Watering" self-esteem also means being good to ourselves in every realm: nutrition, exercise, emotional well-being, creativity, social and romantic relationships, and the family. To accomplish this, we must first become aware of extreme imbalances in these areas. Too many of us live in extremes. In the realm of food, we either punish ourselves for one violation of a strict diet or we overindulge to the point of ill health. In the realm of exercise, we are either couch potatoes or fanatical health-clubbers. In the realm of emotions, we either repress our negative feelings behind a stoic facade, or feel compelled to express every twinge of sadness or anger. In the realm of creativity, we either neglect our artistic impulses or we base our self-worth solely on the world's response to our creative output. In the realm of romance, we either tie our self-worth to the whims of the beloved, or we cut ourselves off because we fear rejection. In the realm of family dynamics, we either stay stuck in old patterns of dependency, or we isolate ourselves in the name of separation.

Thus, being good to ourselves requires that we create balance in all these realms, and that we do so by taking action on our own behalf. Consider the case of Jessica, whose imbalance was in the realm of creativity. A forty-eight-year-old nurse, Jessica had been raised by her family to be an exceptional caretaker, and when I met her she was working full-time as a nurse while tending to her husband and three children. She was anxious, physically exhausted, and frequently sick with a variety of stress-related ailments.

Jessica had always cultivated a "side" activity, music. She had studied the violin as a child and over time she became successful as a professional violinist with local orchestras. But given her work and family responsibilities, she'd never been able to pursue her musical career with the requisite commitment. After participating in one of our mind-body groups, Jessica began to focus on self-care, and she made a momentous decision: she quit her job as a nurse and devoted her career to music.

"All my years as a nurse, taking care of patients, were very fulfilling," she said. "It was work that I really loved. But I just ran out of energy for it. I didn't want to take care of people anymore. . . . Now I feel that I have a better balance, though it still takes work. I have an eleven-year-old, and I want to be helpful to my older daughter and son-in-law and their baby. I'm married, I still have plenty of family. But I do have much more time to devote to this other pursuit, which is the complete opposite of every other part of my life. Music is direct and pure and doesn't involve anybody but you and the composer and your instrument."

Jessica's shift from caretaking to creativity left her calmer, more energetic, and less susceptible to stress-related symptoms.

We may not be in a position to quit our jobs to pursue creative careers.

But we can find ways to express what Lawrence LeShan calls our "foiled creative fire." In her book *The Artist's Way,* Julia Cameron suggests that we take our "inner artist" out on dates. "An artist date is a block of time, perhaps two hours weekly, especially set aside and committed to nurturing your creative consciousness, your inner artist," writes Cameron. "In its most primary form, the artist date is an excursion, a playdate that you preplan and defend against all interlopers. You do not take anyone on this date but you and your inner artist."

Cameron stresses that the artist date should not be an obligatory trip to a local museum. Find experiences that fire your imagination, regardless of whether they fulfill someone else's ideas about art. Take yourself to an old movie, an aquarium, a photography show, an intriguing art exhibit, an ethnic neighborhood for foreign sights, sounds, and tastes. Go to a concert of a type of music that has fascinated you but that you've rarely heard. Or take a long walk on a beach or a country road, and entertain your fantasies about the book you want to write, song you want to sing, part you'd like to play, drawing you wish to render. Start to fulfill those fantasies.

A remarkable thirty-year-long study proved that women who tend to many parts of themselves experience fewer illnesses and live longer than women who do not. Phyllis Moen, Ph.D., Family Professor of Life Course Studies at Cornell University in Ithaca, New York, tracked 427 married women with children who lived in upstate New York. These women, who ranged in age from twenty-five to fifty, were first evaluated in 1956 and followed up to 1986.

Dr. Moen and her colleagues, Donna Dempster-McClain and Robin M. Williams, Jr., found that women who showed remarkably vibrant health over thirty years exhibited two key characteristics: they were members of volunteer organizations, and they took on multiple roles. Over three decades, these women had significantly fewer major illnesses, better mental health, and greater longevity than other women in the study.

The women volunteers got out into the world to help strangers, connecting with members of their community (a point to which I will return in the next chapter). But the fact that they engaged in multiple roles showed that they did not feel restrained in wife and mother roles. They were committed wives and mothers, but they went beyond the 1950s model of the perfect woman by embracing other sides of themselves. Typically, they chose to be socially active in churches and clubs, to spend much time with friends and relatives, and to have jobs outside the home. Moen viewed them as vivacious women who engaged in work and social activities that were both meaningful and enjoyable. Dr. Moen's study, aptly called "The Women's Roles and Well-Being Project," teaches us that women can stay healthier and live longer by exploring many sides of themselves, and by doing so actively in the world.

Lawrence LeShan once said, "We need a fierce and tender concern for all parts of ourselves so that no part of our being is left outside the door, whimpering, 'Is there nothing for me?' " Cultivate this fierce and tender concern for all parts of yourself, and you will become less anxious, depressed, or hopeless. You may reduce addictions to food, drugs, sex, or bad relationships. Your physical health will invariably improve. Water your self-esteem as a daily practice, and you'll ride the roughest waves of stress and change with vigor and with grace.

Seven

♦ ♦ ♦

REACHING OUT TO
FRIENDS AND FAMILY

*T*here are times in our lives when all we wish for is escape. Stress and pressure abound, and running away seems like the only sensible solution. We want to crawl under a rock but we can't, so we crawl under the covers. We eat too much, watch too much television, snap at our partners, kids, or friends. We may fall prey to addiction, depression, or both. Our capacity to experience pleasure in the present dwindles, and our hopes for the future fade.

But escape never provides a solution. It provides only temporary relief from the pain, be it physical or emotional. The same stresses, pressures, or symptoms rear their Medusa-like heads the next day, week, or month. The only way out is to grapple with our pains and problems head on: to find the strength to devise and carry out real-world solutions. In this endeavor, there is only one genuine external comfort, only one outside source for the strength we need to cope, to change, and to grow. That source is human connections—the love and support of friends and family. Social support is the wellspring of our mind-body health, and science has proven it so. The research on the effects of social support on health promotion and disease recovery may be medical science's most important untold story.

In this chapter, I will tell you about the surprising power of groups—whether they offer therapy, mind-body skills, or simply support—to help women cope and heal. But I also emphasize the health benefits of weaving a fabric of support into our lives. Some of us are fortunate to have support networks in place; we may only need to strengthen the connections. But some of us don't have adequate networks. They're lacking essential elements, or they're frayed at the edges because we don't take good enough care of them. Perhaps we have many male compatriots but few women friends, or many women friends but no men other than our partners. Or we have no spouse or partner to provide the kind of intimacy we can't seem to get from close friends. Or our families are so fraught with tension that we don't turn to them at all. Or the quality of our relationships isn't what we wish; there's too much distance, or dependence, or competition, or resentment.

This chapter is about how we can reach out to friends and family to forge the support systems that keep us happy and healthy. Though I run formal groups and believe in their potential, formal groups are not necessary. (I do strongly recommend them, however, to any and all women who have a particular medical problem, because other women going through the same pains and tribulations offer a unique form of support.) We owe it to ourselves to build and buttress our own healing support systems.

Social Support and Health: The Untold Story

*H*ow important is social support to our health and well-being? In 1988, epidemiologist James House, Ph.D., of the University of Michigan, published a landmark paper in which he reviewed a half-dozen studies of a total of more than 22,000 men and women. These studies, conducted in communities all over the map, showed that people without well-established support systems had significantly shorter life expectancies. By contrast, those with rich personal networks had far longer life spans. In fact, people with few friends and supportive relationships had a death rate *two to four times higher* than those with substantial networks.

"At this point, we do not see strong competing alternative explanations for these findings," said Dr. House recently. He had shown that a lack of social support was a critical factor in ill health even after he controlled for every other conceivable factor. In his paper, House writes, "These developments suggest that social relationships, or the relative lack thereof, constitute a major risk factor for health—rivaling the effects of well-established health risk factors such as cigarette smoking, blood pressure, blood lipids, obesity, and physical activity."

House's conclusion is startling. If lack of social support—or, to put it bluntly, loneliness—is a risk factor with even half the pathological power of smoking, then it is time for women and their doctors to pay attention.

In the studies evaluated by Dr. House, the link between social relationships and health was stronger among men than women, though it was still significant among women. Also, marriage appeared to be more beneficial to health for men than for women. Yet women seemed to benefit more from relationships with friends and relatives, which tend to run along same-sex lines. As Stanford University psychiatrist David Spiegel commented ironically to Bill Moyers in the television special *Healing and the Mind,* "This leads me to the unhappy conclusion that having a relationship with a man doesn't do your health much good, regardless of your gender."

Among the most astonishing recent findings is that women with strong support systems may be less likely to develop fatal cancer. Epidemiologists George Kaplan, Ph.D., and Peggy Reynolds, Ph.D., of the University of California at Berkeley, followed 6,848 people for over seventeen years. Women with the fewest social contacts were more than twice as likely to die of cancer than those with many social connections. Socially isolated women were particularly prone to hormone-related cancers, including breast cancer. (In another study of 243 women with breast cancer confined to the breast or regional lymph nodes, those with two or more people they could confide in had a 76 percent survival rate over seven years. By comparison, those with no confidants had a 56 percent survival rate.)

Social support appears to be a key factor in the prevention of many other conditions that commonly affect women. Consider the following findings, each from a different set of investigators:

- Women who sought medical care for menopausal symptoms had significantly less social support than a comparison group of menopausal women who had no such symptoms.
- Working women suffering with menstrual cramps and PMS reported significantly poorer social support than women who were free of these symptoms.
- A study following 1,428 pregnant women turned up "partner support" as one of the most important factors in maintaining pregnancy. (Women with strong partner support not only had fewer abortions, but fewer miscarriages.)
- A review of medical literature showed that the availability of emotional and practical support is strongly correlated with the mother's health during and after childbirth.

Thus, women need social connections to stay healthy and to boost their prospects for recovery from illness. Yet a whole other body of research reveals that the quality of our relationships is as important to our physical health as the sheer quantity. People whose relationships are characterized by hostility or poor communication may have weaker cardiovascular and immune systems than those who can relate to friends and family in a spirit of openness and trust.

Psychologist Janice Kiecolt-Glaser, Ph.D., and her husband, immunologist Ronald Glaser, M.D., are among the leading mind-body scientists in the country. In their lab at Ohio State University Medical School, the Glasers have shown that quality social relationships—in particular, strong marriages and couples with good communication—can strengthen our immune system, the "healer within" that keeps us healthy.

In one ingenious study, the Glasers showed that how we relate and speak to one another has a direct impact on our bodies. They brought ninety male-female couples into their laboratory and monitored their immune systems by drawing blood both before and after they attempted to resolve an issue of disagreement. "Those couples who had the most hostility and negativity during the discussions showed a drop on eight immune measures for the next 24 hours," Dr. Kiecolt-Glaser told the *New York Times*. "The more hostile you are during a marital argument, the harder it is on your immune system." The ramifications are clear: by finding ways to resolve conflicts and communicate without attacking our loved ones, we protect our immune cells, whose job it is to protect *us* from harmful disease agents.

Since 1990, a series of landmark studies have shown that people with life-threatening illnesses experienced physical improvements—including, in some cases, life extension—after participating in group therapy programs. I'll describe these studies shortly, but people who benefited included patients with breast cancer, melanoma (an aggressive skin cancer), HIV, and heart disease. Although these researchers point to several factors that explain these marvelous and unexpected benefits, all of them share one conviction: an essential component with special healing properties was the support of others with the same conditions.

Based on this entire body of remarkable research, we can now say with confidence that you nourish your physical health when you strengthen your loving relationships. Every woman, whether healthy or ill, can benefit by bolstering or expanding her social support system, which encompasses friends, coworkers, neighbors, relatives, parents, children, spouses, and intimate partners. This may seem like an awfully broad prescription, but I will show how you can break down your effort into components you can focus on day to day.

Creating Vital Support Systems

*T*he sleepy hamlet of Roseto, seventy-five miles north of Philadelphia, is nestled in the foothills of the Blue Mountains. To the knowledge of those who've studied Roseto, few if any of its residents have practiced meditation, biofeedback, or group therapy. Through several decades into the mid-1960s, the citizens of Roseto consumed what today would be considered a horrendously high-fat diet. Nevertheless, the town became famous for its surprisingly low death rates, especially from heart disease. There has been only one clear-cut explanation for this finding: the extraordinarily close-knit family and community ties among Roseto's residents.

For the last three decades, Stewart Wolf, M.D., has investigated Roseto, a town settled in 1882 by immigrants from a small town in Italy. For many decades, Roseto remained the exclusive enclave of these immigrants and their descendants. When Wolf and his colleagues discovered that Roseto's death rate was significantly lower than those of three neighboring communities and the country as a whole, they searched for explanations. The citizens' good health and longevity had nothing to do with diet, exercise, or smoking. They ate more fat than, exercised as little as, and smoked as much as their neighbors or the average American. But the researchers observed that the people of Roseto had retained their traditions of familial closeness, intra-ethnic marriages, devoted churchgoing, membership in social organizations, and supportive neighborliness.

Yet Roseto could not retain its cohesive character. Dr. Wolf observed that the social fabric of Roseto began to fray during the sixties, when its inhabitants started to move away, marry outside the clan, abandon cultural and religious customs, and succumb to more material pursuits. As this trend continued, Roseto's death rate from heart disease began to rise. Today, Roseto's mortality rate compares with or exceeds the neighboring townships'.

The Roseto story underscores that our social ties have, over several decades, been shredded by massive social and technological changes. Few of us have the same close-knit communities and extended families that previous generations took for granted.

Depending on our age, our mothers or grandmothers probably had parents living nearby, or right in the house, to help with chores and child rearing. They had close neighbors available at a moment's notice to take the kids. They probably didn't work outside the home, but they had women friends who met together in "coffee klatches" or other informal gatherings.

(Obviously, today's working women have more choices and more independence than their forebears, but they don't necessarily have adequate support systems on the job.) As safety nets of social support have come apart, our emotional and physical health has suffered. While we can't reconstruct a long-gone era, we can resurrect a sense of community and create new forms of extended family.

Just as it's hard to convince a well woman to stop smoking in the name of future health, it can be hard to convince a well woman to seek support in the name of future health or recovery from illness. Many women say their lives are so hectic that they don't have time or energy to expend on social connections. Such thinking is a catch-22 that traps women in their isolation: one of the reasons they're stressed is that they don't take enough time to cultivate relationships.

I've found that many stressed women who use relaxation techniques and cognitive restructuring have more energy with which to pursue relationships. When they're no longer driven by anxious preoccupations, they manage to find the time for soul-nourishing relationships. This creates a positive spiral of increasing well-being.

Every woman's social needs are unique, and we must identify areas of our social lives that require tending. But a few generalizations seem warranted: we can improve our intimate relationships with communication skills, and we can build our social networks by revitalizing old friendships and forging new connections. Women have a particular need for close friendships with other women, as Dr. House's research suggests. I disagree with the notion that we gain little from friendships with men, but I agree that our connections with other women can be especially healing.

One of my patients going through menopause, Barbara, suffered in her isolation. She dared not discuss her flagging energy, vaginal atrophy, decreased sexual interest, or hot flashes with anyone, lest she be met with bemusement or pity. All that changed once she joined our group of menopause patients. She discovered a number of women who experienced similar symptoms and fears. And they'd all been victimized by a harsh social stigma, which says that menopause represents an irrevocable loss of energy, creativity, and attractiveness. Because of this stigma, they responded to each new symptom or bodily change with a creeping sense of dread.

But the group allowed each woman, including Barbara, to reject these punishing thoughts. In isolation, it's hard to say whether Barbara would have been able to shake her negative notions about menopause. But with her female compatriots, she recognized that she was not alone. She was inspired by seeing other women overcome their symptoms and move into a phase of high energy and creativity.

Many patients who undergo multiple miscarriages say that before their first miscarriage they didn't know anyone who'd lost a pregnancy. Once they had their own miscarriages, other women came out of the wood-work to share their experiences. The support they received helped them through the hardest times of grief and loss. I've seen the same phenome-non occur in women with every imaginable medical problem. I've also observed women who are healthy, but who lead lives of continual stress, create networks of support out of old friendships and new contacts. By so doing, they overcome loneliness and reduce the impact of stress on their bodies.

Often, we can develop strong social networks *after* we adopt other stress management methods, including relaxation, cognitive restructuring, and self-nurturance (which is why this book unfolds in the order it does). The reasons are not complex. When we're immensely stressed, we often become hermitlike, wishing only to hibernate in solitude. (Those of us who become severely anxious or depressed may isolate ourselves for weeks or months.) When we feel that lousy, we lack the necessary zest to get out into the world and connect. We'd rather crawl under those proverbial covers. But stress management techniques give us the energy and confidence we need to reach out to friends and family. These techniques also increase the levels of awareness and calm we bring to our intimate relations with spouses and other family members.

Often, we don't have solid support systems because we don't feel entitled to them. Fear, excessive shyness, embarrassment, and feelings of inadequacy disable us from reaching out. If our insecurities are overpowering, we may lose touch with our social needs altogether. In such instances, relaxation can make us more aware of our needs. Then cognitive restructuring enables us to overturn pernicious thoughts that keep us stuck—and isolated—in our fears.

Friendships: Reviving the Old, Forging the New
Reweaving our fabric of support means reviving past and present friend-ships, as well as forging new ones. When we feel isolated, it's usually be-cause stress, depression, or fatigue (or all three) prevent us from seeking out and enjoying our friends, and they prevent us from developing new friend-ships. When our minds and hearts are clouded, we may be unable to over-

come the conflicts or minor grudges that crop up in most friendships. In such instances, we often let go of friendships that could have been saved and strengthened.

Mindy, a patient who was dealing with job stress and pelvic pain, had not spoken to her best friend in over a year. She complained to our group about her friend's insensitivity. "I can't talk to her," she said. With further exploration, Mindy recognized that she used to be able to talk openly with her friend, but that a change occurred after the friend had been through the painful breakup of a relationship. Perhaps the friend had been overwhelmed by her own grief. Once Mindy made this connection, and realized how much she missed her friend, she wrote her a letter. A prompt, positive reply led to a reconciliation that lifted Mindy's spirits.

When I instruct patients to do something good for themselves, some choose to write letters to friends or family members from whom they've separated. They recognize that disconnecting was a form of self-denial; reconnecting is a way of honoring their needs. But reconnecting often means letting go of old resentments. In this regard, forgiveness is a mind-body practice that heals the heart and softens the body. "Through the attitude of forgiveness," writes Joan Borysenko, Ph.D., my former colleague and a leading proponent of mind-body medicine, "we attain happiness and serenity by letting go of the ego's incessant need to judge ourselves and others."

When I encourage women to let go of resentment, I don't tell them to deny anger toward friends or loved ones. Rather, I encourage them to explore and express their anger, so they can move beyond anger toward forgiveness. Stephen Levine, who works with people with life-threatening illness, offers the following advice on forgiveness, advice that can apply to any woman, whether sick or well: "One does not attempt to submerge anger or fear with a forgiveness technique. To force forgiveness, to attempt to touch with forgiveness that which we can hardly approach with a clear awareness, does not further our efforts. The forgiveness technique is most potent when it is used at the appropriate time. First we need to be mindful of our anger, our distrust, our holding, before the enormous power of forgiveness can reach as deep as it is able."

Dr. Herbert Benson quoted a great sage when he told me that people should not judge anyone until they have walked twenty miles in her moccasins. When we genuinely consider the suffering of those who've caused us to suffer, judgment fades. As Levine points out, that does not mean our anger is necessarily invalid. We can explore and express anger (either by ourselves or with the object of our frustration) as a prelude to forgiveness. But it is forgiveness that heals ruptured or neglected relationships.

Forgiveness is not the same thing as condoning hurtful or harmful behavior. We forgive not because another's insensitivity or maliciousness is okay with us. We forgive in order to heal our own wounds and acknowledge the wounds of others.

Though they are exceptions to the rule, some friendships—like some marriages—are so destructive that the only way to treat ourselves kindly is to let go of the person entirely. One of my patients, Camille, became pregnant at the same time as her best friend, Arlene. But Camille had a miscarriage and Arlene gave birth to a healthy baby. Camille complained of Arlene's astonishing insensitivity afterward. Arlene talked incessantly about how happy she was with her daughter and how delighted she was with her life, asking little about how Camille was coping. Camille had another miscarriage, but her friend's self-centeredness continued, and they finally blew up at each other. The fight was so awful that they didn't speak for six months.

In our mind-body group, Camille began to work through her feelings and decided to write to Arlene. In her letter, she said how happy she was for Arlene, but how it was hard to hear about her baby. Camille admitted her anguish over her own losses, and expressed hope that they could see each other. Arlene replied with a brief note thanking Camille for being in touch. But she didn't acknowledge Camille's anguish, and she didn't express the same wish for reconciliation. Camille was deeply hurt, but she told our group that she was glad she'd written, because she could finally put the relationship behind her. She'd spent six months hurting over the split, but now she recognized that Arlene could not be there for her.

Often, however, forgiveness enables us to heal friendships. We can gradually give up the seething and often petty resentments that separate us from people we care about. By the same token, we can overcome insecurities that sap the courage we need to revive old friendships and forge new connections.

As we reach out to friends and family, we ought to remember that most people we care about want to be sought after. So do new friends and acquaintances, most of the time. Phone calls and letters are likely to be received with joy, though of course there will be exceptions. But we should not base our actions (or inactions) on our fear of the occasional cold shoulder. When we do, we live the lives of quiet desperation so aptly described by Henry David Thoreau.

Women, in particular, tend to be delighted to make new connections or revive old ones. In our hectic attempts to juggle work and family responsibilities, we've not only lost community ties, we've lost the time and temperament for play. My stressed patients don't get enough play with other women, the kind of experiences they enjoyed as kids and teenagers.

Do you yearn for those carefree connections—the hanging out, the laughing jags with other girls? If so, you're like my patients and most of the women I know. In recent years there's been so much talk about the inner child. What about the inner adolescent? I'm not suggesting that you regress; rather, that you integrate that "inner adolescent" into your adult personality. Once you admit those desires, you'll find other women with the same needs. Seize opportunities for what several of my patients call a "chicks' night out."

Avoiding Traps That Isolate: Envy, Negativism, and Fear

One impediment to nurturing friendships among women is the competition or envy that can flare up as we settle down in marriages and careers. Some of my patients isolate themselves because they're jealous of friends who seem to have things they desire. They don't want to be around women who've advanced further in their careers, who appear to have conflict-free partnerships, or who possess some physical characteristic they covet.

If envy prevents you from forming intimate ties with other women (or men, for that matter), it's time to restructure your thinking. On first thought, we'd all like to be Christie Brinkley or Princess Diana. But on second thought, we'd reconsider. Would we really accept a life of public fights, painful divorces, and media intrusions in exchange for wealth, notoriety, and perfect skin? Apply the same logic to your friendships. You may focus on aspects of your friend that you envy. But would you be willing to exchange every aspect of your life for every aspect of hers? When you feel one-down with a friend, practice focusing on your own strengths and talents. You'll be able to recognize and accept your friend's assets and good fortune, as long as you never lose sight of your own.

Misunderstandings arise when we harbor false images of friends and loved ones. One of my patients, Mara, was going through a particularly rough patch after her third miscarriage. Soon thereafter, she and her husband, Brendan, stopped to visit a friend on their way out to the movies. The friend's two small children were crying when Mara and Brendan dropped by, but she was not only preoccupied with her babies, she was also fairly rude to the couple. Later, Mara expressed her hurt and annoyance. "Why are these people with kids so obnoxious?"

Mara was admittedly envious of her friend for having children, and that anger clouded her view. In our mind-body group, we asked Mara more questions about the interaction, and she explained that her friend's mood worsened right after she and Brendan declared that they were on their way to the movies. Mara was so focused on her own unhappiness that it never crossed her mind that the friend could be jealous of *her*. The friend probably thought, "If only *I* had the freedom to run out to the movies with *my* husband!" It's a perfect example of women misunderstanding each other's motives and actions because both were blinded by jealousy.

Another common trap, particularly in friendships between women, is what I call the "bitch and moan" relationship. One of my patients, Valerie, had a best friend in whom she could confide. When Valerie finally met the right man, Marty, she dated him for over a year before getting engaged. When she told her friend she was getting married, the friend said, "You're marrying *Marty*? But all you do is complain about him and all your fights!" Valerie was astonished, because she loved Marty and sensed from the start of their relationship that they had a future together. She realized that her friend had gotten a completely distorted view of the relationship, because she only talked to her about him when things were going badly.

It's important to have friends in whom you can confide your anxiety and anger. But what about joy, hope, ecstasy, excitement, and fulfillment? If we can share *only* our bitching-and-moaning sides, our relationships become repositories of unhappiness. To borrow an old phrase from political speech-writer and columnist William Safire, we become "nattering nabobs of negativism." Friendships based exclusively on bad news are as stilted as friendships based exclusively on good news. In all our intimate relationships, we ought to be able to express the full range of emotions, and the many facets of our personalities. In the real world this isn't always possible, but it is a goal worth bearing in mind.

Mind-body pioneer George F. Solomon, M.D., notes that many of us have wonderful friends and families, but we remain lonely because we don't turn to them. We keep them at bay with stoic attitudes about our pains and problems: "But I don't want to upset them." "Why should I lay my trip on them?" "They have so much to deal with; I'll only add to their burden."

Dr. Solomon captured our reticence, and its effect on our well-being, in a recent conversation: "If you have a good friend who asks how you're doing, and you say 'Terrific,' he's likely to say, 'Great. See you next week.' On the other hand, if you say 'I'm feeling really awful,' he might say, 'What can I do to help?' 'What do you need?' If you don't communicate with your support system, then the system isn't supportive."

Reaching Out to Family

If you don't communicate with your family, your family can't be supportive either.

Miriam, a patient with severe stress at her job as a nurse, had the reputation in her family of being a "cold fish." She took that to heart, and began to see herself as a cold fish. Worse still, her parents' and siblings' judgments caused a self-fulfilling prophecy. Since they viewed her as a cold fish, Miriam never felt accepted by them, so she *did* remove herself, but only as a defense mechanism. Miriam hadn't recognized any of this until she joined our mind-body group. With our support, Miriam reframed her self-image.

"The group helped me realize that my behavior with my family was a coping mechanism, a way to protect myself," she said. "It wasn't true. I'm a nurse, and I'm not a cold fish with my patients who are sick. In the rest of my life, I was not a cold fish. But I felt the need to remove myself from my family."

Having gained greater compassion and understanding about her family role, Miriam felt her reticence and resentment begin to fade. She gradually opened up to several family members. It wasn't easy, because her mother had long showed a preference for her brothers and sister, and her father had been distant. But Miriam finally shared her work problems with her mother, and she reconnected with her sister after years of distance. Although she remained guarded with her father and brothers, she no longer held the old grudges.

Reaching out to particular family members helped Miriam heal some deep wounds. As a result, she gained greater awareness and confidence in the rest of her life, including her job as a nurse. Her relations with coworkers improved, her stress levels dropped, and she felt a surge of renewed vitality.

Family ties help us to prevent and recover from illness. But they are less helpful, emotionally and medically, if we don't "use" them in a positive way. That means procuring the support of family members when we need it most, confiding in them, and working through areas of conflict. But women should never feel that they *must* reach out to family members. Some of us have parents, grandparents, siblings, or other relatives who are ceaselessly insensitive, indifferent, or intrusive. We can't simply ignore their behavior and seek their support in a spirit of openness. But many difficult family members are flexible, and we can work through painful conflicts to achieve a healing resolution.

In some instances, particularly when we're suffering with a medical condition, we may consciously choose to set aside old angers in order to have a rapprochement with a parent, brother, or sister. The greater good of familial healing, and the much-needed support of the loved one, take precedence. Ideally, when we come together with a family member under such circumstances, we can eventually broach our conflicts and move to a deeper level of communication. I've seen it happen many times with patients.

Lila was a patient who joined one of my mind-body groups for women undergoing in vitro fertilization (IVF). She'd had eight IUIs, one GIFT procedure, and four IVF procedures, all with no success. Lila had difficulty sharing her experiences with her parents or siblings, because she did not want to cause them emotional strife. Her brother, who had two children, would get upset whenever he heard about her travails. However, when she found out that her brother's wife was pregnant again, and that they hid the news for fear of her emotional reaction, Lila realized that family concealment had gone too far. She wasn't that fragile, she thought. "I told him, I don't want to find out from someone else that your wife is pregnant," she said. "We'd always been close, and it didn't make any sense."

The dialogue between sister and brother brought them closer. "He said to me, 'I wish I could have a child for you,' " recalled Lila. "His wife actually offered to carry our baby to term, but my uterus was not the problem. But the offer really touched me."

Lila had a different problem with her mother, who persisted with probing questions about every detail of Lila's high-tech procedures. "She wanted to know how many eggs I had, how many embryos were fertilized, and so on. I just didn't want to talk about all that stuff." Improving communication with her mother meant drawing up clear boundaries. So Lila told her, in calm tones, that she would share her problems and experiences when she felt like it. Otherwise she would prefer to share other aspects of her life. Her mother complied, Lila no longer had to worry about fending off so many intrusive questions, and their relationship was strengthened.

We all have complex family relationships, and we must tend to each one with care and specificity, because each is unique. But overall, we must both accept each other's needs and respect each other's boundaries. In each case, we can strike a delicate balance between intimacy and separateness—some relationships clearly need more closeness, others need more distance. Cultivating this balance improves the quality of our family relationships, connections we need in order to stay vigorous and well, and to shepherd us through the most difficult times of illness.

Helping Others

We can reach out with compassion just as surely as we can reach out with need. And contrary to popular opinion, not all helping behavior is codependence. Certainly many women get stuck in caretaker roles, particularly in their families, but that does not mean we don't benefit by helping members of our social networks or communities. Recent studies suggest that helping—when carried out as a conscious choice in a spirit of openness—can help the helper as much as the person being helped. Indeed, our physical health may benefit when we engage in regular helping activities.

In the last chapter I mentioned "The Women's Roles and Well-Being Project" conducted by Phyllis Moen, Ph.D., a study of 427 wives and mothers from upstate New York. Dr. Moen followed these women for thirty years and found that women who belonged to volunteer organizations had significantly fewer major illnesses, better mental health, and greater longevity. The astonishing link between altruistic involvement and longevity bespeaks the healing potential of reaching out with compassion.

Dr. Moen also believes that women who volunteered were more "socially integrated," hence less lonely and isolated. Helping others creates social bonds, both with your fellow volunteers and the people who receive your care.

I encourage patients to help others, as long as they don't stretch their emotional and physical resources in the process. One of my cancer patients, Nicole, recovered from her illness after a difficult struggle. Once she got her health and energy back, she decided to volunteer at a local advocacy organization for cancer patients. In addition to defending the rights and needs of patients, the organization ran support groups. Nicole got involved behind the scenes, and when and where possible she met with other patients. Referring to these patients, and the other volunteers, Nicole called them "the loveliest people I've ever met in my life."

If forging social connections only means meeting your own needs, the effort becomes an exercise in narcissism. Forging social connections means paving a two-way street—helping others keeps the traffic flowing in both directions. Find an informal or formal opportunity to volunteer. Allan Luks, author of *The Healing Power of Doing Good*, recommends that you find ways to help that involve personal contact. Writing checks is admirable but it doesn't spark human connections. The choices are many: you can work in a soup kitchen, spend time with needy kids, or help out at your local hospital. Whatever you choose, your altruism may benefit you, emotionally, spiritually, and physically, as much as it benefits the people you help.

Communicating as a Couple

*W*hether your problem is stress, illness, a difficult life passage, or all of the above, it is important to maintain open lines of communication with your spouse or partner, if you have one. His or her support can be vital to your health and well-being.

I've developed guidelines, based on my own and others' research and clinical experience, for communication between partners in a couple. These guidelines apply to marriages or relationships of every conceivable stripe. They are rooted in rather widely accepted principles taught by psychologists, family therapists, and couples counselors. But they are especially important and applicable among couples who face extreme stress associated with life passages or medical conditions.

Here are seven key points, in a nutshell:

1. *Express Your Needs.* Don't expect your partner to read your mind.
2. *Listen, Don't Solve.* Don't expect your partner to fix your problems or vanquish your pain. Likewise, you can't solve his or her problems or pain. Responding to needs does not mean "making it all better." For both you and your partner, it does mean listening, empathizing, and being generally available.
3. *Avoid Blame.* Try not to point the finger at your partner when he or she falls short of the response you hoped for. Experience and express any hurt or angry feelings, but don't blame. (See the next chapter for guidelines on healthy expression of anger.) When you do blame, you reinforce the message that it's his or her job to keep you happy. That sets you up for disappointment and victimhood.
4. *Don't Accept Abuse.* You should not accept abuse or ill-treatment from your partner. Ask yourself whether you're dealing with human foibles and inadequacies, or outright destructiveness. The latter is clearly unacceptable. Learn and adopt the skills of assertiveness to stand up for your rights. (See the next chapter for assertiveness guidelines.)

5. *Step into Your Partner's Shoes.* When you feel you've been wronged, ask yourself what your partner is going through that caused his or her shortsightedness, insensitivity, or egotism. Don't quash your own feelings; rather, resolve them in a healthy way by using the communication skills I've mentioned. Then you'll be able to put yourself in his or her shoes. Recall your own moments of shortsightedness, insensitivity, or egotism, and you'll recognize that your partner has the same infectious disease you have—the human condition.

6. *Turn to Others, Too.* Develop balance in your relationships, so you don't turn to your partner with every one of your needs. Your partner will never be perfect; no one is so well rounded that he or she can respond to every facet of our multifaceted personalities. For instance, if there's an issue you can't discuss, an emotion you can't share, or an activity he or she couldn't care less about, find a friend who can respond.

7. *Resuscitate the Positive.* Share your joys, pleasures, and sense of humor with your partner. Don't let painful issues or negative thoughts and feelings become the sum and substance of your relationship. The life you share with your partner is much larger than the latest crisis.

Learning Each Other's Language

After Serena was diagnosed with breast cancer and had a mastectomy, her relationship with her husband, Jeff, was tested to its limit. Jeff thought that all Serena wanted was reassurance that everything would be okay. In reality, she only wanted him to listen to her fears. "He always talked and tried to help me," said Serena. "But it's hard for men to understand this. I don't blame him. He's not going through it. He'd say to me, 'You're going to be fine.' I'd think, 'How do you *know* I'm going to be fine?' "

Things changed when Serena and Jeff began to practice "paired listening," a technique I teach in my groups and couples sessions. During paired listening, one partner listens as the other speaks for five minutes or more. The partner who speaks can say anything he or she wishes, addressing conflicts in the relationship, expressing emotions, discussing things he or she likes about the partner or their relationship. The partner who listens must remain silent.

Paired listening fostered a deep understanding between Serena and Jeff. He no longer rushed in to reassure Serena before she finished expressing her fears and sadness. She no longer felt that he didn't "get it." Although their communication styles remained different, they learned to respect those differences while making a few basic accommodations that brought them together. Jeff would listen rather than try desperately to fix things. Serena stopped criticizing his responses, and listened more openly to him as well.

"Our relationship is so much better," said Serena. "We have more communication, understanding, and patience with each other. Before I joined the mind-body group, we were losing all of those things. When I would say something, I had the feeling he did not understand it as I meant it. Now I believe he understands."

Serena and Jeff exemplified many of the discrepancies in male-female communication style noted by Deborah Tannen, Ph.D., in her book *You Just Don't Understand*:

> If adults learn their ways of speaking as children growing up in separate worlds of peers, then conversation between women and men is cross-cultural communication. Although each style is valid on its own terms, misunderstandings arise because the styles are different. . . .
>
> Learning about these styles won't make them go away, but it can banish mutual mystification and blame. Being able to understand why our partners, friends, and even strangers behave the way they do is a comfort, even if we still don't see things the same way. It makes the world into more familiar territory. And having others understand why we talk and act as we do protects us from the pain of their puzzlement and criticism.

The guidelines listed on pages 146–47 are meant not to change men's and women's styles, but rather to help us accept each other's differences at the same time that we uncover our similarities. Tannen points out that women (to a great extent) live in a world of connection in which intimacy is paramount. By contrast, men (to a great extent) live in a world of status in which independence is paramount. Many of our stylistic differences in communication have to do with these differing priorities, which are deeply embedded by culture, and, some would argue, by nature. But men also need intimacy and women also seek independence, so it is possible to find a common ground of understanding.

Tannen suggests that we sidestep the trap of believing that we must change men's styles. (Or that men should change our styles, for that matter.) Instead, we do well to learn each other's styles so we can interpret each other's messages more clearly. Certainly many men benefit by expressing their needs for intimacy, and many women benefit by realizing their needs for autonomy. According to Tannen, men can learn from women "to accept interdependence without seeing it as a threat to their freedom," and women can learn from men "to accept some conflict and difference without seeing it as a threat to intimacy." Though we have much to learn from each other, we should not set out to change our partners. When we do, the implied message is, "There's something wrong with you."

When I counsel couples, I often ask them, "How did your parents handle conflicts and express emotions?" The origins of their styles—or their limitations—can easily be traced to their early role models. For instance, my patients frequently complain that their husbands "don't express feelings." When I turn to the man and ask him about his parents, more often than not he describes a father, and sometimes a mother, who could not express emotions. Understanding this clear lineage helps the woman have more compassion, and it helps him have more compassion for himself. Exploring early role models is therefore a helpful antidote to the blame and retribution so common in troubled partnerships.

When we express our needs clearly, listen rather than trying to solve, avoid blame, draw the line at abuse, and empathize with our partners, we create conditions for the understanding we *both* crave. Despite our differences, most men and women want the same thing: to come together in mutual respect and trust.

The Paired Listening Technique

You may wish to jump-start the process of coming together with the paired listening method I mentioned. The ground rules, as stated, are simple. You speak about an issue, feeling, or experience of significance. It may concern your relationship, or it may concern another subject or relationship. Your partner listens without saying a word, and I do mean not a peep. But he or she focuses completely on what you are saying for those five minutes. Then you switch sides and listen to your partner as he or she speaks for five minutes.

I don't suggest that you do this exercise every day forever. Do it for several days or more if you need to. The purpose is to accustom yourself to speaking freely without interruption, interpretation, or argument, and to listen without interrupting, interpreting, or arguing. The sense of being heard and understood grows as you continue to practice paired listening.

After doing this exercise repeatedly, let the method seep into your life. When an important issue arises, take fifteen or twenty minutes to speak while your partner listens, or vice versa. Women often feel that they don't get to communicate feelings or problems to their male partners. Men often feel that their women partners talk incessantly about feelings and problems. When a set amount of time is designated for authentic listening, then both women's need to be heard and men's need for limits are met. In my groups for patients with infertility, I use an often powerful communication exercise taught to me by Steven Maurer, which is designed to resuscitate the positive in partnerships. We set aside one Sunday in which the husbands join their wives for an all-day session of stress management and pleasurable activities. At one point, I instruct each couple to go into a separate office for twelve minutes, for a talk in which each partner speaks for six minutes. I ask them to cover three subjects, two minutes per subject. The first subject is "something you like about your spouse you have never told him/her." The second is "something you like about yourself that you've never told him/her." Finally, each person reveals "something you like about your relationship you've never told him/her."

This exercise demonstrates that when we speak to each other, there is no rule—written or unwritten—that it must be about traumas, tragedies, irritations, grudges, or other unpleasant subjects. (Couples with infertility have often, understandably, spent *years* focusing on anxieties and deep disappointments.) Negative feelings must be aired, but so must positive feelings. Husbands in particular discover that listening to their wives does not have to mean listening to negativity.

The results of this session are remarkable. Typically, both partners in the couple come out of the room floating on air. Many haven't heard such heartwarming expressions from their spouses since the early days of their relationships. If you're undergoing a stressful period—whether due to work pressures, financial hardship, family conflicts, sexual problems, infertility, or illness—try this exercise with your spouse. It may help to shore up your commitment by reminding you what your partnership has been and can be once again.

"News and Goods"

An exercise for resuscitating the positive in everyday life was taught to me by my colleague Margaret Ennis, M.A. It's called "news and goods."

Think about your typical day. How much of what happens in your day (and your resulting mood state) is positive, negative, or neutral? Although the day-to-day variations are enormous, you can roughly estimate an average day. Perhaps 70 percent is neutral, 15 percent is negative, and 15 percent is positive. (That's an answer I hear often.) But what do you focus on most with your spouse when you're home together? If your answer isn't the negative, then you're in the minority.

"News and goods" is a simple antidote to creeping negativity in intimate relationships. When your partner or spouse comes home (or you come home), ask him or her: "What new and good thing happened to you today?" Then he or she asks you what new and good thing happened.

What if nothing good happened? If your definition of "good" is limited to a job promotion, a raise, or a winning lottery ticket, then you'll be able to practice "news and goods" once every few years. The exercise compels you to look deeper into your day.

One of my patients, Leslie, was great at finding small diamonds in the middle of rough days. They were diamonds she offered her husband, Lee, each night. On one day in which nothing good seemed to happen to Leslie, she remembered a moment in the morning when she heard her dog let out a boisterous belch. She searched the terrace and discovered that the dog had eaten an entire tube of sunscreen. On one level, discovering that your dog ate your sunscreen is something new but hardly something good. Yet when it happened, Leslie found it so ludicrously funny that she howled with laughter. When Lee came home, she told him about the dog's misadventure and they howled together. Retrieving that one minute from her day set a positive tone for their evening together, even though the rest of Leslie's day had been a drag.

"News and goods" compels you to hold on to small moments of delight: a pleasant interaction with a coworker, a great joke you heard, or a step forward on a creative project. Something new and good could be as simple as a moment's recognition of beauty while looking at a sun-drenched skyline, a clear morning sky, a flowering tree. Focusing on something new and good forces you to reshape your view of your day. (It's a form of cognitive restructuring for couples.) Moreover, it improves your first contact with your partner. "News and goods" creates an atmosphere conducive to your growth and enjoyment as a couple.

Healing Our Isolation:
The Support of a Group

*F*or more than eight years, I have directed mind-body groups for women. I've led "general" groups composed of people with varying ailments, and I have also led groups of women with specific conditions. In all these groups, I teach mind-body techniques that have been shown to be effective. However, embedded in the background of every group is a healing component that has nothing to do with techniques. It is the quality of support that blossoms when women band together to confront stress and illnesses. That support is an immeasurable contributor to their emotional healing and physical well-being.

Much has been written about the psychological benefits of support groups and psychotherapy groups, so I won't elaborate in great detail. But I will offer a few examples from my clinical experience; a few basic elements of successful mind-body groups; and evidence suggesting that group support yields both psychological and physical benefits to people with serious illness.

Some of that evidence comes from my own studies, already mentioned, which show that participation in mind-body groups reduces emotional distress among women with infertility. (Our preliminary evidence also suggests the possibility of an increase in rates of conception, although we won't have a definitive answer until we've completed our ongoing research.) Because my groups have several components—including the teaching of mind-body methods—there is no way to be certain how much the support of the group, by itself, contributes to these benefits. I do know that the support of other women appears to be an essential element in their overall success.

Other studies have demonstrated the power of groups among women and men with serious, even life-threatening, diseases. In the early 1980s, psychiatrist David Spiegel, M.D., of Stanford University, started a group therapy program for women with advanced breast cancer. Spiegel was quite certain that his program would help these women cope with their illness; he was equally sure that his program would *not* help them live longer. Spiegel was so annoyed by claims that psychological treatments could lengthen life for cancer patients that he set out to prove them wrong. He compared his first group of advanced breast cancer patients (none of whom were expected to survive) to control subjects—women with the same disease and prognosis—who did not participate in his group therapy. After following both groups for ten years, Spiegel was shocked by his own data: the group members had lived twice as long as the women who were not group members. Moreover, only three women had survived, and all three had been participants in his group.

I'll have more to say about Spiegel's discovery in chapter 15, "From Trauma to Transformation." As with my groups, Spiegel's had many components, and it is hard to say which aspects contributed to his patients' improved outcomes. But Spiegel himself is convinced that the emotional support the group members received from each other played a critical part in their psychological well-being and physical fortitude.

Other investigators have shown that group treatments improve outcomes for patients with equally serious diseases. Researchers at UCLA found that patients with melanoma (a potentially lethal skin cancer) who participated in a mind-body group were three times less likely to suffer a recurrence or to die from the disease. At the University of Miami, researchers discovered that patients with HIV who joined mind-body groups maintained stronger immune systems. In a renowned study, Dean Ornish, M.D., head of the Preventive Medicine Institute in Sausalito, California, showed that heart attack patients who followed his program of low-fat eating, exercise, stress management, and group support experienced actual reversal of their heart disease.

Taken together, these studies suggest that group support in conjunction with mind-body techniques can promote emotional and physical improvements among people with serious illnesses, including women with breast cancer.

Groups are powerful not simply because they offer support, but because the kind of support they offer makes us feel less alone with our problems. Reaching out to others with the same pains or conditions, whether they stem from garden-variety stresses or life-threatening cancers, we feel understood. When the atmosphere is right, such groups offer a mirror of compassion in the responses of others who affirm our experiences.

Often, when we isolate ourselves with a life problem or health condition, we feel that there is something wrong with us. We attribute our suffering to the notion that we are somehow inadequate, irredeemably odd, or perhaps even evil. The instant we recognize our pain, our difficulties, our symptoms, or our struggles in someone else's face and words, our perspective changes. Being in a group of women going through the same travails helps to normalize our feelings. We no longer entertain inner voices so punishing that they intensify our suffering, because we've discovered that our thoughts and feelings—no matter how disturbing—are normal.

Often, one of the first things women with common conditions share is the unhealthy shame that torments them. Menopausal women may feel shame about their hot flashes. Breast cancer patients may feel shame about their mastectomies. Infertile women may feel shame about their childlessness. Expressing our shame with others who instantly "get it" has the remarkable effect of diminishing shame. It is as though shame can't survive very long once a caring group of people coax it out into the clear light of day and look at it together. With shame off our backs, we can accept and express our emotional responses to stress, pain, or illness. We no longer wage war on our own minds and bodies, and the process of emotional healing begins.

Nina, a phone company mechanic, joined one of my "general" mind-body groups (for those with various stress-related conditions) because she suffered from anxiety attacks and excruciating migraines. It was clear to Nina, and the rest of us, that feelings of loneliness and worthlessness fueled her underlying symptoms. Because of her insecurities, joining our group had been extremely difficult. Here is how Nina described her initial experiences in our group:

> Whenever you walk into something new, you wonder, What is this going to be like? Are you going to feel strange or awkward? Are things they're going to ask you to do going to be scary? Are you going to feel weird? But I certainly was willing to give it a try, because when you are chronically ill, you get pretty desperate. When I first started, I was going through such hard times that I felt like my emotions would hang out in weird ways. It was because I was trying to sort through so much that has happened in my life. I was concerned that maybe I came across a little strange.
>
> So there I was, feeling like my insides were hanging out on the outside. But after a while I felt comfortable. We were all there because we had stress and illness, and we all knew we were trying to find a way to cope. I came to feel that the group was a safe place to be.

Nina responded to many aspects of the program, including the teachings on relaxation, cognitive restructuring, and emotional expression. They helped her to get a handle on her life and her symptoms. But the fact that she learned these methods in a group of people who shared many of her struggles, and who bonded together in trust, made the process enjoyable. And when other group members shared some small victories, it reinforced

Nina's hope and commitment. Over time, Nina's anxiety and migraine headaches became manageable.

In Appendix B, I provide a list of organizations that offer groups, or that can refer you to groups for your particular medical condition. Use these resources, or any other resources at your command, to find a group that reflects your circumstances and speaks to your needs. If you cannot find such a group, ask your physician. If he or she doesn't know of one, start networking in order to meet (or at least talk to) other women who've had or have the same condition. If you keep your situation to yourself, you'll never meet or speak with anyone who can share your experiences. But if you tell friends and family what's happening, and inquire whether they know others in the same boat, you're going to make those vital connections.

If your condition is relatively obscure, keep networking until you find at least one other similar person. I have "hooked up" women with other women who've had "selective reductions," in which one or more fetuses in a multiple pregnancy is electively aborted. Such women go through a range of painful emotions, most of them tinged with guilt. I've also hooked up infertile women going through an "egg donor" process; women with high-risk pregnancies; and women grieving for babies who have died *in utero*. If you have an open-minded obstetrician/gynecologist, he or she might be willing to connect you with someone who's been through what you're going through.

For women who feel stressed out, a variety of groups are available with different emphases. Stress management groups are popping up around the country, many in hospital settings. Find one near you that suits your purposes. Most of them teach relaxation techniques, including meditation and mindfulness. Some programs, such as "Attitudinal Healing," which has groups nationwide, emphasize emotional and spiritual growth. Twelve-step programs will bring you together with others whose stress leads them toward addiction, be it substance abuse (alcohol, drugs, sex, or the like) or behavioral compulsions (codependence, chronic rage, and so on). Consider these groups when you feel emotionally and/or behaviorally out of control in the face of overwhelming stress and pain.

Remember that group support is only one way to reach out when stress abounds or illness strikes. We also need friends and family. Use the suggestions and exercises to help you weave a strong fabric of supportive relationships.

Many of us pop vitamins, watch the scale compulsively, exercise regularly, and avoid smoking, all in the name of health. But we rarely pay similar attention to our support systems, and neither do our doctors. Eventually, the medical world will recognize that social support is a healing agent as surely as any pharmaceutical. Until then, we can take charge of our health and well-being by tending to our relationships with renewed zest and commitment.

Eight

♦ ♦ ♦ ♦

WOMEN'S ANGER, WOMEN'S JOY:
EMOTIONAL EXPRESSION

Candace was facing major surgery for the second time in her life. Four years earlier, she had undergone a mastectomy after being diagnosed with early breast cancer. Now, after seeing a suspicious mass on a CAT scan, her doctor recommended a hysterectomy. Candace had coped well with the breast surgery. But for some reason—she did not know why—the prospect of this surgery was terrifying. This time, fear grasped her by the throat.

At fifty, Candace, who had two adolescent kids and was beyond the thought or possibility of more children, was not devastated by the loss of her reproductive organs. Yes, it was upsetting, but that was not the crux of her anxiety. Even the possibility of cancer did not devastate Candace, because her doctor was quite certain that surgery would be a cure, even if the mass turned out to be malignant. No, it was the mere thought of general anesthesia and surgery that caused her knees to go weak with fright.

She could not talk to her husband, Sam, about her fears. Whenever she spoke of them, Sam rushed in with soothing words. "He was very supportive, and he meant well," said Candace. "But he would always say the same thing no matter what I said: 'Don't worry about it. It will be okay.' Well, I was worrying about it. He'd say, 'You've been through it before. You can get through it again.' Maybe, but this time I felt different." Sam's reflexive comforting was not what Candace needed just then.

Recognizing her patient's distress, Candace's gynecologist referred her to me. By the time I saw her, she was barely eating or sleeping. To stem the tide of anxiety, I taught her to elicit the relaxation response and I offered to accompany her in the hospital as she was prepared for surgery. Candace calmed down sufficiently to recognize the feelings just under the surface of her panic state. She began to weep in my office, and she then followed a whirlpool of emotion down to the primary source of trouble: her father's death a few years earlier.

Candace had been close to her father, who died suddenly of a heart attack a few months before she was diagnosed with breast cancer. She had not fully grieved this loss, partly because of her own health crisis and partly because her mother, bereft over her husband's demise, required constant caretaking. It had all been too much, and the prospect of hysterectomy brought Candace to her breaking point. Now she needed to allow emotions she had put on hold to come rushing forth.

"I never got my stress out after my father's death," she said. "I held it all in, trying to be strong for everybody, trying not to cry so my mother wouldn't feel so bad."

Candace's fear of surgery was like a young child's fear—a child who needed a loving parent to hold her hand and make it okay. The parent she longed for was her father. By allowing herself to finally grieve this loss, Candace moved beyond the young child's sadness and fear. To get through surgery, she still needed my support, not to mention a prescription from her physician for Xanax, the anti-anxiety agent. But she was no longer gripped by a terror so profound that it threatened her psychological stability.

The mass in Candace's abdomen turned out to be benign. The uterine bleeding she had before surgery, which had been caused by the mass, stopped completely. Her recovery was smooth, and it took far less time than her surgeon had expected. Not only was she relieved, but her entire mental state improved after surgery. She was glad that I had accompanied her in the hospital, right up to the moment she was led into the operating room. (I was glad that she asked for and accepted my support.) Candace was also convinced that grieving over her father had a healing effect on her spirit.

"It still hurts, there is still pain," Candace said recently. "My heart still aches. But now I can talk about it. I will always miss him. But it's gotten much better."

Candace's story illustrates the many benefits of emotional expression. While it is commonly accepted wisdom that expressing emotions is good for our mental health, few people realize that expressing emotions is equally important for our physical health. Three separate European studies evaluated the psychological profiles of women with breast lumps before their biopsy results were known. As it happened, all three studies turned up largely similar results: as opposed to the women whose lumps were benign, the women with breast cancer tended to "suppress their anger" and "avoid conflict and trouble."

These and other studies suggest that expressing negative emotions (such as anger) bolsters the body's defense against disease. But a fascinating study tells another side of this story. While at the Pittsburgh Cancer Institute, Sandra Levy, Ph.D., followed the progress of thirty-six women who had suffered a recurrence of breast cancer. Seven years later, two thirds of them had died. Levy discovered a common factor among the one third who survived: at the beginning of the study, they had expressed more *joy*. This single factor—joy—was a more powerful predictor of survival than several other medical factors that doctors use to determine prognosis. Dr. Levy believes that these women were more hopeful and optimistic.

What can we make of these breast cancer findings? The common denominator is *expression*—of both negative and positive emotions. Women who experience and openly articulate a range of feelings appear to have more psychological and physical resilience.

In this chapter, I explore the importance of expressing emotions to women's psychological and physical health. Based on the above-mentioned studies and my own clinical experience, I don't believe that some emotions are good for our health while others are bad. Indeed, when we stifle so-called negative emotions such as sadness or anger, we may become depressed and hopeless, which *can* be harmful to our health. I must emphasize that depression and hopelessness are not emotions per se; they can be chronic mental states that result from our inability to integrate emotions. Once we acknowledge, express, and resolve feelings such as sadness and anger, we are generally less likely to become depressed or hopeless.

Grief is one example of an emotion that must eventually be expressed and resolved. Have you ever experienced the death of a loved one? If you have, perhaps you understand what Candace went through. Until you can fully cry about your loss, and talk openly about it to someone who empathizes, you carry that grief and it weighs you down. You carry it in different forms—as a fear you can't shake, a lump in your throat, a dark sense of melancholia, a recurring headache, a feeling of emptiness you try to fill with food or drink. You won't free yourself from these manifestations until you confront grief directly. When you do, the weight is gradually lifted and the symptoms disappear. You will feel sad on occasion; you may never completely lose that sadness. But it will no longer sap your spirits or make you sick.

The example of bereavement applies to other emotions. When we harbor anger over some injustice or insult, it will fester, until we find a constructive way to explore and express that anger. When anger festers, it becomes simmering resentment, hostility, even hatred. When we try to wish away primary emotions such as sadness, fear, and anger, they don't disappear; they go underground where they cause chronic states of unhappiness that drag us down.

So we must not judge our basic emotions, splitting them into "good" or "bad," "positive" or "negative." At the same time, we can develop positive ways to manage negative emotions. Spilling our guts to the wrong people or bawling out everyone at work who makes us mad are only two examples of destructive modes of expression. I'll return shortly to the issue of how best to communicate difficult emotions. But suffice it to say that constructive expression can be a boon to women's health. In the words of mind-body clinician Rachel Naomi Remen, M.D., "The only bad emotion is a stuck emotion."

For it is stuck emotions that make it difficult for us to have any emotions. It's not unlike what happens when a car accident during rush hour causes a bottleneck of traffic on a four-lane highway. Ambulances and police arrive, setting up roadblocks that knock the four lanes down to one. Traffic slows to a standstill; at any given time, few cars make it through. Likewise, when we cut off the flow of a "big" emotion such as sadness or anger, we create our own bottleneck. Other emotions, including the positive ones—joy and hope among them—will have trouble getting through to consciousness.

Another way to understand the importance of expression is to view our emotions as the many colors on a palette. When we start erasing bright shades from one end of this emotional spectrum, all we're left with is gray. To be fully human—and healthy—we need access to the full range of emotions.

Writing Out Feelings:
A Health Prescription

One of the most powerful mind-body approaches is deceptively simple. In my groups, I hand participants a piece of blank paper, then ask them to sit quietly and write about one subject only. "I want you to recall the most traumatic event associated with your health condition," I say. "Write about your deepest thoughts and feelings about that event. Write nonstop for twenty minutes, keep your pen moving on the paper, and don't worry about grammar or spelling." The group members sit by themselves, and at first the room is silent, save the scratching and rolling of pens on paper. Soon, however, I hear muffled sobs from women who have let go of all inhibitions in the writing process.

Afterward, we talk about what happened. Some women reveal what they wrote about; others do not. We respect each other's privacy. But those who share their experiences often report that they released grief, fear, or anger that had been frozen in mind and body. The floodgates opened, and they discovered emotions or conflicts they did not know had plagued them.

As a result, these women gained new insight into themselves. And they glimpsed new ways to cope with the stress of their condition. Later, these same patients report that the writing exercise sparked a lasting improvement in their emotional and physical well-being.

I did not make up this approach, and I am not the only one to observe such remarkable responses. It was developed by James W. Pennebaker, Ph.D., a professor in the department of psychology at Southern Methodist University (SMU) in Dallas. Pennebaker has ushered a variety of populations through a similar procedure. He asks them to write their deepest thoughts and feelings about the most traumatic event they can ever remember. Pennebaker has them write for twenty minutes, and brings them back for four days in a row to repeat the procedure.

The people in Pennebaker's studies experience remarkable benefits from writing about traumatic events. They not only feel better emotionally, their physical health markedly improves. Compared to control groups who wrote only about trivial events, the people who wrote about traumas made significantly fewer visits to the doctor and reported fewer symptoms of illness for months afterward. In one extraordinary study, Pennebaker and his colleagues found that the subjects' T-cells—immune cells that lead our internal fight against disease agents—were livelier for six weeks after the experiment.

In study after study, Pennebaker has proven that expressing emotions can enhance physical health. He's demonstrated the benefits of confiding traumas among his university students, unemployed white-collar workers, university staff members, and Holocaust survivors. Pennebaker has found that not only writing but also talking about traumas can be healing. "Just putting upsetting experiences into words," he explained recently, "has profound psychological and physical benefits for our participants."

Why does expressing emotions improve physical health? Pennebaker has shown that holding back thoughts and feelings takes work. By that he means *physiologic* work—our blood pressure, heart rate, and muscle tension increase when we chronically keep emotions locked up. Our immune systems may also suffer when we inhibit feelings. Pennebaker theorized that we lift a great burden from mind and body by confiding long-repressed thoughts and emotions. His studies have proved him right. Whether we write them out or talk them out, expressing emotions not only helps us to feel better, it may strengthen our hearts, our immune systems, and our overall health.

According to Pennebaker, his "journaling" method can be used to heal past traumas, but it can also be used to relieve the stress of ongoing events in our lives. I have tailored his method for women with health problems, asking them to write out feelings about the most upsetting event associated with their particular condition. But I also recommend his approach to women who are simply stressed out: journaling can be an effective adjunct treatment for anxiety and depression.

One of my patients, Brenda, an office manager, felt unable to handle minor conflicts on the job and in her marriage. Her stress levels were skyrocketing, and she began to have physical symptoms, including headaches and severe menstrual cramps. On my suggestion she started to write out her feelings about her problems. After a few writing sessions she got substantial relief from her distress and her ailments.

Brenda continued the writing process, and the experience deepened for her. She realized that she had never fully grieved the loss of a dear friend, Patricia, who had died of cancer a year earlier. Patricia had been a soul mate, the one person with whom she could share all her angers and sorrows. After Patricia died, Brenda felt helpless, as though a gaping void in her life could never be filled. She finally wrote out her grief, and the tears flowed freely.

After a few sessions she called "cathartic," Brenda's writing changed yet again. Instead of writing *about* her loss of Patricia, she wrote *to* Patricia. She would confide her ongoing frustrations, saying things she couldn't to anyone else. Writing to Patricia had the uncanny effect of making Brenda feel less alone.

Many of my patients who do this writing exercise experience a catharsis that makes them feel relieved almost immediately. They gain greater insight into their current stresses and symptoms, and they feel that they've put their emotional house in order. But some do not have this experience. In fact, I've had patients who tell me they feel worse, as though a Pandora's box had been opened and that nothing they do puts the lid back on. Many of these patients cry when they write, but the wound that is exposed doesn't seem to heal.

I've learned from experience why this happens. When I first employed Pennebaker's method in my mind-body groups, I would instruct patients to write out their emotions during one of our weekly sessions together. I did not always counsel them to continue writing for several days afterward. I soon realized that these women had only scratched the surface of deeply buried and very painful emotions, and of course, they were left with exposed wounds.

But when I began counseling women to continue the process for several days—as Dr. Pennebaker had in his studies—the results were much better. By writing for twenty minutes over three or four days, the women were able to work through their sadness, anxiety, and anger. By the second or third writing session, a change would occur. Having gotten the feelings out, they began to better understand the effect that a particular trauma or stressor had had on their behavior and their lives. As with Brenda, the changes that occurred over several writing sessions represented a healing process in which emotional catharsis gave way to insight, acceptance, and resolution.

Dr. Pennebaker points out that people often resist writing in journals because they know they will confront painful problems and emotions and they can't see beyond the initial discomforts. In a recent conversation, he addressed this issue: "In the back of their minds, some people think, 'I don't want to write in my journal today. It'll make me feel bad.' And you know, they're right. If we just write for one day we are going to feel worse." All of Pennebaker's studies show that a commitment to writing for three or four days is necessary for the shift from anxiety to acceptance to occur. Working out past traumas can't be accomplished in one sitting.

Guidelines for the Writing Exercise

If you believe that this exercise will help you to handle emotions that impede your mental and physical well-being, follow the instructions discussed above. If you are physically healthy, write about the most stressful event or ongoing problem you face in your daily life. If you believe your current problems are primarily the result of past events, write about the traumatic circumstances in your past. Write about what happened, and how you felt or feel about it. Don't stick exclusively to facts or to feelings—write about both. (Pure facts without feelings won't be liberating. Pure feelings with no facts won't help you to understand your experiences. This process involves both emotional catharsis *and* insight.) Repeat this twenty-minute process for at least three or four days, and keep going for as long as a week if you find that the exercise continues to be fruitful. If you've covered one traumatic event or stressful circumstance and there are other ones pressing, move on and explore them as well.

If you have a medical condition that causes emotional distress, write about the most traumatic event or stressful aspect of this condition. Then follow the same guidelines given above, and continue the exercise every day for at least three or four days.

"Unfreezing" Emotions

These days, psychiatrists and psychologists often refer to posttraumatic stress disorder, or PTSD, in which people repress memories and feelings associated with a traumatic event and are left with scars and symptoms that persist for years. Some of us have milder forms of PTSD that may not require psychiatric treatment, but they involve a similar mental dynamic. An event or series of events from the past, involving, say, parental neglect, may be too painful to accept when it occurs. We put those emotions and memories "on hold," and they remain sequestered in a part of our psyche. Our experiences are frozen in time, and so is our full capacity for emotional experience. The same process can occur with more recent events, such as those associated with the breakup of a marriage, the loss of a job, a cancer diagnosis, a struggle with infertility, multiple miscarriages, or chronic pain.

Many of us seal away these memories and emotions where they remain intact yet locked away until we liberate them from sequestration. Yet some of us do talk with friends and family about our hurts and angers but are still not liberated from memories and emotions stuck in time. Indeed, it is possible to talk incessantly without much relief, because we have not processed the feelings in a deep-going manner. (For instance, when Candace talked to her husband, Sam, his rush to comfort was well intended, but it did not help her get to the bottom of her troubles.) One way to process emotion is to enlist the help of a professional therapist who knows exactly how to help you "unfreeze" experiences stuck in time. Indeed, the writing technique should *not* be used as a substitute for psychotherapy. If you are chronically anxious or depressed, consult your doctor for a referral to a mental health professional.

With or without therapy, you can use the writing exercise to melt defenses and unfreeze emotions. When you stick with the process, writing becomes a journey that naturally wends its way from deep feeling to insight to acceptance. It's like following a yellow brick road from the source of trouble—a traumatic event or situation—to a healing resolution rooted in awareness, forgiveness of self, and, in some cases, forgiveness of others.

The writing process has also helped many of my patients reach various kinds of decisions. For infertile patients, writing out emotions can help them achieve a clearheaded state that enables them either to move forward with medical treatments, adopt, or choose not to have children. For patients with early breast cancer, or menopausal hot flashes, or PMS, it can help them decide what medical treatments make sense for them, especially when doctors offer a variety of options.

Repressed grief and anger, in particular, can cloud our consciousness and prevent us from moving forward with clarity and conviction. Once we become fully aware of these emotions, we can thoroughly sort them out, which enables us to make almost any important decision. Sound decision making is based on conscious consideration of the callings of the head *and* the heart, with balance and perspective.

The writing exercise, as one way to process difficult emotions, can also help us to make transforming life passages. Consider the case of Viola, who came to see me on an individual basis because of a low-grade depression that affected her entire quality of life. A successful thirty-eight-year-old corporate middle manager, Viola was happy with her work, but she had never married. She yearned for a man she could love and marry, but years of dating had not turned up the right fellow. In Viola's mind, her inability to find a life partner was the overriding cause of her unhappiness.

I recommended to Viola that she practice the writing exercise on a regular basis. She immediately began to "let 'er rip" on paper, and what instantly emerged was profound anger—at her situation, and at the men she had dated. She also explored and exorcised her feelings of loneliness. "It felt like a great unloading, a kind of dumping out on the page," she said. In a strange way, the writing process itself eased her loneliness. "I had my companion when I came home," commented Viola. "It was the notebook I wrote in every night."

The writing process allowed Viola to let off steam, but it also allowed her to regain her bearings. At my request, she spent time writing down things she liked about herself, helping to rebuild her self-esteem as she simultaneously let go of deep-seated resentment and alienation toward men.

Nine months after Viola began the writing process, she met and became involved with Allan, an accountant with whom she shared many interests. One year later, they married. Viola is obviously ecstatic with this turn of events. Although the writing process had no bearing on the crossing of paths that enabled her to meet her future husband, she does believe that it profoundly changed her attitude and aura, which made her more attractive to Allan. "I had left my baggage at home," she explained.

Viola pointed out that "people know whether you are a happy person, an anxious person, or a depressed person. And they are not necessarily going to be receptive to someone who is anxious or depressed. When I met [Allan], I wasn't carrying around that burden with me all the time. I had this time and place for unloading, and it was my journal at home."

Whether women are lonely, angry, struggling in their careers and relationships, or beset by medical conditions, they can use the writing process to get on with their lives with confidence. It is a remarkably effective and illuminating approach to mental, emotional, and physical well-being.

Anger as Your Ally

Generalization though it may be, most women have trouble with anger. In my experience, a majority are afraid of expressing anger, even in the most constructive ways. And a significant minority have the opposite trouble: they get mad at the drop of a hat, expressing anger in often destructive ways. Women of the former group can't work themselves up to a steady boil; women of the latter group can't stop themselves from exploding like a pressure cooker left sitting on a high flame.

Since most of my patients have trouble expressing anger, I focus my teachings on the positive aspects of anger and the constructive ways of channeling and communicating it.

Positive aspects of anger? In her marvelous book *The Dance of Anger*, psychologist Harriet Goldhor Lerner, Ph.D., helped to redefine and demystify anger for women:

> Anger is a signal, and one worth listening to. Our anger may be a message that we are being hurt, that our rights are being violated, that our needs or wants are not being adequately met, or simply that something is not right. Our anger may tell us that we are not addressing an important emotional issue in our lives, or that too much of our self—our beliefs, values, desires, or ambitions—is being compromised in a relationship. Our anger may be a signal that we are doing more than we can comfortably do or give. Or our anger may warn us that others are doing too much for us, at the expense of our own competence and growth.

If anger is a signal worth listening to, why do so many women fear, suppress, or talk themselves out of anger? Parental and social teachings have made women feel that anger is unladylike. The message we've gotten is that our anger is inappropriate, perhaps even shameful. It's an emotion that has been largely reserved for men, while women are given more leeway to be sad and fearful.

It's an imbalance we must rectify within ourselves, both by our individual efforts and with the help and support of other women. The first step is to recognize the positive aspects of anger. As Dr. Lerner points out, anger is a signal that carries useful information about our needs, our relationships, our environment. It is also an energizing emotion, one that can often lift us out of depression and hopelessness.

In her book *Maps to Ecstasy*, Gabrielle Roth captures healthy anger: "Proper anger . . . is quick, clear, needs no explanation. It's the bared teeth of a bitch protecting her litter, the arched back and hiss of a cat threatened by a coyote. There's nothing cleaner, more effective than appropriate anger. Authentic anger is specific and justified, and its direct expression exposes impropriety and defends integrity in a way that benefits everyone."

Have you ever been deeply wounded by a romantic partner or a friend? When you respond passively, you may collapse into a state of insecurity or despair. When you respond actively, you rise to defend yourself with energy and determination. Healthy anger is a protective emotion. It says to one's self and others: "I am worth defending. My needs and feelings should be respected."

Women with medical conditions are often angry at their bodies. At menopause, they are angry at their bodies for causing hot flashes and vaginal atrophy. With PMS, they are angry at their bodies for losing control. With chronic pain, they are angry at their bodies for causing nonstop misery. With cancer, they are angry at their bodies for producing a tumor. With infertility, they are angry at their bodies for not producing a baby.

Here's what you can do when saddled with anger associated with these conditions. First, acknowledge your anger; it does no good to pretend it doesn't exist. Then use cognitive restructuring to change relentless negative thoughts about your body to more realistic, positive ones. Yes, you feel betrayed by your body. But your biology must be allowed its imperfections; you are not a robot.

When you are relentlessly mad at your body for its perceived failures, you betray and abandon your body. But you can gradually heal the mind-body split. Stephen Levine, author of many books on healing, offers the most basic example of this split. What happens, he asks, when we stub a toe? We send anger into that toe. The pain throbs, and we send hatred into the pain. But what if we sent kindness into that toe? Rather than fighting the sensations, what if we accepted them with mercy and compassion? Perhaps the pain would subside more quickly.

Without kindness, mind and body are forever at war. One way of expressing that kindness is to meet your body's need for relaxation. Use the relaxation methods in chapter 3 to ease back into a calm body, a body capable of some pleasure and gratification.

Women with constant stress at work or in relationships may carry chronic resentment toward others. So may women with medical conditions, who resent hurried doctors, or friends who have the health or the children they wish they had, or spouses who just don't get it. This kind of resentment is not clean anger. It is not the open, direct expression and resolution of a useful emotion. Resentment is blocked anger that hangs around like an uninvited guest, causing trouble.

Joan Borysenko once likened the person with chronic resentment to someone carrying a hot coal around in her hands, waiting to toss it at the individual who made her feel bad. The question is, Who gets burned?

If you carry resentment like a hot coal, use the writing process to keep from getting burned. In your writing, ask yourself these questions: What does your resentment feel like? Is the person you resent the only cause of your agitation? Does your resentment remind you of how you've felt in other situations? What is the basic anger beneath your resentment? Can you imagine letting go of resentment? Use journaling to release your anger, and to discover deeper layers of emotion and experience that contribute to your chronic state of resentment.

You may also need to communicate underlying anger directly to those who have caused you pain. But it helps enormously to process these emotions first through writing or talking to a friend or therapist, because you'll approach the person with greater clarity and conviction. You'll be less likely to explode irrationally, or otherwise behave in ways you will quickly regret. When you do communicate anger, there are certain guidelines for healthy expression that I offer in the upcoming section "Assertiveness."

For women who tend to explode irrationally, these assertiveness skills, along with cognitive restructuring, are essential. I teach these women how to manage anger and communicate needs and feelings effectively without alienating people. And I teach them to change negative thoughts that fuel ceaseless cycles of blame and retribution. By contrast, when I treat women who fear and repress anger, I try to validate their underlying emotions, letting them know that anger is a human reflex that cannot be ignored.

For both groups of women, I teach certain exercises for a balanced awareness and acceptance of anger. You can use these exercises when anger creates difficulties in everyday relationships, or in a struggle with a medical condition.

Exercises for Awareness and Acceptance of Anger

The following exercises, which include a guided imagery practice, were taught to me by Joan Borysenko. They are designed to help women develop greater awareness of anger, and to manage and express it more effectively. First, use the following two fill-in questions to help you gain focus:

1. It makes me angry when _____.
2. When I get angry, I'm afraid that _____.

When filling in the first blank, try to find an underlying theme in your response or responses. Does it make you angry when a friend or family member says or does something hurtful or unfair? When someone close insults you? Neglects you? Does not meet your needs? Ultimately, what factor or factors trigger your anger? Usually, these triggers are one or several of the following: lack of support, unfairness, disrespect, or outright abuse. Don't use this exploration to reinforce a sense of victimhood. Use it to find out what relationships and situations cause your anger; where you are responsible for creating these circumstances and where others are responsible; and how you can communicate your needs and rights with greater force and clarity.

In filling in the second blank, again look for underlying themes. If indeed you are afraid to express anger, what is the real source of that fear? Are you convinced that the person to whom you express anger will dismiss, reject, or abandon you? Are you concerned that once you let anger out of the bag, it will never stop coming? Are you worried that you will lose control and hurt someone emotionally or physically? Are you anxious that your anger will destroy a relationship?

Women who are afraid of their own anger usually express one or several of these fears. Some of them are rational. (If you allow yourself to have a violent temper tantrum, you may indeed harm a relationship.) But many of these fears are irrational. More often than not, appropriately expressed anger will not cause others to reject or abandon you.

You won't be able to accept the healthy, positive aspects of anger until you confront your fears about anger. Take a look at your answers to this fill-in question, and you'll realize how ingrained these fears are—and how many of them are irrational. Many of us were taught from a young age that anger is a wrong, bad, crazy, out-of-control emotion that does not befit a young girl, or, for that matter, a mature woman. Given these early teachings, our belief that anger will invariably yield destruction or abandonment should come as no surprise.

So we must tease out the rational from the irrational fears. You will discover just how many of these fears are baseless. Moreover, you set the stage for the next level of learning: that you can manage and express anger in positive ways that do not involve blaming, destructive outbursts, or violence.

Here's an imagery exercise to help you explore the roots of your relationship to anger. Sit in a comfortable chair, and imagine that you're walking through a beautiful field of flowing grass. Now walk to the edge of the field where a forest of tall oaks and pines begins. Find a small pathway into the depths of the woods, and walk for a little while amidst the trees until you come to a cave. Stand and watch quietly as anger emerges from the cave. Anger can be any image—a person, an animal, a big hairy monster, a mythic figure, a ball of fire, an amorphous black cloud. Allow your imagination to conjure any image of anger that feels right to you.

Now imagine that you approach your image of anger, and take it by the hand. Walk with anger out of the woods and into the field. Sit down in the field with anger, and hold a conversation. Find out about your anger with an exploratory spirit. Be open to the idea that, as a child, your anger protected you. It defended you from insults, hurts, and ill-treatment. If you discover anger's protective quality, thank anger for serving this purpose for you. Thank anger for being there.

Talk to anger about what it has done for you. Recognize that anger has protected you, but that you have emotions and coping strategies other than anger that can also protect you. As an adult you have other resources—assertiveness, conviction, control, articulation. Talk to anger about what it can and cannot do for you now.

When you are finished conversing with anger, stand up, walk back to the edge of the field, and say goodbye to anger. Head back out into the field. Then turn around to see what has happened to anger. Did anger return to the cave, or is it still standing at the edge of the woods? Once you have an image of anger, continue on your way, strolling across the field.

This exercise helps to reduce women's fears about anger. Often, the moment a woman takes anger by the hand, the big monster becomes a friendly Frankenstein; the ball of fire shrinks; the huge frightening bear becomes smaller and fuzzier, like a children's storybook character. For one woman, a gigantic hairy monster turned into Cousin Itt from the Addams Family. (Indeed, I wonder if the success of the '60s sitcom *The Munsters* had something to do with its transformation of famous angry monsters into lovable characters kids could warm up to.)

The purpose of the exercise is to inculcate the message, on an imaginal rather than intellectual level, that anger is an ally, not an enemy. Yes, anger can get out of control and we need skills to harness it. But we are capable of anger for a reason, and every woman can recognize that her anger, at its source, is a natural part of her emotional repertoire—one that has helped her to deal with stress, insults to her integrity, threats to her well-being. It's not enough to know that anger is an ally; many women need to feel it on a gut level. The dialogue with anger helps to reestablish a "friendly" connection with anger, calming their fears that anger is an enemy capable of harming others and swallowing themselves. Many women have insights during this imagery exercise. One patient, Geraldine, waited for quite a while for anger to emerge from the cave. When it did, its personification frightened her: anger was her mother. But this led Geraldine to a series of realizations about her immense fear of anger. She was so scared of becoming like her mother—a ball of rage capable of sudden, frightening outbursts—that she gradually shut down her own relationship with anger. She sacrificed her own self-protective mechanism because she'd come to associate it with her out-of-control mother. The exercise helped Geraldine to unravel problems in relationships and work that had plagued her for years.

After the exercise, I ask women how the image of anger changed from the time it emerged from the cave to the time they turned around to see where it ended up. Typically, anger changed radically, though in stages. While anger started as an outsized, often monstrous image, it became smaller and friendlier when taken by the hand, and smaller and friendlier still by the end of the dialogue. For one woman, a frightening apparition gradually transformed into Casper the Friendly Ghost. For most, an image of danger soon becomes protective, communicative, sometimes even cuddly.

When you practice this imagery exercise, do not dwell upon how you think it should turn out. Although the above-mentioned response patterns are common, every woman has her unique response. Follow your intuitions, explore your responses, and evaluate your thoughts and feelings afterward.

Since anger is a message that something is wrong in our internal or external environment, it is our task to pay attention. The way to reduce anger is not to deny its existence, but rather to heed its call—to find out what needs are not being met, what rights are being violated. Once we properly interpret anger, we can use our knowledge of its messages to communicate, to make changes, to right wrongs, or to rectify imbalances in our relationships.

Assertiveness: Making Constructive Use of Anger

Once we become aware of anger, interpret its messages, and defuse its fury, we can use anger as an agent of change, particularly in our relationships. Using anger as an agent of change means one thing: learning to assert ourselves.

Assertiveness is the appropriate behavioral channel for anger. It is a style of relating that enables us to use anger constructively. When we assert our needs and rights in a clear and balanced manner, we vastly reduce the chances that we will alienate people in our environment, be they coworkers, friends, or family members.

Of course, assertiveness is a sign of psychological health. But asserting our needs may also strengthen and balance our immune systems. Thirty years ago, George F. Solomon, M.D., studied women with rheumatoid arthritis (RA) and their sisters who did not have the disease. Since both sisters had the same genetic inheritance—which can play an important role in RA—Solomon wondered if psychological differences between the sisters could explain why one got sick and the other didn't. He used role-play exercises and psychological tests in one study comparing the women with RA to their healthy sisters. "In every single case," said Solomon, "the healthy sibling was more assertive than the sister with arthritis." In later research, Solomon showed that HIV patients who are more assertive may live longer and that assertive elderly people are more likely to stay vigorous and healthy.

Here's another one of those generalizations that is true, but only because of social indoctrination: most women have greater difficulty with assertiveness than most men. Despite the great strides women have made toward equality between the sexes, social hierarchies still discourage women from speaking out on their own behalf. And family conditioning, in which girls are typically given less freedom than boys to show anger or draw sharp boundaries, often thwarts maturing women's assertiveness. They've learned that anger is wrong, assertiveness is wrong, and people will reject, abandon, or even loathe them for daring to speak out.

Women can begin to cultivate assertiveness by learning exactly what it is—the opposite of passivity, but not unbridled anger or aggression. Assertiveness means directly stating your needs, feelings, and opinions without blaming, erupting, or lashing out. The following chart, from behavioral scientists Edward A. Charlesworth, Ph.D., and Ronald G. Nathan, Ph.D., compares passive, assertive, and aggressive behaviors:

Passive	*Assertive*	*Aggressive*
You avoid saying what you want, think, or feel. If you do, you speak in such a way that you put yourself down. Apologetic words with hidden meanings, a smoke screen of vague words, or silence are used frequently. Examples are, "You know," "Well," "I mean," and "I'm sorry." You allow others to choose for you.	You say what you honestly want, think, and feel in direct and helpful ways. You make your own choices. You communicate with tact and humor. You use "I" statements. Your words are clear and objective. They are few and well chosen.	You say what you want, think, and feel, but at the expense of others. You use "loaded words" and "you" statements that label or blame. You employ threats or accusations and one-upmanship. You choose for others.

Assertiveness is the balanced, appropriate way of channeling anger and frustration. Recognize your own passive responses and work to transform them into assertive ones. This effort will call upon your willingness to stand up for yourself. Likewise, recognize your own aggressive responses, and work to transform them into assertive ones. This effort will call upon your willingness to privately explore your aggressive impulses while publicly taking a clear, nonblaming, nonviolent stand on your own behalf.

For many women, *no* is a four-letter word. But *no* is a word that draws boundaries, affirms your autonomy, lets others know where you stand. *No* protects you from undue self-sacrifice and stifling obligations. Learning to say no is therefore a first tenet of assertiveness.

In groups, I use an exercise I learned from mind-body practitioner Matthew Budd, M.D., to help my patients say no. I have patients go off in pairs and sit facing each other. I hand each pair a list of twenty-five questions. Each question is a request that would be hard for anyone to turn down. One person in each pair ask the questions, and her counterpart has to say *no*. Then they change roles and perform the exercise again. Included are questions such as: Can I borrow a quarter for a phone call? Would you have dinner with me tonight? Could you give me the name of your hairdresser? Could you move your chair a bit closer so I can hear you better? It's not socially acceptable for people to decline such requests, and is therefore enormously hard to say no to them, even in a role-play situation.

During the second phase of the exercise, I tell the respondent to make up any conceivable reason for her "no," and I tell the questioner to keep pursuing her request. Sometimes the answers are hilariously preposterous. In one instance, a woman asked her partner if she could spare a quarter for a phone call. The partner said no. The questioner said, "But I see you have a pocketful of change." The partner replied, "But I have plans for every one of these quarters, dimes, and nickels." Although the toughest questions force partners to come up with bizarre excuses, other questions are not so tough and the explanations are more reality-based. Many women turn down dinner requests because they have previous plans.

During the third and final phase, I tell the respondent to say no but offer alternative strategies. In the case of the woman who asked her partner for a quarter, the partner said, "I only have one quarter for a phone call, and I have a beeper that could go off any minute. But let me give you a dollar. There's a convenience store down the street that can give you change."

This exercise teaches that there are three ways to say no: (1) a simple no; (2) no, because . . . ; and (3) no, but how about . . . Then I ask my patients to practice these three approaches, which offer women alternative ways to protect themselves from requests that impinge upon their needs, boundaries, or energy reserves. The "no" exercise reinforces women's sense that they have options—ways to say no that don't inflict hurt or devastate relationships. It also points out that there *are* times when a simple no is necessary and sufficient. When a coworker asks you out repeatedly, bordering on harassment, a simple no takes the strongest stand. Too much explanation gives such a person room to engage in a struggle with you—just what you don't want.

Often, however, our need to please and protect others means that a simple no can be painfully difficult. In these instances, we can draw up boundaries without causing ourselves and others undue anguish. If necessary, we can combine an explanation (approach 2) with an offering of alternatives (approach 3). We can say, "No, I can't make dinner tonight because I'm exhausted. But let's reschedule." "No, I can't move my chair closer to yours because of severe back trouble. Can you move yours closer to mine?" "No, I know you love my chicken recipe, but I'm too bushed tonight to make it. Why don't we just go out for pizza?"

Here's a strange but logical paradox: the more assertive we are, the less angry we are. Why? Because our anger builds internally when we keep saying yes even though we desperately want and need to say no. When awareness and expression of anger are minimal, our snowballing anger goes underground, where it can wreak emotional and even physical havoc. Yet we keep saying yes, and our anger may leak out in little digs, covert rebellions, chores and good deeds carried out with barely concealed frustration. This veiled expression of underground anger is commonly known as *passive aggression*. Given few outlets for legitimate anger, many of us become passive-aggressive martyrs, and we should understand the origins of our behavior rather than feeling shameful about it.

Recognize your own passive-aggressive behavior, and change it by directly asserting your needs and rights! When a yes is heartfelt, by all means say yes. Don't look for opportunities to say no to prove your assertive mettle. This practice is not meant to reinforce a closed-hearted stance in the world. But watch for telltale signs that you're selling yourself out with any given yes—a creeping sense of dread, exhaustion, or resentment. In some instances, to quote my colleague Ann Webster, saying no to someone else is saying yes to yourself.

Finally, standing up for your needs and rights without blaming others may be the signal aspect of good assertiveness skills. Harriet Goldhor Lerner has developed the clearest possible guidelines. Here are her critical points, adapted from her book *The Dance of Anger*.

- *Don't use "below-the-belt" tactics.* These include blaming, interpreting, diagnosing, labeling, analyzing, preaching, moralizing, ordering, warning, interrogating, ridiculing, and lecturing.

- *Do speak in "I" language.* Learn to say, "I think . . ." "I feel . . ." "I want . . ." instead of "You don't . . ." or "You are . . ." A true "I" statement says something about the self without criticizing or blaming the other person and without holding the other person responsible for our feelings or reactions. Watch out for the disguised "you" statements or pseudo-"I" statements. ("*I* think *you* are controlling and self-centered.")
- *Do recognize that each person is responsible for his or her own behavior.* Don't blame your dad's new wife because she "won't let him" be close to you. If you are angry about the distance between you and your dad, it is your responsibility to find a new way to approach the situation. Your dad's behavior is his responsibility, not his wife's.
- *Don't tell another person what she or he thinks or feels or "should" think or feel.* If another person gets angry in reaction to a change you make, don't criticize his or her feelings or deny him or her the right to be angry. Better to say, "I understand that you're angry, and if I were in your shoes perhaps I'd be angry, too. But I've thought it over and this is my decision."

Apply these skills to your relationships with employers and coworkers, husbands and partners, children and parents, siblings and friends. When you have a medical condition—particularly a chronic one that requires many encounters with doctors and health-care personnel—rely on assertive communication to stand up for your rights as a medical consumer and a human being. Surviving a hospital stay, in particular, calls upon your skills of assertive communication. Doctors and nurses don't want to be blamed any more than husbands and partners do, so state your needs and rights with clarity. Seek information but don't lecture or ridicule. In order to take responsibility for your own health care, you must firmly and respectfully demand involvement in every medical decision that affects your well-being.

Spanning the Spectrum of Emotions

*A*ccess to the full spectrum of emotions in our human repertoire is a worthy goal, one that translates into a richer and a healthier life. But sometimes the process is extremely difficult. The exercises and approaches I've recommended will help you make progress, but you may need the aid of a therapist to explore the unique reasons for your particular blocks or difficulties. You can also make your own explorations. Ask yourself: Which emotions can I express? Which ones can't I express? Where did I learn or develop these tendencies?

In mind-body groups, I have participants call out every emotion they can think of. Then I write them on a blackboard: anger, joy, love, hate, anxiety, fear, sadness, grief, jealousy, disgust, hope, ecstasy, and so forth. Invariably, the list includes many negative and many positive emotions. I ask participants to think back to their childhoods, and ask themselves: Did my parents express these emotions? Did I have good role models for expression? As a child, was *I* allowed to express positive and negative emotions?

The answers are diverse, but few women have parents who modeled appropriate expression of the full range of negative and positive emotions. It is no wonder that women (and men, in somewhat different ways) have so much trouble with expression. Without those early models, they can't expect themselves to readily express emotions. It's an exercise that gives women insight into their current-day patterns, and it helps them to understand their limitations. Women who are sick may find themselves beset by intense feelings—especially grief and anger—that they cannot handle. If you find yourself in such a bind, use this simple exploration of your history to cultivate awareness and, most importantly, compassion for yourself. When it comes to expressing emotions, we ought to view our limitations with little surprise: we were never taught how. If anything, many of us were taught to stifle anger, sadness, fear, or joy.

One of my menopause patients, Janice, had a rather typical family configuration with regard to emotional expression. She grew up in a household where her father could express anger but her mother could not. As a young child, neither parent allowed her to express anger. Today, as she faced the "change of life" with many symptoms, regrets, and conflicts with the medical world, Janice found herself angry—at her body, her younger friends, and her doctors. But she did not know how to handle her anger.

When Janice took a hard look at this family legacy, a sense of recognition washed over her. She experienced what I call the "ah-hah" phenomenon— a moment of realization, in which connections between our early upbringing and our current troubles come suddenly into sharp focus. "Now I know why this has been so damned hard for me," she said.

When fathers express anger but mothers do not, the implied message to young girls from their gender model—Mom—is "keep a lid on it." But every family is different, and a myriad of configurations exist. If mother was a rageball, daughter may be afraid of her own anger. Alternatively, she may herself become a rageball, and develop the opposite problem: Type A explosiveness. She may express anger in a distorted manner, while being unable to express other emotions, such as sadness or joy. When fathers are violent or abusive, daughters may grow up with the fear that any expression of anger—even mild irritation—will provoke someone's dangerous wrath. So they spend the better part of a lifetime stifling even the slightest twinge of frustration or dissent.

In some families, the prevailing atmosphere makes it impossible for female children to acknowledge fear, sadness, anger—any "unpleasant" emotion. The parents' explanation is often, "I don't want to hear that whining." In other families, the prevailing atmosphere makes it hard for girls to show unmitigated joy, to celebrate victories, to evince pride in their accomplishments. The parents' explanation is often, "I don't want to hear that bragging."

When we make such "ah-hah" connections, we can begin to overthrow the tyranny of old teachings. These teachings were not only constraining, they were based on false assumptions. Our authentic expressions of fear, sadness, or anger are not whining. By the same token, our authentic expressions of joy, pride, and celebration are not bragging. But we internalize these teachings so completely that we banish emotions from our repertoire, and even from our consciousness. The late British psychiatrist R. D. Laing understood how we block awareness and expression of emotions. "First we forget," he said. "And then we forget that we have forgotten." Perhaps we can liberate ourselves from this bind by finally remembering how it all got started.

We can also use relaxation techniques to reduce the surface anxiety that keeps emotions at bay. Once anxiety melts, layers of emotions are exposed. Often what emerges first is sharp anger about past or present insults or traumas. Once that anger is recognized and expressed, the next layer is often sadness. For when we've been repeatedly hurt, stressed, or traumatized, our initial defense is fury. But beneath that fury is grief—the sense of loss we feel when basic needs for love, nurturance, and respect have gone unmet. We can combine mind-body techniques to help us peel away these layers.

The stresses and traumas that cause a buildup of negative emotions may be associated with early childhood events, ongoing difficulties in work or relationships, and, of course, medical conditions. Many of my patients have been twice traumatized—first by life events, then by their medical conditions. These patients often peel away the layers of emotion, reaching a core that is once again capable of tranquility and joy. As Joan Borysenko once said, "Our essential core is peaceful and whole. The work of healing is in peeling away the barriers of fear and past conditioning that keep us unaware of our true nature. . . . Discovering our peaceful inner core in turn brings the body back to wholeness and allows us to live well, in spite of our physical limitations."

Reaching deep into themselves, these women have acknowledged their pains and been liberated from their grasp. In so doing, they have avoided the trap of victimization. They did not let family mistreatment, work troubles, marital discord, physical symptoms, or even medical nightmares destroy their emotional lives. They regained control by honoring—rather than denying and splitting off—their inner experiences.

As you embark on a path toward emotional healing, be gentle with yourself. Do not create false or unreasonable expectations. Use the writing process, the anger exercises and imagery, and the assertiveness teachings as guideposts in a gradual but rewarding growth process. Although moments of revelation occur, they are not pills that work overnight. Nor are they time-release capsules that offer a predictable course of change. Every woman's emotional healing is different, with unexpected developments, down times, and joyous spurts of catharsis and insight. In fact, if the road isn't bumpy, you might be heading in the wrong direction. There is no quick-and-easy path to emotional health and physical well-being.

One of my patients struggling with infertility, Holly, said it better than I could. "I'd love to be the television hero who gets the feelings all in the right order," she said. "That's the problem with the TV generation we've been brought up in. We're given these unrealistic, almost moralistic ideals. But life does not work that way. I'd like to think of myself as being this terrific hero who has the right feelings at the right time in the right order. But I know that *my* life does not work that way."

Holly did not follow a TV script, but she followed her own bumpy road with enormous courage. At the outset of what was to be this new phase of her life, she quit her lucrative job, deciding that she would raise her child and, eventually, go to graduate school in a completely different field of endeavor. But her elaborate plans and hopes for a family and a new career were dashed when she could not get pregnant after years of high-tech treatments. Family relations were badly strained when siblings with children did not understand the kind of sensitivity Holly needed.

But she entered our mind-body group with a fierce commitment to work through her profound disappointment, to come out the other side with renewed hope and vigor. Holly did just that. She and her husband are considering adoption, but right now, she just wants to live a full life. She's finally granted herself "permission to feel what I'm going to feel," come what may. Despite everything that's happened, all the twisty turns and dashed hopes, Holly has found something she never expected to find—her peaceful inner core.

Nine

◆ ◆ ◆

MINDFUL EATING,
MODEST EXERCISE

The significance of diet and exercise for women goes beyond issues of nutrients, metabolism, cancer prevention, and cardiovascular fitness. What we eat and how we move our bodies have a momentous impact on how we think, feel, cope, and function. These mental states, in turn, influence our health on another level—through the biological corridors of the mind-body connection. When we are miserable about food and weight, and we don't get sufficient exercise, our negative moods are bound to compromise our health. When we are at peace with food and our weight, and we get daily exercise, the positive moods that result are bound to uplift our well-being, our physical vitality, and our capacity to resist illness.

Countless books bespeak the importance of sound nutrition and exercise for a healthy body, and I agree with much of what has been written. Women in particular must educate themselves about how diet and exercise can keep them fit through all stages of the life cycle, preventing heart disease, cancer, osteoporosis, and other maladies. But women are also affected psychologically by an unsound diet, an unhappy relationship with food, an obsession with weight, and a lack of physical activity. That is why I teach mindful eating and modest exercise as a health prescription designed to be as nourishing to the soul as it is to the body.

To embark on a sensible nutritional program, it is necessary to reorder our often disordered relationship with food. Over the course of a lifetime, women are subjected to a ceaseless barrage of conflicting cultural information about food and weight: advertisements tempt us with high-fat foods; the media regale us with images of stick-thin beauty; and magazines and books shower us with ever more miraculous fad diets. What's a woman to do? The more anxious we are about our body images, the more vulnerable we are to scarfing down excessive amounts of high-fat food to comfort ourselves. The more weight we gain, the more we need diets to conform to those images of beauty. And we now know that traditional diets generally don't work, so the moment we fail and regain weight, we're thrust right back onto the merry-go-round.

Round and round we go, until our health suffers and some of us are beset by eating disorders. I'll discuss the medical and psychological ramifications of eating disorders—and the role of mind-body medicine in their treat-ment—in chapter 14. Though most women don't develop clinically diag-nosed eating disorders, a vast number of us have disordered relationships with food and weight—we eat too much, or too little, or nutritionally imbalanced diets. Many get caught in the yo-yo cycle of dieting and weight gain. When these problems continue unabated, they eventually become full-blown eating disorders.

For many of us, diet and weight are stressors as profound as marital problems, family conflicts, job pressures, or physical illnesses. We lose our sense of control—that key marker for psychological well-being—in the face of food cravings and weight fluctuations. We must finally learn that we can't recapture control by traditional dieting. In fact, nutritionists and behavioral psychologists have pegged dieting as the actual *cause* of many eating disor-ders. After a few transgressions from a traditional weight-loss diet, women often feel so guilty that they throw in the towel and start binging. Young women who suffer from anorexia—which involves extreme food depriva-tion—often develop the disorder as a result of dieting.

How, then, do we develop healthy control over food and weight? First, by finding more soul-satisfying ways to exert control in our hectic lives than through eating. Second, by alleviating, through relaxation techniques and coping skills, the anxiety that causes compulsive eating. Finally, we must adopt a balanced diet that includes healthy foods, essential nutrients, and a flexible approach that rejects the restrictive logic of dieting. We can develop this dietary pattern (not a *diet*) by making gradual changes rather than by artificially imposing on ourselves a painful and often unnatural form of restraint.

I call these changes "eating transitions," and they involve small steps and achievable goals. Through a behavioral approach I will describe shortly, women can substitute one healthy food for one unhealthy food over a period of weeks and slowly build on their successes with new eating transi-tions. Through this method, many of my patients have transformed their eating habits over time, which is a far healthier and more enduring way to maintain a reasonable body weight. This approach circumvents the yo-yo cycle of crash and fad diets, and it limits the guilt women feel the moment they transgress with some forbidden nosh or nibble.

Some women ought to lose weight because obesity increases their risks of heart disease, hypertension, diabetes, arthritis, and certain cancers. (Women who weigh 20 percent more than their ideal body weight are considered obese.) For them, a steady commitment to change may be necessary, but this can still be achieved through gradual eating transitions. But many women don't need to lose as much weight as they think, or they don't need to lose weight at all. For them, the motivations for dietary change can be to achieve:

- A healthy capacity to self-nourish
- An intake of healthy foods for optimal energy and psychological well-being
- A properly balanced diet with the nutrients needed to prevent disease and maintain vigor

Meeting these goals requires a balanced effort, one in which guilt is replaced with self-compassion and the plan itself is not destined to fail. For this purpose, I have created an easy-to-follow program of sound nutrition that takes the stress out of eating. It is a blueprint for a sane relationship with food, one that can last a lifetime. Moreover, the program is designed to help prevent heart disease, high blood pressure, osteoporosis, and, according to some studies, breast and gynecologic cancers.

The 80/20 Plan: Keeping It Simple

The conspicuous culprit in weight gain and disease risk is a high-fat diet. Most of us know this basic fact, but we have an excruciatingly hard time making the needed changes. There is no longer any question that a high-fat diet—with over 30 percent of total calories coming from fat—is a major risk factor for heart disease and cancer, the number one killers of both men and women. The saturated fats from animal sources (primarily derived from meats and dairy foods) are the worst, driving up cholesterol levels and contributing to atherosclerosis and heart attacks.

Yes, media reports of nutritional research do confuse us with seemingly contradictory evidence. Some studies implicate a high-fat diet in breast cancer, while others do not. Some studies say that saturated fats are the worst, while others implicate the polyunsaturated fats found in vegetable oils. But no body of research has called into question one incontrovertible fact: *We must cut down on our overall fat intake*, regardless of whether the sources are animal fats or vegetable oils. The average American woman gets 36 to 42 percent of her calories from fat, and that is far too much. Even if high fat turns out not to be a major factor in breast cancer, isn't it enough that excess fat makes us susceptible to colon cancer, obesity, diabetes, hypertension, high cholesterol, and heart attacks?

Perhaps we surrender to confusion because it's easier to throw in the towel than to change addictive eating patterns. "Every day I hear a different recommendation," goes the refrain I hear repeatedly. "These scientists can't make up their minds. I'm just going to eat whatever I want." Many of us use these conflicting reports as a rationale for rebellion against constraints we simply can't stand, especially when our comfort foods are being attacked. On the other hand, some prescriptions for fat-cutting are so rigid that we rightly rebel against them. The perfectionism rampant in our culture is foisted most cruelly upon women in the realm of diet: one false move and we feel like failures whose punishment is either disease or a lifetime of self-loathing about our bodies.

The solution to this bind is not complicated. We can and should cut back on fat, no question about it. But we must also avoid extremism and self-punishment in the name of health. Not only do we suffer emotionally under that kind of regimen—which itself is a health risk—but we usually fail anyway, abandoning our efforts until self-hatred prods us back onto the merry-go-round. The answer is a simple method for fat-cutting and healthy eating that sets aside obsessiveness and dietary terrorism. (When we feel we have to watch every morsel—as though a single cookie or one slice of roast beef could destroy our self-image or clog our coronary arteries—we live in an intolerable state of fear about food.)

The simple overall guideline I recommend I learned from two nutritionists who presented this plan at a lecture I attended in 1986. Their approach, called the 80/20 plan, made so much sense that I've been teaching it to my patients ever since. If 80 percent of what you eat is healthy, low-fat, nutritious food, then you can allow yourself to indulge in modest portions of foods you enjoy for the other 20 percent. Some of these foods will contain more fat than is desirable, but in the context of an 80/20 plan, your overall percentage of fat calories will drop and remain relatively low.

The American Heart Association, the American Cancer Society, and the government's National Heart, Lung, and Blood Institute all recommend that we reduce the percentage of calories from fat to 30 percent or less. However, there is some evidence that we significantly reduce our risk of heart disease and certain cancers by cutting our fat intake even more, to 25 percent, 20 percent, or even less. Some of my patients can go the extra mile to 25 or 20 percent of total calories from fat, and women who choose vegetarianism may go even lower. But many women have trouble cutting it that drastically in a short period of time, and I am concerned that they will abandon all efforts to reduce fat because the goal—and the means to that goal—is not feasible.

The problem is compounded by the difficulty in keeping track of the percentage of our calories that come from fat. You must have a fat counter, a willingness to check fat grams on every package or jar of food you consume, and the time and commitment to add the figures and determine what your overall percentage of fat is each day. I applaud women who can follow through on this, but I don't know many who can keep up this practice for very long.

The 80/20 plan is not as precise in its fat-cutting potential, but I have found that women who stick to these parameters invariably cut down significantly on fat. The key here is that women *can* adhere to this plan more easily than they can adhere to one requiring too many calculations.

What are the healthy foods that should constitute 80 percent of our diets?

- Skinless chicken, fish, lean meats, legumes, and soy products as sources of protein
- Complex carbohydrates, including fresh fruits, vegetables, and grains
- Starchy complex carbohydrates, including breads, cereals, potatoes, and pasta
- Nonfat or low-fat dairy foods, including milk, cheese, and yogurt

The 20 percent of foods that don't fit this category may include sources of fat, including oils, margarine, and butter; whole dairy products; red meats; and baked goods and snack foods. I don't advocate that you use the 20 percent to indulge in every super-high-fat food. If you do, you'll probably gain weight and undermine your efforts to eat more healthfully. Rather, use the 20 percent as a form of leeway—it's okay, for example, to have an occasional hamburger or steak, some butter on a potato, olive oil and garlic on your pasta, and modest desserts.

The 20 percent gives you flexibility and it keeps you out of food prison, a place none of us care to be. I tell my patients that if they've just had a low-fat lunch of skinless grilled chicken over greens with a glass of seltzer, a bowl of sherbet with fruit is certainly fine on occasion. On the 80/20 plan, you will never feel that an occasional cookie is a punishable sin. And the 80 percent is an attainable goal for the introduction of more healthy foods into your diet.

Other straightforward goals are part of the 80/20 plan—goals based on the reduction of recognized risk factors for disease and the maintenance of optimal health. In addition to an overall reduction in fat intake, these goals include:

- A reasonable balance among protein sources, complex carbohydrates, starchy carbohydrates, and dairy
- Use of olive and canola oils for cooking, salad dressings, spreads, dips, and so on, whenever possible
- A low to moderate intake of refined sugars (in most desserts, muffins, pastries, certain breakfast cereals, ice creams, and the like)
- Salt and sodium in moderation
- Caffeine (in coffee, teas, sodas, and chocolate) in moderation
- Alcohol in moderation

These goals are widely recognized as essential for a healthy diet, but several offer specific health advantages for women.

A high intake of refined sugars—mainly found in sweets and snacks—is a problem primarily because it contributes to obesity, which is itself a risk factor for women. (Sugary foods also tend to be loaded with fat.) Studies have linked obesity with hypertension, diabetes, and heart disease. One long-term study led by the American Cancer Society indicated a link between obesity and higher mortality rates from breast, endometrial, and cervical cancers. Sugar does not appear to directly cause these diseases. But a high sugar intake can lead to significant weight gain, which *can* contribute to disease. And sugar does play a role in diabetes or hypoglycemia; women with these conditions know they must watch their intake.

Though starchy carbohydrates like bread, pasta, and white rice are low in fat, many nutritional experts now believe that excessive amounts of these foods can cause some people to overproduce insulin, the hormone produced by the body to process simple sugars and starches. The more insulin your body produces, the more likely it is that you will convert calories into body fat. Not everyone is subject to this problem, but for those who are, too much starch and sugar contribute to insulin resistance, high levels of blood lipids, excess weight, and an inability to lose weight. A sensible course for many women is to moderate the intake of starches while eating more grains and fresh fruits and vegetables.

We absolutely need some fats in our diet, especially the "essential fatty acids" such as linoleic acid. Several recent studies suggest that a diet too low in linoleic acid can create conditions for hardening of the arteries. The answer? Make certain to eat green leafy vegetables, some seeds and nuts, fish, soybeans, and canola oil—all of which are high in essential fatty acids.

A reduction in salt and sodium is particularly important for women at or beyond menopause, that time when their risk of heart disease increases exponentially. Certainly women with family histories of hypertension should consult their physicians about restricting salt and sodium intake.

Excessive alcohol intake compromises almost every one of our biological systems, causing gastrointestinal disorders, liver disease, and brain and heart problems. Among women, alcoholism can cause menstrual irregularities, early miscarriage, and complications of pregnancy. The infants of women who drink during pregnancy may develop birth defects, known as fetal alcohol syndrome. A high intake of alcoholic beverages increases the risk of hypertension, and recent research suggests that we increase our risk of breast cancer as we increase our intake of alcohol beyond one or two glasses per day. (More on the alcohol–breast cancer link in chapter 15.) It is true that light to moderate drinking may benefit cardiovascular health, but excessive drinking is unquestionably bad for our hearts.

Women should not overdo caffeine for a variety of reasons. More than a few cups per day can increase anxiety. Women with mitral valve prolapse, a benign heart condition, may be susceptible to non-life-threatening but nevertheless disturbing heart arrhythmias, which can sometimes be exacerbated by excess caffeine. (If you have this problem, try cutting or eliminating caffeine slowly, and see if it helps. The best way to reduce caffeine without withdrawal symptoms is to cut back by half a cup a week.) Also, a high intake of caffeine can impair the quality of bone, so menopausal women concerned about osteoporosis should consider moderating their intake.

Much has been written about the supposed link between caffeine and breast pain and cystic breasts (so-called fibrocystic disease). In her wonderful book *Dr. Susan Love's Breast Book*, Dr. Love reveals that the data on this link do not stand up to scientific scrutiny. But she acknowledges that some women do report benefits from reducing their intake. Though every woman responds differently, cutting down on or giving up coffee, tea, and chocolate is worth a trial run if you are really bothered by these symptoms.

Overall, the 80/20 guidelines, including the above-listed goals for disease prevention and good health, provide clear parameters but lots of breathing room. Notice that I do not advocate *elimination* of saturated fats, sugar, salt, caffeine, and alcohol. If you are genuinely motivated to do so in the name of health or commitment to a particular lifestyle or spiritual tradition, I support your efforts. (One caveat: We do need *some* fats in our diet. Consuming less than 10 percent fat can be bad for our health.) But I don't believe that all women should be subjected to the mentality that even small amounts of these food substances must be avoided as if they were highly toxic poisons. (One clear exception is alcohol intake during pregnancy, which can cause serious birth defects.) In large amounts, such foods can certainly be harmful to our health. But it is also harmful to our health to feel constantly that our inability to live up to impossible standards means that we are weak-willed, shameful, or worse.

Eating Transitions:
Victory in Slow Motion

*I*n place of a highly restrictive diet, I offer my patients a road map for slow transformation, a means to the goal of an 80/20 diet. This change in eating habits is eminently doable because it does not require them to enter a fortress of self-denial.

Eating transitions are small changes carried out over time that reinforce our sense of control over food, and allow us to develop a healthy mastery of our eating patterns and our weight. The primary focus of eating transitions is a move from high-fat to moderate-, low-, and nonfat foods. For example, one of my patients, Louise, used whole milk in her coffee and her cereal at breakfast. Eight ounces of whole milk has a hefty 8 grams of fat, and it is largely saturated fat. I asked Louise to consider changing to 2 percent milk, which has 5 grams, for the following week. The week after that, she shifted to 1 percent milk, which has only 2.5 grams of fat. Finally, by the end of the month, she moved to nonfat milk. By the time Louise began drinking nonfat milk, the change did not seem so drastic, as she had accustomed herself to the taste of milk with decreasing amounts of fat. I validated for Louise that this was a meaningful change worth feeling good about, even if she had not suddenly transformed decades of eating patterns. She was able to continue making small changes until eventually she had cut her overall fat intake substantially.

Table 9-1 lists many of the eating transitions I typically recommend. If this lengthy list does not include a particular high-fat food that you like, create your own transition to another food in the same food group. For instance, if you love creamy gelato and have it twice a week, substitute nonfat, refreshing fruit-based gelato. And once or twice a month, indulge your desire for creamy gelato.

For each of the following transitions, take two weeks or as long as one month to make the substitutions before moving on to another eating transition. This "small steps" approach enables you to target one high-fat, high-calorie food at a time, without feeling majorly deprived. Notice that in many instances the transition involves two steps—from a high- to a moderate- to a low-fat choice. If the third step does not seem like one you can sustain, progress only to the second step. (For instance, if you can't stand brown rice, stay with white rice as a transition from Chinese fried rice.)

Remember, the ultimate goal here is not to cut all fat from your diet over the course of months or years. The purpose is to meet the overall goals of the 80/20 plan to the best of your ability. Here are examples of eating transitions you can make. Home in on those foods you eat most and would like to cut back on.

Start with a transition from a high-fat food you eat frequently. Make one transition per month to allow this process to be as doable as possible, and so you don't feel deprived. If a particular food is extremely hard to give up, start with one that is easier. Once you've made a switch over several weeks or as long as a month, you may move on to another transition. Over time, make as many transitions as you can, with the goal of a balanced diet that fits within the 80/20 plan and reduces your fat intake to a level that is right and achievable for you. Do not set goals for more transitions than you can accomplish in a given period of months.

Most importantly, allow yourself to feel good about every single eating transition you make. Don't judge yourself by the standards of the weight-loss industry, which suggests that the only diet worth sticking to is one where you shed poundage in a matter of days. This "eating transitions" approach is based on principles of behavioral medicine, which indicate that we human beings can make small changes incrementally over time *when we get positive feedback from ourselves and others.* Consider this book as the voice of "others" who affirm for you the value of each transition. Now look within for positive feedback from yourself as you cultivate healthier eating patterns.

One other recommendation as you make these transitions: eat mindfully. That is, be mindful of what you eat and how you eat. Make your selections not out of anxiety, but out of awareness. And when you eat, chew slowly, tasting each morsel. Enjoy each taste sensation; don't gobble down more

TABLE 9-1

Eating Transitions

FROM	TO	TO
Meats, Chicken, Fish		
Hamburger	Lean hamburger	Ground turkey
Tacos/chili with ground beef	Tacos/chili with ½ ground turkey, ½ ground beef	Tacos/chili with all ground turkey
Steak with excess marbling	Steak with minimal marbling	Lean roast beef
Hot dogs	Reduced-fat hot dogs	Chicken, turkey, or fat-free hot dogs
Fried chicken with skin on	Grilled chicken with skin on	Grilled chicken without skin
Fried salmon with hollandaise sauce	Fried salmon without hollandaise sauce	Poached salmon with lemon
Fried codfish	Broiled codfish with butter	Broiled codfish with lemon
Fatty meats or chicken every dinner	Lean meats and skinless chicken every dinner	Low-fat fish or meatless protein source two or three times per week
Fats and Oils		
Butter, margarine	Olive oil, canola oil	Jams, jellies on breads or bagels; cooking spray on nonstick pans
Dairy		
Whole milk	2% milk	1% milk, then nonfat milk
Full-fat yogurt	Low-fat yogurt	Nonfat yogurt
Sour cream	Low-fat sour cream	Low-fat or nonfat yogurt
Hard cheeses	Low-fat cheese alternatives	Nonfat or skim cheeses
Whole-milk mozzarella	Part-skim mozzarella	Skim mozzarella
Cream cheese	Low-fat cream cheese	Nonfat cream cheese
Cottage cheese	Low-fat cottage cheese	Nonfat cottage cheese
Cheese spreads	Low-fat cheese spreads	Jams, jellies instead of cheese
Premium ice cream	Low-fat ice cream	Sorbet

FROM	TO	TO
Premium ice cream	Low-fat frozen yogurt	Nonfat frozen yogurt
Premium ice cream	Sherbet	Frozen fruit juice bars

Breads, Cereals, Pastas,
Baked Goods, Nuts

White breads and rolls	Rye breads and rolls	Whole-wheat breads and rolls
Croissants	English muffins	Whole-wheat bagels and rolls
White pastas	Spinach pastas	Whole-wheat pastas
Chinese fried rice	White rice	Brown rice
French fries	Baked potato with butter	Baked potato with nonfat yogurt
High-fat, high-sugar breakfast cereals	Low-fat, moderate-sugar breakfast cereals	Nonfat, low-sugar breakfast cereals with high fiber
High-fat muffins	Low-fat muffins	Bagels or fat-free muffins
Buttery crackers	Wheat Thins	Cracked-wheat crackers
Cakes, cookies	Reduced-fat cakes, cookies	Fresh fruits
Nuts roasted with oil and salt	Raw nuts with no salt	Fewer nuts, more fruits

food until you've swallowed the last bite and given yourself a moment to breathe. Indeed, practice the mindfulness exercise on page 62 in chapter 3, in which you eat a chocolate Kiss slowly and mindfully (you can also eat a raisin or an orange). Let this practice carry over into your daily eating habits.

Eating too quickly and mindlessly is part and parcel of our use of food as a stress-reducer, an attempt to quell anxiety or fill an emotional void. The problem is that food does offer momentary comfort but it can't solve problems that cause anxiety or emotional voids. Mindful eating can break this cycle, as it reminds you that you eat for pleasure and nourishment, not to block unpleasant feelings or thoughts. You may also find that mindful eating awakens new tastes for healthier foods, including vegetables, fruits, and grains.

When you adhere to your eating transitions, you eliminate from your life: (1) the stress of unhealthy eating and weight gain; (2) the stress of dieting itself and the fatigue associated with the yo-yo cycle; and (3) excessive fears of diseases linked to a high-fat, high-calorie diet and obesity. As such, this victory in slow motion is not so much about weight loss as it is about self-nurturance, self-esteem, health promotion, and peace of mind.

Vitamins and Minerals for Women

*F*oods are certainly the best sources of vital nutrients, as nutritionists and nutritional biochemists are the first to say. But as most of us know, we can't always get optimal amounts of certain vitamins and minerals from food alone, either because we simply don't eat enough fresh foods in a given day, because we travel or eat out frequently, or because our processed foods don't contain enough of them. Certain vitamins and minerals are particularly important for prevention and alleviation of conditions that affect women, and supplementation can sometimes be a sensible adjunct to healthy eating.

Vitamin A and Beta Carotene

Vitamin A and its biochemical precursor in the body, beta carotene, which is found in dark green, yellow, and orange fruits and vegetables, are essential for healthy immune systems. Beta carotene (one of the so-called carotenoids) is a powerful antioxidant, which means that it protects our cells from damage caused by free radicals, those unstable molecules that result from normal metabolic processes. Population studies reveal that people with hefty intakes of foods rich in beta carotene and other carotenoids have a lesser incidence of many cancers. That's why many nutritional experts recommend that you increase your intake of these foods, which are now linked to both cancer prevention and heart health. The best food sources of beta carotene and other carotenoids are the dark green leafy vegetables, carrots, red peppers, asparagus, and sweet potatoes.

Population studies have shown that people with an insufficient intake of foods high in vitamin A and beta carotene are at increased risk for a variety of cancers, including cervical cancer. These studies support the recommendation for food sources, but they don't prove whether it is also helpful to take supplements of vitamin A or beta carotene. What do we know about the utility and safety of such supplements?

A few studies—most notably, one from China—suggest that beta carotene pills help to prevent cancer. Yet a recent Finnish study showed that beta carotene supplements did not prevent lung cancer among long-term, heavy smokers. (In fact, the smokers taking beta carotene had a slightly higher incidence of cancer.) This study remains controversial, since its design has been questioned, and a wealth of data supports the value of beta carotene.

Research now under way at Harvard Medical School and elsewhere will offer more definitive data on whether beta carotene pills can prevent various cancers. But this same group has already produced a surprising finding in its follow-up of 22,000 male doctors: those taking a supplement of beta carotene suffered only half the expected number of heart attacks and strokes.

Until we have more information, vitamin A or beta carotene supplements cannot be recommended as surefire cancer preventatives. Food sources remain the most sensible approach. However, if you do choose to supplement, 25,000 IU of beta carotene is considered safe. But be careful with vitamin A supplements. A recent study showed that daily vitamin A supplementation over 10,000 IU can cause birth defects in women who are pregnant. Indeed, vitamin A pills in the weeks and months *before* conception can also be risky to the future fetus. Moreover, a large intake of vitamin A supplements can trigger serious side effects. By contrast, beta carotene is converted by the body into vitamin A only at levels that are required and can be tolerated.

B Vitamins

All of the B vitamins are necessary for our health and vitality. Their roles in the body are manifold, but certain of them are particularly helpful for women's conditions. In general, women with high estrogen levels may require more B vitamins, since the liver needs B vitamins to break down and inactivate estrogen metabolically. Women with PMS may naturally have higher estrogen levels, and menopausal women on HRT are taking pills that increase their estrogen. For these women, B-complex pills, or a multivitamin with B-complex, is an option to consider.

Specifically, a few studies have shown that vitamin B_6 is beneficial for women with PMS, relieving some of the symptoms (see chapter 10). Vitamin B_6 is also crucial to our maintenance of healthy immune systems. But don't take supplements of more than 200 mg, because they can cause side effects.

Folic acid, one of the B vitamins, has emerged as a nutrient of special importance for women. At least one study has shown that folic acid supplementation could slow or reverse precancerous changes in women with cervical dysplasia, a condition that, left untreated, can become cervical cancer. Researchers have found that expectant mothers with a folic acid deficiency have a greater likelihood of having babies with birth defects, including neural tube defects and spina bifida. Many nutritional experts now recommend folic acid supplements before and during pregnancy, at a dosage of 400 mcg. And, since our diets may not provide sufficient folic acid, all women may consider a daily supplement of 400 mcg, which is the U.S. RDA. Recent investigations have offered tantalizing hints of yet another benefit: the prevention of atherosclerosis that can lead to heart attacks.

Good food sources of B vitamins include whole grains, grain cereals, brewer's yeast, beans, peas, meats, fish, poultry, liver, eggs, and milk products.

Vitamin C

This most hotly debated of the vitamins is famous for its supposed capacity to prevent and alleviate the common cold. Although this evidence continues to be a bone of contention, there is no question that vitamin C is a multi-armed nutrient that keeps us healthy on several fronts. It is a powerful antioxidant, immune stimulant, antiviral, and detoxifier. It is essential to collagen synthesis and repair, which is crucial as we age. A high intake of vitamin C from food sources is associated with resistance to various cancers, most especially to cancers of the stomach, esophagus, colon, rectum, bladder, mouth, and larynx.

For women, eating a variety of foods containing antioxidant nutrients, including vitamin C, has been shown to prevent and sometimes to reverse cervical dysplasia. Though it remains theoretical, vitamin C's antiviral properties may be helpful in combating cervical cancer, which can be caused by certain strains of human papilloma virus (HPV).

Fresh fruits and vegetables are the best food sources of vitamin C. At the top of the list are citrus fruits, cantaloupe, strawberries, asparagus, broccoli, dark green leafy vegetables, cabbage, cauliflower, brussels sprouts, red and green peppers, sweet potatoes, and tomatoes. Some nutritional experts suggest vitamin C supplementation of between 500 mg and 1,000 mg per day. Others advocate much higher doses, but the evidence to date is insufficient for me to make such a recommendation. It is true, however, that water-soluble vitamin C appears to have few side effects, though large dosages can cause "bowel toxicity"—namely, diarrhea that goes away if you cut down on your intake.

Vitamin D

The highest incidence of colorectal and breast cancers occurs in geographic areas where people get the least exposure to natural light, which is essential for the formation of vitamin D in the body. It appears that vitamin D, which is necessary for calcium transport and absorption, does help to prevent these cancers, though we don't yet have data to suggest that taking vitamin D pills will, in fact, ward off colon or breast cancers.

Vitamin D's role in calcium transport and absorption means that it also plays a part in preventing osteoporosis. Fortified milk products and cereals are good sources; so are liver and fatty fishes. But if you don't get enough of these foods, and you don't go out in the sun that often (whether due to climate, disinclination, or concerns about sun exposure and skin cancer), it is not a bad idea to supplement with 300–400 IU of vitamin D, but no more, since higher dosages can cause side effects.

Vitamin E

In the 1960s vitamin E was hailed as a virtual cure-all. In the wake of the inevitable disappointment, vitamin E has gradually emerged as a micronutrient with great potential for disease prevention and health maintenance, especially among women.

Two recent studies by investigators at the Harvard School of Public Health and Brigham and Women's Hospital in Boston followed more than 120,000 men and women taking supplements. They found that people with the highest daily intakes (100 or 200 IU) of vitamin E developed heart disease at a rate about 40 percent lower than comparable men and women whose intake of this vitamin was lowest. Since postmenopausal women have increased risks of heart disease, they may want to consider vitamin E supplementation. The Harvard researchers say they're not ready to make broad recommendations, and they caution against megadoses. But they do note that people take 400 IU of vitamin E with no known side effects. At least one reasonably well-designed scientific study shows beneficial effects of vitamin E in the treatment of menstrual cramps, PMS, and fibrocystic condition of the breasts. Some clinicians report improvements when menopausal patients with hot flashes take vitamin E supplements. Though intriguing, these data and clinical reports do not yet add up to strong evidence. That certainly could change over the next several years.

Vitamin E is found in whole grain cereals, wheat germ, dark leafy vegetables, liver, walnuts, almonds, peanuts, and vegetable oils. Vitamin expert Patricia Hausman, M.S., who has reviewed all the safety data on supplements, says that a supplement of 400 IU of vitamin E is "a good, safe dose."

Calcium

Calcium is essential for bone health and the prevention of osteoporosis in women. The sooner you increase your intake of food sources and take supplements, the better your chances of warding off the decrease in bone quality and the accompanying symptoms, including diminished height, curvature of the spine, back pain, and hip and backbone fractures.

We also need calcium for heart health, nerve transmission, and muscle contraction. Given the difficulty in getting adequate amounts of calcium, I recommend both dietary sources and supplements. The foods replete with the most calcium include low- or nonfat dairy foods; dark green leafy vegetables such as collards, broccoli, and kale; soybean products; canned salmon and canned sardines; shrimp; figs; and rhubarb. Many nutritional experts suggest calcium supplements of between 1,000 and 1,500 mg to prevent bone loss. Certain types of calcium supplements are more readily absorbed, especially calcium carbonate or calcium citrate, both of which should be taken with food to avoid stomach upset. Women taking calcium should consider adding magnesium supplements, which also contribute to bone health. (See chapter 13 for more information on magnesium and the prevention of osteoporosis.)

Iron

Younger women often need more iron due to the depletion that occurs when blood is lost during menstruation. These women may or may not require supplementation; depending on the severity of the loss, food sources of iron may be sufficient. Red meats, chicken, fish, liver, spinach and other green leafy vegetables, kidney and pinto beans, and whole grain products are rich in iron. (Foods with high levels of vitamin C may also be needed, since this vitamin facilitates the absorption of iron.) Supplements of 10 to 15 mg may be considered if your iron depletion is substantial, contributing to anemia.

Pregnant women need more iron, and iron-deficiency anemia affects about half of all pregnant women. Food sources are unlikely to be sufficient, so supplementation during pregnancy—especially during the second half of pregnancy—is considered a good idea by many obstetricians and nutritionists.

Postmenopausal women generally need less iron, and it may therefore be best to avoid iron supplements, even in multivitamin and mineral combinations. In general, iron supplements ought to be avoided by women who don't need them. Recent studies suggest that excessive stores of iron may compromise our immune systems, and contribute to coronary artery disease. We are also learning that iron overload is a far more common problem than previously suspected. In sum, use iron supplements only when you have reason to believe that you are anemic or iron-deprived, and then only after you've consulted your doctor.

Selenium

This mineral has been found to play an important role in cancer prevention. While selenium supplements have yet to be proven to prevent breast cancer, Japanese women with a naturally high intake of selenium have a low incidence of breast cancer. When they emigrate to the United States, which has fewer dietary sources of selenium, their breast cancer rate dramatically increases. (Higher fat intake is another reason for this shift.) In various animal studies, rats or mice given selenium supplements developed fewer breast tumors. A 1983 Harvard study analyzed blood samples from healthy human volunteers and followed their medical status for a decade. Those who started out with the highest levels of selenium were half as likely to develop cancers, when compared to those with the lowest blood levels.

Most nutritional experts consider between 100 and 200 mcg of selenium to be a safe supplemental dose. Fish, wheat products, grains, asparagus, mushrooms, and garlic are rich food sources of selenium.

♦ ♦ ♦

You may consider this option to simplify your vitamin-taking regimen. Take one multivitamin and mineral supplement with adequate dosages of vitamins A, C, and E, and the B vitamins. Add only your calcium supplements. Finally, if you are trying to conceive or if you are pregnant, make sure to take your folic acid.

Exercise: Boon to Health, Balm for the Soul

"If exercise could be packaged into a pill, it would be the single most prescribed and beneficial medicine in the nation," said Robert N. Butler, M.D., of Mount Sinai Medical School in New York.

Some of the physical benefits of exercise are fairly well known: it can lower cholesterol, reduce the risk of heart disease, lower blood pressure, curb insomnia, control blood sugar, facilitate digestion, improve strength and flexibility, and, lest we forget, help you to lose weight.

But other benefits relevant to women are less well known. Exercise plays a key role in bone health and the prevention of osteoporosis; women who exercise regularly may be less prone to cancers of the breast, uterus, vagina, ovary, and cervix; and exercise is now considered a bona fide antidepressant.

All of the above are true, and here is some of the supporting evidence:

- Many recent studies have proven that regular exercise can increase bone mass before and after menopause.
- Dr. Rose E. Frisch, Associate Professor of Population Science at the Harvard School of Public Health, analyzed 5,398 women who graduated between 1925 and 1981. Athletes who got consistent exercise were two and a half times less likely to develop cancer of the uterus, ovary, cervix, and vagina than their more sedentary counterparts, and nearly two times less likely to develop breast cancer. This proved true regardless of whether the women used birth control pills, estrogen replacement, smoked, or had family histories of cancer.
- A series of studies led by psychiatrist John Griest, M.D., at the University of Wisconsin has shown that exercise can be as helpful as psychotherapy in the treatment of mild depression. Other investigators have turned up similar results.

The evidence that exercise helps to prevent osteoporosis and female cancers continues to build. But consider the role of exercise as a stress reducer and antidepressant, and it becomes clear that physical activity has a healing influence on multiple levels. Several studies have shown that exercise reduces anxiety; one experiment using fifteen subjects showed that a fifteen-minute workout reduced anxiety to below preexercise levels. Kenneth Cooper, M.D., M.P.H., author of *The Aerobics Program for Total Well-Being*, cites studies to buttress his belief that aerobic exercise mitigates our body's reactions to stress and the fight-or-flight response.

"Better cardiovascular fitness tends to put a 'governor' on the effect that the adrenal gland's secretions can have on the heart," says Cooper. These secretions—the stress hormones, including adrenalin—are released in the bloodstream during situations that arouse anxiety, fear, or anger. They stimulate the heart to beat faster, but exercise can moderate this effect, leading to a lower heart rate during stress.

When we overreact emotionally, our hearts overreact, pumping and working harder. Stress hormones can also cause coronary artery spasm and increased blood clotting, both of which contribute to atherosclerosis and heart disease. By buffering these effects, exercise helps to protect our hearts from the ravages of stress.

We now have evidence that exercise can stimulate the immune system—particularly the "natural killer cells," known as NK cells, which play a critical role in protecting us from viruses, bacteria, and cancer cells. NK cells are like freelance assassins capable of knocking off invading pathogens without help from any other subset of immune cells.

More and more doctors and fitness experts now prescribe exercise to relieve mild to moderate depression, and numerous studies support their recommendation. I have found exercise to be enormously helpful for my depressed female patients, whether or not they have another medical condition. It certainly is not a cure; psychotherapy, and in some cases, medication, is essential. But exercise has indirect psychological and direct physiologic effects that help to alleviate depression. Regular physical activity can improve mood, enhance vigor, heighten self-esteem, and sharpen mental faculties.

The mood-enhancing benefits of aerobic exercise may be due to changes in brain biochemistry. Researchers have uncovered evidence that exercise causes the pituitary gland to release more endorphins, powerful painkillers and mood-enhancers that are chemical cousins of synthetic morphine. Habitual runners in particular seem to benefit from surges of endorphins, which relieve muscle soreness and arouse feelings of euphoria—the so-called runner's high. Indeed, regular joggers report symptoms similar to withdrawal if they stop their routine, symptoms that suggest that they are genuinely addicted to regular rushes of endorphins.

Given the capacity of exercise to relieve stress, anxiety, and depression while enhancing mood and self-esteem, we can now say that exercise is not only good for our muscles, bones, and hearts. It is good for our psychological and even spiritual well-being, which, in turn, carries other widespread, untold benefits to every bodily system.

Exercise: What to Do?

*W*omen are often resistant to the idea of regular exercise. The reasons they give are manifold: too little time, shame about their bodies, a fear of strenuous activity, worry about injury, or a supposed inability to change "at my age." Happily, there are ways to circumvent these obstacles to exercise while retaining its benefits.

Regular exercise does require commitment, but many women are turned off by media images of marathon jogging, nonstop aerobics, heavy weight lifting, intensive physical training, or hours on the StairMaster or Nordic-Track. The good news is that you don't have to do any of these to get the essential biological and psychological benefits of exercise. A few years ago, the Centers for Disease Control and the American College of Sports Medicine announced that recent research showed that moderate exercise a few times throughout the day conferred many of the same benefits as formal exercise carried out for long periods of time. If you walk or run up and down stairs for ten minutes three times a day, you'll get the same physiologic effects as if you had worked out intensively for a half hour.

So don't be browbeaten into believing that moderate exercise does little to promote your health and well-being. Any transition you make out of a sedentary lifestyle is worthwhile. Once you make exercise a regular part of your routine, the evident improvements in your energy levels, mental acuity, and self-esteem will prompt you to continue. The positive results may also motivate you to ratchet up your commitment and activity level by several notches. I must add, however, that you should check with your doctor before embarking on *any* exercise program.

Much has been written about the need for aerobics. Aerobic exercise is any sustained activity that requires oxygen and that elevates your heart rate into what is known as the target zone. Fifteen to twenty minutes of jogging, brisk walking, race walking, swimming, or biking can raise your heart rate into the aerobic arena, and women motivated to improve cardiovascular fitness should therefore consider aerobics. But I have two caveats. Don't dismiss all physical activity just because you do not choose an aerobic program. And, if you wish to do aerobics but you're not in great shape or are unaccustomed to an exercise regimen, you can very gradually work your way up to aerobic levels. For an excellent discussion of aerobic exercise, as well as a calculation to determine the target zone for aerobic activity, I recommend the chapter "Move into Health," by James S. Huddleston, M.S., P.T., in *The Wellness Book*.

Anaerobic exercise, which does not require oxygen, is high-intensity activity of short duration. Any exercise begins with a short burst of anaerobic activity, but when you sustain the activity at certain levels of intensity, it becomes aerobic, which not only confers cardiovascular benefits but also helps to burn fat. Women who wish to lose weight are therefore encouraged to work up to aerobic levels. But anaerobic activity, which burns stored glucose (sugar), builds muscle. Here is a list of aerobic and anaerobic exercises.

Exercise Choices

Aerobic	Anaerobic
Walking	Weight lifting
Jogging	Short-distance
Rowing	sprinting or swimming
Swimming	Calisthenics
Biking	push-ups
Aerobics	sit-ups
Cross-country skiing	pull-ups

Specialists in exercise recommend that you try to get 70 to 80 percent of your exercise from aerobic activity, and the remaining 20 to 30 percent from anaerobics. Recent research suggests that aerobics plus weight training in particular increases the ratio of muscle to fat more effectively than either approach alone.

Furthermore, women at menopause can strengthen their bones and help to prevent osteoporosis with weight-bearing exercises, which include any exercise in which you carry your own weight, such as walking, running, dancing, NordicTrack, and, to an extent, cycling. The purpose is to maintain weight on bones, including your hips, pelvis, and spine. Weight lifting increases bone density. It also contributes to muscular strength, which in turn can prevent some of the falls that result in broken hips and backbones among elderly women. The use of small weights or hand-squeezers strengthens your wrist bones, which are particularly susceptible to fractures.

For women with arthritis or joint pain, for whom walking or running is difficult or impossible, swimming is a wonderful option. Water supports and cushions the muscles and joints, reducing stress and facilitating movement. Water aerobics are superb, classes usually are not expensive, and they are recommended for anyone, with or without disabilities. But swimming and water aerobics do not constitute weight-bearing exercise, and should not be the activity of choice for women who want to prevent osteoporosis.

I encourage aerobics, but I know that many women need to build up slowly to the intensity and duration of activity needed for them to reach their target heart rate. You can start by engaging in moderate activity every day, *even if only for a few minutes*. Arguably the best moderate exercise is walking.

Walking: Springboard to an Active Life

With the exception of women who have severe arthritis, injuries, heart disease, or other disabilities, every woman can walk, and the potential joys of walking cannot be overstated. You don't need to join an expensive health club, and you don't need equipment, a trainer, a competitor, or a partner. If you are one of those women who feels she can hardly find time for leisure, consider this meager commitment: five to ten minutes per day of walking. Walk around your block, or down your street, taking in the sights and sounds and smells. If you are at home with children, take them with you. Remind yourself that even these five to ten minutes hold health benefits.

After doing this every day for a month, walk for fifteen minutes, extending your route a few extra blocks or an additional stretch of country road. Over the course of several months, or longer if that is comfortable, do your best to build up to thirty minutes of walking every day. Eventually, you may even be able to walk forty-five minutes per day, your schedule permitting.

As you continue this walking ritual, try increasing the briskness of your walk until you can really feel your heart beating, a sign of aerobic activity.

To save time and add another dimension to physical activity, you can actually incorporate the relaxation response into your walking or other exercise ritual. Be mindful of your breathing and your environment. Repeat your focus word or phrase as you breathe and walk. If anxious thoughts distract you, gently return your focus to your breath and movement. The rhythmic repetition of walking—or of other exercises, such as jogging, swimming, or biking—lends itself to mindful relaxation and focused breathing.

In order to successfully integrate walking into your daily life, I strongly suggest that you avoid unreachable expectations. Take the "small steps" approach and build from there. Inject as much fun into your routine as possible; if you can, find a walking partner you thoroughly enjoy. I often find that women who walk together will lightly chide each other into sticking to their routine—a positive form of guilt inducement when it comes from a good friend.

I encourage walking because it is so simple that women are far more likely to keep up the routine. You can walk whenever and wherever you want, and the psychological and physical benefits are literally instantaneous. As you increase both the duration and intensity of your walking, the short- and long-term benefits only increase, and you will know it.

◆ ◆ ◆

Give exercise a try. Consider it a mind-body therapy of the highest order, one that may reduce your risks of heart disease and cancer; ease the menopausal transition; bolster your immune system; quicken your energy; alleviate stress and depression; and raise your mood and self-worth. As with the relaxation response, exercise is a coping strategy you can use to enhance control. When the world within or without threatens to send you reeling with helplessness, moving your body is an antidote with immediate positive effects. It also helps to do exercise that you enjoy, for when exercise is about pleasure, self-regulation, and self-esteem, it becomes integrated into your life out of choice. When that happens, motivation becomes a moot issue, commitment is natural, and the wide-ranging benefits to mind and body can hardly be measured.

Part II

· · · · · · ·

WOMEN'S CONDITIONS, WOMEN'S TREATMENTS

NOTE TO THE READER

In Part II each chapter concentrates on a different common women's health condition. The comprehensive approach offered for each condition consists of a custom-tailored combination of the mind-body techniques described in chapters 2 to 9 of Part I. For basic instructions on each of these mind-body methods, please refer back to the appropriate chapters. (In certain instances, page numbers are provided for your convenience.) This approach provides an integrated, fully realized program for each condition.

Ten
• • •

THE STORM BEFORE
THE CALM: PMS

*E*ach month it's the same. About eight days before the onset of your menstrual cycle, anxiety creeps up on you, threatening your sense of ease and balance. Every day until your period starts, you feel alternately agitated and exhausted. Your temper is short and the fights with your mate begin, even though you've been getting along fine for weeks. When you're not anxious or angry, depression nips at your heels—everything is tinged with bleakness. Your stomach is bloated and your breasts are achingly tender. You're seized at a moment's notice by cravings for sweets and salty snacks. If anyone wants to talk to you about your feelings, well, you wish they'd just get lost.

The day your period hits, these dreadful feelings and symptoms disappear like clouds after a cleansing thunderstorm.

If you've experienced similar symptoms, than you know firsthand about premenstrual syndrome, or PMS. This particular cluster of conditions is from a typical case file of a PMS patient. Although the complex of symptoms varies from woman to woman, millions have some verifiable form of this condition. By some estimates, 5 percent of American women have PMS so severe that it literally incapacitates them. And a far larger number have some difficulty with PMS: between one third and one half of adult women under fifty experience psychological and physical discomforts prior to menstruation. In other words, some ten to fourteen million women are troubled by PMS.

Women with PMS are often the butt of jokes, but the condition itself is no joke. Humor can cast a refreshing light on PMS symptoms, but we shouldn't forget that the syndrome is real, and it can seriously impair women's quality of life.

PMS is a vexing condition. It can be difficult to treat, and we still don't know its exact causes. We do know that PMS, which ranges from mild to severe, is a group of signs and symptoms that occur during the late luteal phase of women's menstrual cycles, usually during the week prior to the onset of menses, though it can occur two weeks before a period, and sometimes it continues for a day or two after menstruation. The most common symptoms are psychological: irritability, anxiety, and depression. Also common are physical symptoms such as nausea; diarrhea; headaches; swelling in the joints, breasts, and genitals; skin problems; food cravings; weight gain; and fatigue.

Mainstream medicine offers help to women with PMS, but that help is limited. There is no "magic bullet" for this condition. By themselves, dietary changes and exercise can sometimes be effective. But various medical treatments, including vitamins, certain hormones, and antidepressant drugs, have failed to demonstrate predictably good results. Only recently have scientists shown that the newest class of antidepressants—headed by Prozac— offers some relief to a sizable percentage of PMS sufferers. A 1995 study in the *New England Journal of Medicine* suggests that Prozac reduces symptoms in more than half the women with PMS.

But here is the billion-dollar question: How many women want to take Prozac every day for years or decades to prevent symptoms that occur one week out of the month?

The Hippocratic oath tells doctors, "First do no harm." In other words, we should apply the safest treatments that have a good chance of working before moving on to treatments that are either invasive or risky or carry significant side effects. Prozac is not terribly risky, but it is expensive and it does have potential side effects.

Fortunately, we do have one highly effective approach to PMS that carries no side effects whatsoever: mind-body medicine. Along with myself and Herbert Benson, M.D., my colleague Irene Goodale, Ph.D., who passed away in 1994, proved that eliciting the relaxation response brings about significant reductions in the symptoms of PMS. In our study, published in 1990 in the journal *Obstetrics and Gynecology*, we found that women with severe PMS experienced a 58 percent reduction in their symptoms.

How does relaxation compare to Prozac for PMS? It is difficult to make absolute comparisons, because ours is the only study of relaxation for PMS, and many Prozac studies have been conducted. But the 1995 *New England*

Journal study, using three different measures and two different dosages, showed that the patients experienced, on average, between 39 and 52 percent reductions in symptoms.

Other investigations of Prozac for PMS have turned up varying results: some showed poorer response rates and some showed better response rates than those of the *New England Journal* study. Overall, Prozac undoubtedly helps many women with PMS. Indeed, I support its use for women with severe PMS *for whom other treatments have failed.* But I believe that we should offer women a safe method to reduce their symptoms—one that costs little or nothing and carries no side effects—*before* we offer a costly drug with potential side effects.

How effective can relaxation be? Tracy, a paralegal, married with a young son, came to me because PMS was wrecking her life. She would function and feel well until ten days before the onset of menstruation. Then she would come apart at the seams. Though exhausted, she could not get any sleep. Tension headaches plagued her. She became so bloated that she could not fit into most of her clothes.

But Tracy's worst symptoms were emotional. She became extremely moody and irritable, flying off the handle at her husband and son. She not only lost interest in sex, she barely spoke to her husband. Although Tracy's mood would radically improve the day her period began, the damage had been done: the family tensions did not disappear as magically as Tracy's symptoms. The distance between herself and her husband grew, and their marriage was in trouble.

I met with Tracy, told her about the relaxation response, and taught her several methods: breath focus, body scan, and progressive muscle relaxation. I gave her audiotapes to guide her practice at home. Tracy was so distraught about the effects of PMS on her life that she became absolutely committed to the relaxation response. She undertook this new approach in a methodical, organized fashion.

Tracy's commitment paid off. After eight weeks of regular practice, Tracy's premenstrual symptoms were markedly relieved. She still experienced some mood changes, but she was no longer so irritable and short-tempered. Her breast tenderness and bloating lessened noticeably.

Most importantly, Tracy's relaxation practice broke the vicious cycle of out-of-control behavior with her family. She would make it through those ten days without any major, destructive episodes with her husband or son. As a result, the emotional tenor of her marriage improved. Over time, Tracy and her husband regained their sense of togetherness.

Tracy's story illustrates what relaxation techniques can often accomplish for women with PMS. She also benefited from cognitive restructuring, and some basic instructions in anger management. But relaxation was the primary focus of her mind-body treatment.

In my clinical experience, the most effective nondrug treatment for PMS includes the following combination of elements:

- *Relaxation:* First and foremost, a regular practice of eliciting the relaxation response
- *Stress management:* Other mind-body methods, including cognitive restructuring, anger management, self-nurturance, and social support
- *Nutrition:* A relatively low-fat, low-sugar diet with high intake of complex carbohydrates—fresh fruits, vegetables, and some starches
- *Exercise:* Regular exercise that is not too strenuous or demanding, such as walking

Remember, we already know that relaxation alone, when practiced regularly, results in a significant reduction of PMS symptoms. Combining it with these additional elements, in what mind-body clinicians call a "package," is even more effective. Studies support the helpful role of sound diet and exercise in managing PMS, and the other mind-body methods make simple sense. Women who cannot control their moods or anger can clearly benefit from cognitive restructuring and anger management.

I will return to each of these elements shortly, in what is a comprehensive mind-body treatment for PMS. But first, let's review a few facts about this syndrome, and the research that supports a mind-body approach.

PMS: Facts, Signs, and Symptoms

While much about PMS remains a mystery, some facts are certain. PMS can occur to women anytime from menarche (the onset of menstruation) to menopause. However, most women who go to their doctors for serious premenstrual symptoms are thirty- to forty-year-olds, and the disorder often worsens with increasing age. PMS is more likely to occur in women with a history of depression or anxiety. (As many as 57 percent of women with PMS have a prior history of emotional disorders.) But PMS is not depression or anxiety; it is a distinct syndrome that may overlap certain psychological conditions and can be worsened by these conditions. In other words, women who've had emotional disorders may be at increased risk for PMS, and their PMS may be more severe.

What causes or contributes to PMS? Possible factors include hormonal imbalances, dietary deficiencies, and emotional stress. Although stress may not be the primary cause for most women's PMS, it appears to be a contributor for many. In three separate studies, women who reported more stressful life events also had more of these premenstrual symptoms: negative emotional states, water retention, pain, and interference with day-to-day functioning.

Recently, the American Psychiatric Association distinguished between garden-variety PMS, which consists of relatively mild versions of the syndrome, and something called PDD, "premenstrual dysphoric disorder." Women with PDD are the 5 percent with specific premenstrual symptoms so severe that they interfere with day-to-day functioning. The woman with PDD may not be able to work, sleep, or relate to others as she normally does, creating a ripple effect that harms her overall quality of life.

The following checklists describe symptoms common among women with PMS and PDD, the only difference being that the symptoms of PDD are more severe:

Physical PMS Changes

- breast tenderness
- Bloating, weight gain of several pounds
- abdominal cramping
- change in appetite
- weakness, fatigue, lethargy
- headaches (including migraines)
- change in sleep pattern
- joint and muscle pain

Emotional or Psychological PMS Changes

- anger, irritability (often the most common emotional symptoms)
- anxiety, panic, nervousness
- mood swings, outbursts
- intolerance, impatience
- pessimism
- tearfulness, depression, withdrawal
- poor concentration, forgetfulness

Use these checklists as a guideline to determine the nature and severity of your premenstrual symptoms. Also, keep track of all your symptoms every day for two months. Create a simple chart of the days of the month, leaving room for notes on your psychological and physical discomforts. You will learn exactly when they arise during the luteal phase of your cycle, and which ones are most troublesome. (If you notice psychological symptoms *throughout* your cycle, that's a tip-off that PMS is not the key to your troubles, and you should consult a mental health professional.) This chart will enable you to be more specific in your discussions with health professionals, and in your treatment decisions.

It also makes sense to determine whether you have PDD, the more severe version of PMS. If you do, your treatment plan is especially important, because your ability to fully function and enjoy life may depend on getting relief. But remember, there is good news about this syndrome. If you do have PDD, as determined by the specific guidelines below, your commitment to a mind-body treatment program offers the prospect of real improvement.* And so do medications such as Prozac, when other methods don't work.

The American Psychiatric Association puts out the *Diagnostic and Statistical Manual (DSM-IV),* which allows mental health professionals to diagnose specific disorders accurately. For PDD, the guidelines are clear: if you have five of the following eleven symptoms, and they interfere with your normal functioning, then you have PDD. These symptoms should also arise during the week or two before your period, and stop pretty abruptly when your period comes. Consider which of these feelings or problems interfere with your daily life during that time†:

1. Markedly depressed, hopeless, or self-deprecating
2. Highly anxious, tense, keyed up, or on edge
3. Suddenly sad, tearful, more sensitive to rejection than usual
4. Markedly or consistently angry, irritable, or prone to personal conflict
5. Decreased interest in usual activities such as work, hobbies, friendships, or school
6. Finding it hard to concentrate
7. Lethargic, easily fatigued, weak
8. A significant change in appetite, a tendency to overeat or specific food cravings

---

* Our study of relaxation and PMS showed particular benefits for women with severe PMS, though it should be noted that our criteria for severe PMS were not exactly the same as those now used for PDD. I suspect, however, that there is significant overlap.

† This list is an adaptation from T. C. Semler, *All About Eve: The Complete Guide to Women's Health and Well-Being* (New York: HarperCollins, 1995).

9. Needing to sleep more, or the inability to get to sleep
10. A sense of being overwhelmed or out of control
11. Physical discomfort, such as breast pain, breast swelling, headache, fatigue, bloating, joint or muscle pain

If you are uncertain about whether you have PMS or the more severe PDD, talk to your internist, obstetrician/gynecologist, or mental health professional. If need be, he or she will also help you distinguish your symptoms from other problems such as depressive disorders, anxiety, or panic attacks.

From this point on, I will simply use the term PMS to include both PMS and PDD. Although the distinction is important from a medical viewpoint, the treatment plan I recommend is essentially the same for both. Importantly, if you don't "qualify" for PDD, you may still have troublesome PMS, and you can greatly benefit by the practices I recommend. The main reason for making the PMS/PDD distinction is this: if you think you have the more severe PDD, and nondrug approaches do not offer sufficient improvement, discuss the possibility of medication with your doctor.

Though we don't understand the exact mechanisms of PMS, the trigger may be sex-hormone fluctuations that occur during the luteal phase—the time between ovulation and menstruation. These hormonal fluctuations may, in turn, cause imbalances in various brain chemicals, thus altering our emotional states. Stress appears to play a role in this process. Women have been shown to be more physiologically sensitive to stress during the late luteal phase. They respond to stressful stimuli with greater surges in heart rate, blood pressure, and stress hormone secretion than occur during other times of the month.

Consider this finding: several days before their periods begin, women become more responsive to the negative effects of one particular stress hormone, noradrenalin. Noradrenalin is well known as a hormone associated with certain emotional states, namely, irritability, anxiety, and anger. Add stress to the equation, and women's sensitivity to noradrenalin could trigger those familiar PMS episodes of emotional upset.

Why is this finding so important? Recall the research (cited in chapter 2) of Dr. Herbert Benson and Dr. John Hoffman, which showed that *the relaxation response can reduce people's sensitivity to noradrenalin*. This finding provides one powerful explanation for relaxation's ability to alleviate PMS. The PMS patient who regularly practices relaxation may be reducing her own sensitivity to noradrenalin, which is one biological factor in her irritability, anxiety, and anger. Though this theory remains unproved, the studies I have cited all point in this direction.

Whatever the mechanisms, which titillate us researchers and lead us down new paths, one thing is certain: *Relaxation can help relieve both the physical and psychological symptoms of PMS.*

Relaxation and PMS: The Evidence

*W*omen with PMS don't need studies to tell them that stress plays a part in their condition. But they do need studies to encourage them to do something about stress and its effect on their sensitized physiology and emotional state in the days before menstruation.

For the 1990 study mentioned earlier, my colleagues recruited forty-six women with documented PMS and randomly assigned them to three groups. The first group simply charted their symptoms throughout their menstrual cycle. The second group read leisure materials twice a day. The third group practiced the relaxation response twice a day. In addition to their twice-daily practices, the latter two groups also charted their symptoms.

Why these three groups? As careful researchers, we had to be certain that any benefits discovered in the relaxation group occurred because of the relaxation practice itself. By including the other groups, we could see whether women benefited just by charting symptoms or taking time for *any* activity, such as reading. During the five-month study, all three groups kept careful records of their symptoms and filled out symptom assessment forms.

After completing the study, we discovered that:

- The women who practiced relaxation showed significantly greater improvement in the physical symptoms of PMS than women in the charting or reading groups.
- Women with severe PMS who practiced relaxation experienced significant improvements in emotional symptoms, and became less socially withdrawn. The same marked improvements were *not* seen in the reading or charting groups.
- Women with severe PMS who practiced relaxation showed a 58 percent improvement in all PMS symptoms, compared to a 27 percent improvement in the reading group and a 17 percent improvement in the charting group. (The change in the charting group was no surprise; behavioral research has repeatedly shown that mere observation and awareness of symptoms offers some benefits, probably by enhancing the

sense of control. But the improvement in the relaxation group was significantly greater.)

The 58 percent improvement among women practicing relaxation is as good as or better than the results seen in most studies of Prozac for serious PMS. The fact that the results were so much better than those found in the reading and charting groups demonstrates that the relaxation response has special qualities, above and beyond self-monitoring or taking time out for a leisure activity.

The study adds weight to our theory that relaxation practice may reduce women's sensitivity to norepinephrine, the stress hormone that appears to contribute to emotional and physical symptoms during the premenstrual phase. We also found that relaxation is particularly effective in women with severe symptoms, offering medical options and hope for those who suffer the most with PMS and PDD.

Mind-Body Medicine for PMS

Although eliciting the relaxation response should be the cornerstone of mind-body treatment for PMS, the most powerful approach combines relaxation with other mind-body methods, nutrition, and exercise. Indeed, in 1994 Australian researcher Robert J. Kirkby published the results of his study comparing a mind-body treatment for PMS with movement therapy and a control group. All three groups benefited, but the mind-body program—which emphasized cognitive restructuring and included relaxation and other coping skills—was significantly better. Patients in mind-body treatment experienced an impressive 60 percent reduction in PMS symptoms.

Include these elements in your practice, emphasizing those that speak to your needs and symptoms: a relaxation practice that works best for you; cognitive restructuring to replace negative thought patterns; coping skills for better communication and emotional expression; anger management; and a healing focus on family issues associated with your PMS.

Relaxation Practices for PMS

"Do what works for you" is my motto in suggesting relaxation techniques for women with any medical condition. (Remember the "Chinese buffet" concept? Sample relaxation methods from chapter 3, and stick with those that feel right. Move to another method when your needs and symptoms change.) However, in this chapter and all subsequent chapters, I share my experience regarding which techniques *tend* to work best for a particular condition. Take my recommendations as loose guidelines, not hard-and-fast prescriptions. I probably can't repeat often enough the dictum that every woman is unique.

Interestingly, I've found that women with PMS have success with certain techniques during the "follicular" phase of their cycle (from menstruation to ovulation), and with entirely different techniques during the "luteal" phase. The reasons are not complicated. During the follicular phase, women do not experience PMS symptoms. It is easier for them to do "quiet" relaxation methods, such as meditation or mindfulness. My PMS patients can generally calm their minds enough to benefit from these approaches, which require focus and attention.

However, when these patients are in their late "luteal" phase—and PMS symptoms such as irritability and physical discomfort appear—the situation changes. They often need techniques that provide *them* with a focus, so they don't have to work so hard to overcome their agitated minds—techniques that offer specific instructions to keep the mind focused as the body relaxes. Thus, the agitated mind is kept busy with something other than its own agitation. As the process continues, the relaxing body brings the mind along for the ride.

When your symptoms are at their worst, don't struggle with quiet meditations, unless they happen to do the trick. Use progressive muscle relaxation, which gives you instructions for tensing and relaxing each part of your body. Or use guided imagery, which is particularly helpful for women with PMS-related fatigue. Or do yoga, which gets you out of your head and into your body. When your symptoms abate, use whatever techniques work, including the "quieter" relaxation techniques such as meditation. You may not need to change techniques as the follicular phase gives way to the luteal phase, when symptoms arise. But if you do, know that you are responding to the shifting rhythms of mind and body.

You may wonder, "Why would I need to do relaxation during my follicular phase, when I have no PMS symptoms?" The answer is simple—you won't get the same benefits during your luteal phase, when PMS can hit like a sledgehammer. Our study and my own experience confirms that significant relief from PMS comes when you maintain a commitment to relaxation and other lifestyle changes throughout your cycle.

I can't overemphasize the issue of motivation in mind-body treatment. I've had many patients who lose inspiration as soon as their period hits and their symptoms vanish. Thinking "But I feel fine!" they abandon relaxation and every other approach they've implemented. As a result, they don't get the long-term stress reduction that is essential for alleviation of PMS. Then they think, "I guess this mind-body stuff isn't working." The only options left are suffering or medication with possible side effects. That is why I encourage my patients to stick with mind-body methods throughout the month. Within a few months, they find out whether a committed effort will bear fruit. Most often, it does.

Think of your efforts as having two phases. The first phase occurs when you are suffering with PMS and need relief, so you maintain your relaxation and other practices. The second phase occurs during the rest of the month, when you have no PMS. During this time, you maintain your practices to feel better—more relaxed and confident—in every phase of your life and health. The payoff may include prevention of severe PMS.

Iris was a PMS patient I saw some years ago. A partner in an esteemed Boston law firm, Iris was a high-powered, high-stress woman. Her Type A traits—including impatience and anxiousness—seemed to take a toll on her well-being. She had severe PMS symptoms each month for five days, and the rest of the month she felt "normal." But "normal" for Iris was a speedy treadmill—overworking and overdoing.

In the hopes of slowing Iris down so she could ground herself in her senses and her body, I suggested that she do something—anything—mindfully. Iris chose to take a shower. It was a perfect choice. This was a woman who got up at 6:00 A.M., was in the bathroom at 6:01, in the shower at 6:02, out of the shower at 6:08, and dressed by 6:15. For Iris, the shower was six minutes of necessary hygiene—nothing more, nothing less.

When I next saw her, she was giddy with enthusiasm. "I could not believe how enjoyable the shower has become," she said. "The shampoo smells so great. The warm water against my skin is energizing, reviving. I feel blood moving to the surface of my body. Then, I towel-dry slowly, feeling the cotton towel rubbing across my skin. The whole experience is different now."

Before, when Iris took showers she did not exist in the present. Her mind was racing forward to meet her day, with plans, schedules, strategies. Meanwhile, her body and senses got left behind. Now, Iris had transformed six minutes of frenzied mental activity to fifteen minutes of pure, unadulterated relaxation.

This practice, and other relaxation techniques, helped Iris get a handle on her PMS. Her monthlong change made the days before her period much easier. It also transformed her approach to life. She brought mindfulness into her day, taking time to appreciate sensory experience, to put work and relationships and ordinary pleasures into better balance.

Transforming the PMS Mind-set

Women with PMS clearly feel out of control, and they worry that their behavioral symptoms will wreck their relationships, and perhaps even their careers. Cognitive restructuring can help women change the negative thoughts that worsen PMS-related depression and anger. However, during the most intense symptomatic period, it may be hard to restructure your thoughts. In that case, do your best before and after the onset of PMS to transform your negative mind-set. These efforts will help make you calmer when PMS strikes.

Specifically, remind yourself—as I remind my patients—that you can and will get help to alleviate PMS. Mind-body methods, diet, and exercise stand an excellent chance of offering relief, but if they are insufficient, you can turn to medication. Tell yourself repeatedly, as if a mantra, "PMS will not ruin my life. I will be able to control my symptoms."

Tracy, the paralegal with PMS, constantly thought, "My husband will leave me." When I helped her restructure this thought, I did not say, "Don't worry, your husband will never leave you." That would have been false. Rather, I asked her to consider this replacement: "I can begin to control my PMS. Once I do, I'll be able to revitalize my marriage, and my husband won't *want* to leave me." Tracy embraced this thought, and it became a positive self-fulfilling prophecy. She did control her PMS, and she did revive her marriage.

A common negative thought among PMS patients is "I'm fat, I look terrible." These are women subject to anxiety, intense cravings, and water retention. Add up these factors and you get overeating and rapid weight gain. Most of these women are not extremely obese; they may be only a few pounds overweight.

If you suffer from this mind-set, restructure your negative thinking. Stop mentally punishing yourself for being subject to physiologically based impulses and cravings. Then recognize that you can make the gradual but steady changes in diet that will help you shed the poundage that causes you so much misery. (Refer to chapter 9, "Mindful Eating, Modest Exercise.")

Transforming the PMS mind-set also means investigating and expressing negative emotions. Repressed or denied sadness, fear, and anger may burst forth during those premenstrual days of heightened sensitivity. Some PMS patients are able to wrest something positive from the depression, anxiety, and anger that erupt during this time. They use writing and other personal approaches to explore these emotional states, and make discoveries about themselves they might not otherwise have made.

When the Cycle Gets Vicious: Anger Management

Although emotional expression is helpful for PMS patients, one emotion— anger—can readily get out of control. Those of you who become irritable or explosively angry during the days before your period are all too familiar with the consequences. Marriages, family relations, and friendships may be strained to the hilt. When it's happening, you know you're losing control but you feel helpless to stop what you're doing. Blame becomes the order of the day, as both you and your partner enact a volatile dance of accusation and retaliation. It's a phenomenon that led comedian Richard Lewis to call jokingly upon harried husbands and boyfriends to start a PMS telethon. I'd add one caveat: women are even more anxious for a remedy than the men in their lives.

While there is no "cure" for premenstrual anger, we do have one solid recommendation: anger management. When you follow the guidelines for anger management given in chapter 8, you have a clear sense of when you cross a line from steam blowing to flame throwing. Although premenstrual physiologic changes can make it difficult, *you can still exercise a degree of control.* My PMS patients are comforted by the knowledge that they can prevent their irritation and anger from spiraling to the point of destructiveness. Remember, too, that your relaxation practices will help to douse free-floating anger at its source.

Pay careful attention to Harriet Goldhor Lerner's guidelines for appropriate expression of anger and assertiveness (see pages 175–76). To the best of your ability, avoid vitriolic exchanges and the language of blame. Communicate your desires clearly, using "I want . . ." or "I feel . . ." instead of "You never . . ." and "You always . . ."

You may wonder, "But what do I do with all that boiling rage?" First, find out what aspects of your needs and anger are rational. Take a deep breath or a time-out to make this determination. Communicate real needs and frustrations with as much clarity and as little blame as possible. Then, take your boiling, out-of-control rage into a private space, and write it out on paper. You can also dance it out to music or pound on pillows. Find a private mode of expression that is safe and effective. If need be, share your fury with a counselor or therapist. But make a separation between your rational anger with others and your irrational fury that, in truth, has nothing to do with "them." Work on each level separately, with consciousness and care, and you will defuse the most potentially disruptive symptom of PMS.

Often, PMS is a total family affair. The woman's symptoms affect not only husbands or lovers, but children as well. Her angry or tearful outbursts can have a powerful impact on loved ones, and a spiral of resentment can turn an otherwise healthy family into a dysfunctional family.

That is why PMS treatment centers around the country are beginning to treat the "PMS family." Both the patient and her loved ones benefit greatly from counseling from health professionals, who explain what's going on. The entire family learns that their experiences and feelings are quite typical. As it is common for a woman with PMS to become emotionally distraught, and sometimes to lash out, it is also common—and normal—for her loved ones to feel guilt, worry, confusion, fear, and resentment.

Educational support for "PMS families" can go a long way toward healing this spiral of hurts. Mere knowledge of these dynamics helps women and their families to feel much better. Counselors or therapists also teach many of the methods I have suggested here—anger management and coping skills that enable family members once again to communicate in a language of understanding.

Nutrition and Exercise for PMS

Diet and exercise are key elements that work together with mind-body methods in a total treatment plan for PMS. The degree to which dietary treatments can influence PMS is hotly debated. But dietary change does help many women, and in my experience, it works best in the context of other self-help measures. We must bear in mind that what happens during the late luteal phase affects how we feel the rest of the month, and if PMS cravings cause us to put on poundage, we struggle with that extra weight all the time. We must therefore find ways to manage PMS cravings so that we don't compromise our health or gain more weight than is comfortable for us.

Nutrition
Thankfully, the diet prescription for PMS is directly in line with basic nutritional recommendations for a healthy heart, preventing overweight, immune strength and balance, and psychological well-being. Following are the key points to remember.

EAT MORE COMPLEX CARBOHYDRATES, LESS SUGAR. Research has shown that women with PMS crave carbohydrates for a reason—they stimulate biochemical changes that reduce their emotional distress. Carbohydrates seem to spark a chemical chain reaction that leads to an increase in brain serotonin, a neurotransmitter that helps us maintain emotional stability. Indeed, Prozac and other similar medications are effective against depression because they allow serotonin to do its job in the brain. For the same reason, they can sometimes be effective against PMS. Though they work differently, carbohydrates also influence serotonin in a positive way. In other words, when you crave sweets and starchy snacks, you are unknowingly trying to medicate yourself!

But there is a problem. Eating lots of sweet snacks containing simple carbohydrates—refined sugars—causes rapid rises and falls in blood sugar, which only increases fatigue and irritability. And most sweet snacks—candy bars, ice cream, cakes, and the like—also contain loads of fat. So you gain weight, which can be damaging to both your physical health and your self-esteem. Fatty and sugary foods also contribute to water retention, the source of many uncomfortable PMS symptoms. Moreover, high fat has been linked to the excess estrogen and lowered progesterone that can also contribute to PMS.

Fortunately, there is a fairly simple solution. Complex carbohydrates, including starches such as breads and pastas, and the vast cornucopia of fresh fruits and vegetables, appear to have the same positive effect on brain chemicals and mood states as sweet snacks, without the downside. You don't have to grab chocolate bars to feel better; instead, you can grab lots of veggies and enjoy pasta dinners.

One caveat: recent studies suggest that a high intake of starchy carbohydrates can trigger weight gain. While I recommend that you increase your complex carbohydrates, I would lean toward fresh fruits and vegetables. Enjoy your breads and pastas, but exercise some moderation there.

You may not be able to rid yourself of sugar cravings. Having a cookie when you crave one won't harm you. But it's important to make conscious selections; do your best to replace sugary and fatty snacks with low-fat ones. Revisit the last chapter to remind yourself how to make such choices. Even if you only replace ice cream with sorbet, or potato chips with low-fat pretzels, you will be taking a positive step forward.

MODERATE INTAKE OF MEATS. Some studies also suggest that you lower your overall protein intake, eating less red meat, chicken, and fish than you normally would. In one recent study, women who normally ate less protein experienced higher levels of well-being before and during their periods. Too much protein also tends to increase your fat levels. Based on the current state of research, I would not recommend drastic reductions in protein, but I would suggest that you moderate your intake of red meats, which, in any case, contain much saturated fat. Also, as you begin eating more fresh fruits and vegetables, you'll simply have less room for meats.

DRINK LESS ALCOHOL AND COFFEE. Some women use alcohol in an attempt to relieve emotional symptoms of PMS, but clinicians know that alcohol only makes things worse, emotionally and physically. Excess alcohol lowers blood sugar, and it can trigger anxiety, irritability, dizziness, and headaches. Too much coffee can also worsen anxiety, irritability, tension, and insomnia. If you can't stop, exercise restraint: gradually reduce your coffee intake down to one or two cups a day.

WATCH OUT FOR EXCESS SALT. Too much salt causes water retention, which is why so many women complain of bloating during the premenstrual phase. Water retention also contributes to the breast tenderness that affects so many PMS sufferers. Salty foods and even spicy foods can worsen these symptoms, so watch your intake carefully.

◆ ◆ ◆

A variety of nutrient supplements have been recommended in the treatment of PMS. Overall, the evidence in favor of these supplements is sketchy, but some reports are positive. Use caution as you consider these supplements.

VITAMIN B_6: Many studies have evaluated vitamin B_6 (also known as pyridoxine) in the treatment of PMS, with decidedly mixed results. A few studies have shown clear improvements in mood and other symptoms in women who took between 100 and 500 mg of B_6, whereas women taking a placebo did not experience the same benefits. In the final analysis, B_6 may help some women and not others. If you do try this supplement, be careful about dosages: doses of greater than 200 mg are not recommended due to possible neurologic side effects, such as tingling, dizziness, and headaches.

CALCIUM: Of course, calcium is a must for women to prevent osteoporosis. But it may also help with PMS. In one study, women who got 1,000 mg of calcium carbonate experienced an improvement in mood, water retention, and pain. More studies are obviously needed, but since calcium makes sense in any event, consider calcium supplementation in addition to nonfat or low-fat dairy foods.

VITAMIN E, MAGNESIUM, AND EVENING PRIMROSE OIL: Holistic health practitioners recommend all three of these nutrient supplements as useful in the treatment of PMS. The scientific evidence for all three is thin—few positive studies suggest significant benefits from taking vitamin E, the mineral magnesium, and the essential fatty acids contained in evening primrose. Very modest supplementation probably can't harm you, and it might help. Each nutrient certainly carries other benefits: vitamin E is a powerful antioxidant, magnesium is needed for healthy heart functioning, and essential fatty acids are vital to certain biochemical interactions in the body. But don't expect miraculous improvements in your PMS, and consult your physician or a registered dietitian before taking any nutritional supplements.

Exercise

The evidence that exercise helps reduce PMS is strong. Several studies support the positive effects of moderate to vigorous exercise, particularly of the aerobic variety. Exercise produces sweat, which helps to offset water retention. It promotes blood flow, eliminates toxins in the body, and increases endorphins—brain chemicals that improve mood, reduce depression, and lessen pain. On its own, exercise promotes weight loss and improves psychological state—obvious pluses for women with PMS. Finally, the proof is in the pudding: regular exercise has been shown to alleviate a spectrum of PMS symptoms.

Extremely strenuous exercise is not indicated; it can have some negative effects on your menstrual cycle. Also, many women feel they can't meet the demands of a rigid exercise regimen. I recommend that you start with a program of ten to fifteen minutes of walking each day. Gradually increase your speed and duration over the course of several weeks.

Drug Therapy for PMS

As mentioned, Prozac can be effective for patients with PMS. By some estimates, it helps many (not all) women with PMS obtain about a 50 percent reduction in symptoms. Some patients experience near-complete remission of PMS.

But Prozac and its antidepressant cousins (e.g., Zoloft and Paxil) should, in my view, be methods of last resort. They are expensive, and some people experience significant side effects: loss of sex drive, nervousness, insomnia, headaches, and dizziness among them. It may not make sense for women with mild PMS symptoms to use these drugs throughout the month. And, based on our study, women with *severe* PMS stand a very good chance of benefiting from relaxation techniques. That is why Prozac and its cousins should be therapies of last resort.

However, if you have severe PMS, let the fact of Prozac's availability be a source of comfort. Should all your nondrug efforts fail to stem the tide of your symptoms, you can turn to this medication and your chances of improvement are quite good.

I can't say the same for other medications that have been tried for PMS. Antidepressants other than Prozac have a very poor record of success. For many years, doctors prescribed progesterone products. But clinical trials have shown that progesterone does not yield significant benefits. It also causes side effects, such as irritability, spotting, and erratic menstrual cycles. Some clinicians prescribe so-called natural progesterone products, and they claim good levels of success. But we still don't have scientific studies to back these claims.

Anti-anxiety drugs such as alprazolam can be useful in PMS, but they should be used with caution because of the withdrawal symptoms that can occur after long-term use is finally discontinued. Diuretics reduce water retention, but they, too, carry a downside: possible dehydration, lethargy, and potassium depletion. Drinking lots of water and getting sufficient exercise may allay the need for diuretics.

Be open with your doctor about your concerns about medications for PMS. Make informed choices, and don't feel guilty if you end up choosing Prozac or another form of drug therapy. There's no shame in turning to mainstream approaches; no woman should suffer needlessly. But most of the women I treat and know are sensible in their approach. They'd rather take matters in their own hands, using mind-body medicine, diet, and exercise to achieve results before they turn to medication.

Marta's Story:
On the Road to Recovery

I leave you with the story of one patient who wove together her own mind-body approach for PMS. Her story illustrates the intimate linkage between our emotional life throughout the month and the symptoms we experience during the days before menstruation. Marta was a thirty-two-year-old film editor who joined one of our mind-body groups at the Deaconess Hospital, led by my colleague Cynthia Medich, R.N., Ph.D. The week before her period was invariably a dark time of depression, anxiety, and underground anger. Before Marta joined the group, she'd begun a process of emotional recovery through psychotherapy and participation in a twelve-step group. Early abuse had cast a shadow over her life for as long as she could remember. She was exquisitely sensitive to people's ill treatment or manipulativeness, which created difficulties for her at work. Her vulnerability also made relationships difficult. She had not had a romantic involvement in years. But Marta was working hard to take responsibility for her own healing, to transcend the hurts of the past and discover her strengths in the present.

Marta was often depressed the entire month. She was also dogged by headaches, burning sensations, and severe menstrual cramps. But the worst came during her premenstrual days, when all her emotional and physical symptoms would dramatically worsen. Psychotherapy and her twelve-step program had helped, but these were stubborn conditions. "I needed more tools to help me deal with PMS," she said.

So Marta joined the mind-body group, and she found the tools she needed. She listened to our meditation tapes every day, using body scan to ease her physical tensions. She loved yoga, and began a regular practice five times a week. Mini-relaxations helped Marta when an emotional or physical symptom arose in the midst of her day.

Her relaxation practice worked in tandem with her psychotherapy and twelve-step commitment. Intense emotions—especially a deep sadness—would arise in her therapeutic work, and relaxation helped her to tolerate and accept these feelings. "When I first started, I was in a lot of emotional pain. Emotions came up that were scary. The meditation helped me with that fear."

Marta discovered that her burning sensations were directly linked to early physical abuse. Her depression, anxiety, and sense of vulnerability originated in a family environment where she never felt safe. As she began to heal emotionally, she used relaxation and yoga in a different way—to culti-vate peace of mind. "In recent months, my meditation and yoga is mostly calming and soothing," she said.

She also uses meditation to distract her from PMS symptoms. "I can distance myself from the distress," she said. "It doesn't always go away completely. It depends on what's happening in my life at the time. But I know that for half an hour I can completely distract myself. When I get the relaxation response, something happens physically and mentally—it's like a spiritual connection. I feel this whole physiological change. That's when it helps with PMS."

Marta maintained a marvelous sense of balance in dealing with her PMS symptoms. On some occasions, distraction was what she needed. On other occasions, it helped to simply be mindful of her discomforts. "I realized that sometimes, the best thing I can do with emotional and physical pain is just sit with it." Often, being mindful of her pain, Marta would notice its fluctuations until it began to subside.

She skillfully combined mind-body approaches in her efforts to heal PMS. For instance, Marta used cognitive restructuring to alter her most damaging negative thought: "People are out to get me." Once she recog-nized the early roots of this thought, new light was shed on her current interactions. She recognized that people were *not* out to get her. They were simply out for themselves. This recognition removed the sense of threat from Marta's work relationships. She became more assertive, confronting her boss when he was verbally abusive. On one occasion, she worked up the nerve to confront him after he publicly excoriated her for not finishing a task that she had, in fact, completed.

A few months after completing our mind-body program, Marta met a young man with whom she started a relationship, her first in years. She believes that the strengths she gained through therapy and mind-body medi-cine made this possible. "I realized that this was good for me!" she said. "He treats me well, he's a nice guy. But I know he's not going to solve any problems for me. I'm doing that."

Marta's work had freed her, not to see herself as a victim of abuse but to rise above victimhood, to take responsibility for herself and her growth. She doubts whether her relationship, which continues to be a source of happi-ness, would have gotten off the ground if she'd still been searching for someone "to rescue me."

Marta says that all of her symptoms have improved. The burning sensa-tions and headaches have all but ceased. Her depression and anxiety have eased considerably. Although her PMS symptoms have not completely disappeared, she has a newfound sense of control over them. Moreover, with each passing month, her emotional life and physical well-being keep getting better.

"When I first came to the mind-body clinic, most of my life was a mixture of anger, anxiety, and depression," she said. "There were very few moments I would remain calm. But I could recall those few moments, and I wanted them back. Well, now I've got them back."

Eleven

• • • •

RECLAIMING YOUR LIFE: INFERTILITY

Naomi and Arthur wanted a child so badly that nothing else mattered. Yet their efforts to become parents weren't getting anywhere. On the road to biological parenthood, Naomi and Arthur were stuck in a gridlock so dense they could not move in any direction. Not only weren't they making progress toward procreation, they were stalled in their careers and their sex life. With their hopes slipping and their despair and anger rising, Naomi and Arthur's marriage was on the brink.

The couple's experience mirrors that of so many others dealing with infertility. Naomi was thirty-five when they began trying, and she expected no problems: she had twice before gotten pregnant and had abortions. Arthur's sperm analysis showed no significant problems. One year later, they were confused by their lack of success. Naomi went to a fertility specialist who suggested a laparoscopy to find out whether she had tubal scarring from endometriosis or any pelvic infection. She did have some scarring, and her surgeon successfully removed it all. Her specialist's prognosis was straightforward: "Now you should have no trouble getting pregnant."

When they did have trouble, the couple's bewilderment only grew. For the next year and a half, they did everything they were supposed to do. They kept temperature charts to determine when Naomi was ovulating, and they timed sexual intercourse each month to the best of their ability. This led to a familiar problem among infertile couples: Their sex life lost spontaneity, and not just around the time of ovulation. The baby-making mind-set sapped their passions throughout the month.

Worse still, the monthly waiting and hoping played havoc with their emotions. Naomi and Arthur would do everything right, then nervously anticipate the possibility of pregnancy, only to be gravely disappointed the moment her period hit. This roller-coaster ride of rising expectations and dashed hopes left the couple anxious, depressed, angry, and exhausted.

"This monthly cycle is devastating on a relationship, and it's devastating on yourself," remarked Naomi. "You even start wondering if you're with the right person. You're so out of control that you question everything."

A friend of Naomi's had heard about our Mind-Body Program for Infertility at the Deaconess Hospital, and so had Arthur. Both encouraged her to give it a try. Naomi was considering high-tech hormonal treatments, but it was a choice she personally preferred to put off for as long as possible. Hoping to ease her despair, and to allay further medical treatment, Naomi signed up for our program.

"I told my husband, 'I'm going to forget about everything for twelve weeks—my temperature, when we make love—everything. I'm so stressed out that I can't handle this anymore. For the next three months, I will concentrate on reducing my stress. Then we can discuss what we're going to do.'"

What Naomi found when she started our program surprised and ultimately delighted her. She learned from day one that our program was not designed to increase her odds of pregnancy. Indeed, our program was designed to get her mind *off* pregnancy. The purpose was to get her life back—to take her off the roller coaster of rising expectations and dashed hopes. Naomi was both angry and depressed, and our program would help her manage the anger and relieve the depression. She committed herself to our process, and she began to regain control over her life.

The group support was especially helpful to Naomi. "I had started to think that I was mentally unbalanced," she said. But after spending time in the group, "I finally realized that not only was I normal, but the way my husband was responding was normal, and that we really did need help coping with this."

The couple's sex life finally got back on track. "I had for years been watching when I made love, only doing it when we had to." Then, two months into the program, Naomi and Arthur made an effort to have a romantic dinner together on Valentine's Day, something they hadn't done in ages. They drank champagne, went home, and made love. "I had no idea whether or not I was ovulating," said Naomi. "The thought did not even enter my mind."

Naomi came to our last group session and announced that she was pregnant. She realized in retrospect that she had conceived on Valentine's Day, the only instance of lovemaking near her time of ovulation. Naomi and Arthur's daughter is now four years old. Their marriage has been strengthened, and Naomi continues to use mind-body methods as "a life tool."

Naomi and Arthur's story illustrates, first and foremost, that a comprehensive mind-body program can help women to reclaim their lives from the maelstrom of infertility. We know that infertility causes stress, depression, and anxiety, and we have proved in our research that our program relieves all three. But their story also begs the question, Can mind-body methods help infertile women to give birth?

We do not have a final answer to this most intriguing question. However, that has not been our primary goal, which is the emotional health and well-being of infertile women. Our main focus has been to evaluate whether and how our interventions reduce the distress of women with infertility. But we are also involved in an ongoing evaluation of whether this approach will increase rates of conception.

I have spent nine years developing and researching this mind-body approach to infertility. I am convinced, based on our scientific findings, that mind-body medicine empowers women with infertility to reclaim their lives. Evidence is also building that it can increase the odds of conception. In my view, these developments offer hope to countless couples at a time when rates of infertility are on the rise.

Today, one in six couples—15 percent—are infertile. Approximately ten million Americans are impacted in some direct way by infertility. I've repeatedly heard the comment from women, based on their experiences with numerous friends, that "there must be an epidemic out there." There is no epidemic, but the numbers are increasing. The evident rise in infertility rates appears to have several causes: Medical advances entice more couples to seek treatment, who are then counted among the infertile. Environmental pollutants may affect both men's and women's fertility. Many women of the baby-boom generation have pursued careers with great passion, only to wake to the ticking of their biological clocks in their late thirties and early forties. They've put off childbearing for longer stretches than previous generations, increasing the incidence of age-related infertility. Also, there's the epidemic of sexually transmitted diseases such as chlamydia, which can cause pelvic inflammatory disease (PID) and can lead to tubal scarring, a factor in some cases of infertility. Finally, to the extent that stress may influence infertility, our stressful times could modestly contribute to our high rates of infertility.

With recent breakthroughs in high-tech fertility medicine, infertile couples who once had no hope for biological children now have hope. But 50 percent of the couples who seek medical treatment for infertility still do not conceive. Those who do conceive often endure a long, expensive journey to parenthood. Couples on the high-tech roller coaster need support and coping skills, whether or not they succeed in their efforts.

Mind-body medicine offers that help. When I started the Mind-Body Program for Infertility, there were no other similar programs in the mainstream academic world. Support groups have long been available, many run by RESOLVE, the marvelous nationwide network for infertile couples. But I have not been aware of other programs that teach mind-body methods tailored for women with infertility. Within the past two years, I began training health-care professionals in various cities to offer mind-body infertility programs, and my eventual goal is for women throughout the country to have access to this approach. Already, we have established mind-body programs for infertility in New York, New Jersey, and Texas.

As I've said, given the current state of evidence, I cannot tell patients who enter our program that they are definitely more likely to get pregnant by virtue of their participation. But there is another reason I do not make such claims. They are counterproductive to patients' health and well-being! As with Naomi and Arthur, the emotional damage wrought by infertility comes largely from the cycle of rising expectations and dashed hopes. My patients often say they live in twenty-eight-day cycles, anxiously hanging on test results, ovulation times, the first signs of their periods. If the mind-body program were perceived as just one more desperate effort to conceive, it would only add to my patients' stress.

I knew from the outset that my program would be designed to lead women gently out of the infertility trap. The only sensible approach was to remind them, in every way I knew how, that there was life *beyond* infertility. The mind-body program would not be another little cul-de-sac in the labyrinth of hope and hopelessness. It would be an exit door.

Yes, they would talk about their infertility and their treatments, and the effects on their marriages and their lives. But the expressed purpose would not be another search for a magical solution. The purpose would be to express feelings, achieve understanding, reach resolution, and learn relaxation techniques—all so they could reclaim joy and meaning in their daily lives and relationships. Without the relentless focus on their menstrual cycles, hormone levels, tests, and treatment schedules, these women could once again live in the present, with mind, heart, and senses fully engaged.

Certainly many of my patients harbor hope that their participation will increase their chances of pregnancy. I certainly could not and would not talk any woman out of her hope! But I suggest that women gently put their hopes off to the side, as if in abeyance, while they concentrate on getting their lives back.

Before I describe the Mind-Body Program for Infertility and how you can apply its lessons on your own, I will first share with you the scientific evidence on the links among stress, depression, and infertility, along with our program's record of success.

Stress, Depression, and Infertility

*T*wo questions predominate in the ongoing debate about psychological aspects of infertility: First, does infertility cause stress and depression? Second, do stress and depression cause infertility?

The first question is less controversial and easier to answer. Common sense dictates that infertile women experience stress, and that they often become anxious or depressed. As one of my patients, Delores, said, "I feel that my life has been on hold for eight years." It's sad enough to face the prospect of being unable to have children when you want them. It gets worse when the rest of your life starts to fall by the wayside.

After following several large groups of patients who participated in the Mind-Body Program for Infertility, I found that they were indeed depressed and anxious when first entering the program. By the time they completed the program, their scores on standard tests for depression and anxiety had dropped significantly—proof that the mind-body program was working.

Given these findings, I wanted to explore whether we could intervene to prevent serious depression altogether in women with infertility. So I went to speak with representatives at the National Institute of Mental Health (NIMH), the government agency that funds this type of research. They asked, "To begin with, how do you know that women with infertility are more depressed than other women?" Though the answer seemed obvious to me, the fact remained that no one had proved that this was true. Before I could take my research idea further, I had to show that infertile women were in fact very depressed.

My colleagues and I recruited a group of 338 women who were being treated for infertility, and a control group of 39 healthy women who were going for routine Pap tests. We tested them on several measures of depression, and—no surprise—the infertile women were significantly more depressed than the control group. Specifically, the infertile women were twice as likely to be depressed as the others, and their depression levels peaked after two years of infertility.

Naive scientist that I was at the time, I returned to NIMH with hope and a gleam in my eye. I said, in essence, "Look, these women really are depressed. Now can we investigate whether mind-body treatment can prevent the depression that afflicts women after a few years of infertility?" The head of my study section at NIMH posed yet another question. "Okay, they are depressed. But how do we know they are depressed because of infertility? Perhaps they're just depressed because they have some medical condition."

At the time, I did not know how to answer his question. I went to Harvard Medical School's library in search of studies that might have compared infertility patients to other medical patients. I found nothing. By sheer coincidence, when I returned to my office from this fruitless endeavor, I found several printouts on my desk from a colleague, statistician Patricia Zuttermeister. On a whim, she had decided to compare the psychological test results of our infertility patients with those of other patients in our behavioral medicine programs—women with cancer, heart disease, hypertension, chronic pain, and HIV, the virus that causes AIDS.

What I saw amazed me, and Patricia and I put together a paper that demonstrated our findings. We found that the infertile women had depression scores that were basically indistinguishable from those of women with cancer, heart disease, hypertension, and HIV! The only patients who were significantly more anxious and depressed than the infertile women were those with chronic pain. (See Figure 11-1 for a clear comparison of the distress scores—anxiety, depression, and other negative states of mind—of women with infertility and other serious medical disorders.)

Our conclusion was unequivocal: the psychological toll of infertility can no longer be underestimated. Depression was far more prevalent among infertile women than among fertile women. These infertile women were as depressed as women with cancer, heart disease, or the AIDS virus. Our study was published, and in 1994 I received a five-year grant from the NIMH to study the effectiveness of our mind-body program as a treatment for infertile women.

This clinical trial will reveal whether mind-body treatment reduces stress and depression better than a standard support group or a control group. We will also find out, definitively, whether mind-body medicine increases conception rates. If it does, then we can reasonably assume that stress and depression contribute to infertility.

We already have clues that stress and depression do contribute to infertility. On the female side, emotional upset has been shown to cause tubal spasms, irregular ovulation, and hormonal shifts, all of which can impact fertility. On the male side, stress has been associated with significant drops in sperm counts and quality. (One patient told me that at the start of treatment her husband's sperm count was a fabulous one hundred million. A year and a half into the stress of fertility treatments, his count went down to fourteen million—low enough to cause trouble.)

Why these linkages? As I emphasized in chapter 1, the hypothalamus, that nugget of brain tissue that controls the flow and timing of reproductive hormones, also regulates our emotional responses to stress. Stress can alter the way the hypothalamus orchestrates these hormones, leading to irregularities that interfere with fertility. For instance, stress may affect the levels of

FIGURE 11-1

Comparison of Distress Scores Among Behavioral Medicine Patient Populations

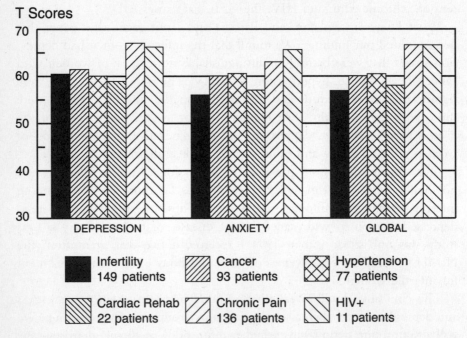

Source: Domar, A. D., P. C. Zuttermeister, and R. Friedman, *Journal of Psychosomatic Obstetrics and Gynecology* 14 (1993): 45–52.

women's estrogen (essential for normal ovulation) and progesterone (necessary for an embryo to implant).

Thus, scientists searching for a mind-body link in infertility have homed in on cases where the apparent cause is hormonal imbalances. One such investigator, Samuel Wasser, Ph.D., a reproductive biologist at the University of Washington in Seattle, gave a battery of psychological tests to a group of thirty-eight infertile women, before medical workups revealed the possible causes of their condition. Afterward, he found a striking pattern. Women whose infertility was caused by hormonal factors had significantly higher psychosocial stress levels than women whose infertility was caused by anatomical factors, such as scarring of fallopian tubes. The women with hormone-related infertility also had fewer social supports to help them cope effectively with stress.

The findings fit Wasser's hypothesis perfectly: Stress would *not* be involved when the problem is anatomical, as with blocked tubes, but stress and emotional factors could play a role when the problem is a hormonal imbalance. The women with hormone-related infertility were more anxious, angry, and frightened. They also had less solid social support, including a best friend they could always rely upon.

And a few small studies have addressed a key question: If stress and emotional upset contribute to infertility, can psychological treatments bring about conception? In one study in the early 1980s, a researcher in Bogota, Colombia, studied fourteen infertile couples. Only seven of these couples received individual training in how to manage stress and anxiety. Within three months, four of the seven who received counseling got pregnant; none of the others did.

In another study, at Yale University, Alan DeCherney, Ph.D., now president of the American Fertility Society, studied nineteen infertile couples. Ten of them met with a therapist to work through emotional issues associated with their infertility, while the others served as a control group. After a year and a half, six of the ten couples achieved pregnancy. Only one of the nine control-group couples was able to conceive.

These studies offer tantalizing hints that psychological treatments can help couples whose infertility is caused or exacerbated by stress and emotional factors. But they were too small to offer rock-solid proof. When I first began working with infertile couples, I hoped to provide more substantial evidence to answer this question: Can psychological treatments reverse infertility?

The Mind-Body Program for Infertility

I began the Mind-Body Program for Infertility under the auspices of Deaconess Hospital's Division of Behavioral Medicine, with the help and support of Herbert Benson, M.D., and infertility specialist Machelle Seibel, M.D. The program included all the elements described in Part I of this book: relaxation techniques, cognitive restructuring, emotional expression, coping and communication skills, and the support of a group of women undergoing the same trials and tribulations. It was a ten-week program, with new lessons and methods taught during each two-and-a-half-hour weekly session. The average group was composed of fifteen women who came together to reclaim their lives.

The only scientific way to reach my goals of finding out whether the mind-body program reduced stress, anxiety, and depression, and whether it could possibly improve conception rates, was to conduct a controlled clinical trial. I had to assign infertile women randomly to a treatment group and a control group, and compare the results over time. I had just begun interviewing infertile women to include in our study when my best-laid plans fell apart. As it happened, the first three were randomly selected to join the control group. The problem was, I could not get them to stop crying long enough to fill out the necessary forms. They knew that others would be enrolled in a stress management program, and they were so desperate for help that they were inconsolable at the thought of being bypassed.

At that time, I felt that I could not deny an opportunity for relief to so many women who felt so miserable and out of control. I put my study plans on hold. Instead, I would recruit women to join the program and follow their psychological improvements from start to finish. I'd observe their conception rates, but without a control group I could not prove whether mind-body medicine improved the odds of pregnancy. But I could show whether mind-body medicine enhanced their psychological well-being.

In our first study, we followed a group of fifty-four women who participated in the program, measuring their mental and emotional states before and after completing it. These patients experienced significant reductions in anxiety, depression, and fatigue, as well as increases in vigor. When they began, many had severely high scores in depression, anger, and anxiety. Afterward, their scores plummeted into the normal range.

These were women who, on average, had endured infertility for well over three years. Within just six months of completing our program, about one third—34 percent—had become pregnant. We were struck by this surprisingly high figure.

Encouraged by these findings, we conducted the same study again with a new group of fifty-two women. Again, the women's levels of depression, anxiety, and anger dropped precipitously. Remarkably, within six months of completing our program, nearly one third (32 percent) had again become pregnant.

Without a control group, we could not say whether the pregnancies were a result of participation in our program. But we had a hunch that our one-third pregnancy rate was very high, a hunch confirmed by a study conducted by Dr. John Collins and Dr. Timothy Rowe from McMaster University and the University of British Columbia. Among a similar group of infertile women who did not participate in a mind-body or relaxation program, 18 percent conceived within a six-month period.

Year in and year out, I am astonished by how many of my patients leave our program and resolve their infertility within a short time span. They either get pregnant, adopt, or choose to get on with their lives without children. Most do end up with children, and my office walls are lined with pictures of both biological and adopted babies. I have no greater professional and personal thrill than getting news of a patient who, after years of struggle, has finally become a mother.

Recently, we tabulated the results for 284 infertile women, the total number of women for whom we have complete data during our first seven years. Here is what we discovered about this large population of participants:

- Women experienced significant decreases in depression, anxiety, hostility, and fatigue. Generally speaking, their levels dropped from high down to normal after our ten-week program.
- Within six months of completing our program, 42 percent of the women had gotten pregnant. A total of 36 percent went on to give birth.
- The women who were the most depressed, anxious, and stressed out upon entering our program were the ones most likely to get pregnant within six months of completing our program.

Note that our psychological findings hold up in a large population of 284 women, and that the overall pregnancy rate—42 percent—is even higher than we found in our two earlier, smaller studies. But the last finding is perhaps the most interesting. Why would women who were the *most* stressed out and depressed at the outset be most likely to get pregnant?

In fact, this finding dovetails with our hypothesis. We know that our program successfully reduces stress and depression. These women were extremely distraught, and once they got our treatment—which made them cope and feel better—a large percentage got pregnant. We can deduce that for these women, stress and depression had contributed to their infertility. Once their emotional state improved, many became fertile. Among the women who were *not* so stressed out and depressed, physical factors could have been the main reasons for their infertility, and mind-body treatment would therefore be less likely to spur conception.

How high was the pregnancy rate among women who entered our program feeling profoundly upset? Using one series of tests, the figure approached one half (between 45 and 49 percent). More recently, we began using a standard measure for depression (the Beck Depression Inventory) that is considered quite sensitive. The last 115 women who joined the mind-body program received this test. Among women with the highest scores in depression—the top one fourth—a whopping 57 percent got pregnant within six months!

What can we learn from these findings? I believe that depression—often in response to chronic stress—can indeed play a part in infertility. For some infertile women, depression may be an initial "triggering" factor. For others, their struggle with infertility may itself cause depression, which then feeds a cycle of increasing emotional upset that further reduces their chances for conception. In both instances, depression may hinder one or several biological factors crucial to fertility, including maturation of the egg, ovulation, and implantation. When we effectively treat women's stress and subsequent depression, we stand a chance of helping them become fertile.

I must add one caveat. While I know that mind-body medicine relieves stress and depression, and I believe that this relief has a positive influence on reproductive health, there are other possible explanations why women who join our program have higher-than-expected pregnancy rates. Women who feel better might have sex more often with their husbands or mates. They may be more aggressive in seeking medical treatment, and indeed, many of my patients do become more active. My current hunch is that these factors have contributed to our results, but that mind-body factors have also contributed. As I have emphasized, our current five-year study will provide more definitive answers.

For now, we do know that mind-body medicine relieves the distress of infertility. For a substantial number of women, this relief correlates with pregnancy. But mind-body medicine is no certain remedy. As with other major medical conditions, infertility is complex—it cannot be reduced to one factor. Mind-body methods will never be cures, but someday they will be recognized as an integral part of treatment for infertility.

We know that many stressed-out women get pregnant. We also know that some calm, well-adjusted women are infertile. There are no simple answers and no easy fixes. But we've begun to understand how the mind and the reproductive system are linked, and we've developed an approach that helps women to enhance their emotional and reproductive health simultaneously.

When I talk about the Mind-Body Program for Infertility, people often ask, "What is your success rate?" They're taken aback when I reply, "Oh, about 98 percent." They say, "You mean that 98 percent of your patients get pregnant?" "No," I respond, "ninety-eight percent of my patients leave the program with major psychological improvements." That is my goal—to help patients reclaim their aliveness, their joy, their capacity to live life to the fullest. I consider motherhood, however it's achieved, to be a wonderful—and not infrequent—side effect.

The Program: From
Relaxation to Reclamation

The women who enter the Mind-Body Program for Infertility are from many walks of life, but they share stunningly similar emotional responses to infertility. All of them are seeing doctors or specialists for their problem, but they vary widely in their place on the continuum of high-tech treatments. Some have had no treatment at all; others have just begun high-tech methods such as IVF (in vitro fertilization); still others have been through numerous cycles of IVF or other assisted reproductive technologies such as GIFT (gamete intrafallopian transfer) and ZIFT (zygote intrafallopian transfer).

I meet privately with every woman who applies to our program. I want to know the women who will comprise our groups, and I want to make sure that they are right for the program. Very few women are not good candidates. I consider myself blessed, because the vast majority of the hundreds of women who have joined our program have been highly motivated and committed. They do their "homework," practice some form of relaxation regularly, participate in exercises, forge bonds with the other women, and show great initiative and spirit.

They are women like Nancy, who joined our Mind–Body Program for Infertility after pursuing pregnancy for a solid ten years. She had tried every imaginable medical treatment, including three unsuccessful IVF cycles. Now, after a decade of emotional zigzags that would have laid anyone to waste, Nancy felt like a shell of her former self. Her marriage was suffering, and her work as a technician in a biotech laboratory no longer satisfied her. After joining our group, she began to reclaim her sense of humor, her hope, and her bearings. At the last group, Nancy informed us that her most recent attempt at IVF—her fourth try—had been successful. Nancy was pregnant!

She and her husband, Cal, were beside themselves with rapture, and the tensions between them melted away. Then, five weeks after finding out she was pregnant—on the verge of happiness and a sense of completion—Nancy's life seemed to unravel. Her mother called to say that her sister, who'd recently fallen ill, had suddenly died. Nancy took a week off to attend the funeral and to spend time with her family. She returned home only to be hit with another shock, this one delivered by mail: a letter from her company telling her she'd been fired due to belt-tightening. A month later, Cal got into an accident on the job that caused him to miss a month's work, and that left him with chronic pain, dampening his energy and his spirits.

How did Nancy, finally pregnant after so many years of struggle, cope with this sudden, overwhelming turn of events? She turned within, calling upon the coping skills she'd just learned. But she also turned without, to the new friendships she had forged in our group.

Even though our ten-week program had ended before Nancy's sister died, most of the group members continued to meet. This particular group of thirteen women had been especially close, and the quality of their support for other was extraordinary. Nancy turned to them with her grief, and her fears about being pregnant while her world was coming apart at the seams. Their care and concern, she felt, helped her to persevere. This disparate group of women, who shared with each other their vulnerabilities, strengths, and the breadth of their experiences, became her touchstone of sanity and coherence in the midst of chaos.

Nancy also came to me for several individual sessions to help her deal with depression. She worried that her emotional state was pathological, and I reassured her that her feelings were normal, given what she had endured—and continued to endure. I supported her decision not to seek another job right away, because she felt that her mind-body health, and that of her child, required that she preserve her emotional and physical energies for the rest of her pregnancy and the months that followed. (It would be a financial strain, but she and Cal decided it was worth it.) My work with her and, most important, the ongoing group meetings helped Nancy maintain her balance. "The coping skills I learned in the group were essential," said Nancy. "But the group's support saw me through."

With that support, and a growing capacity for both grief and transcendence, Nancy was able to appreciate the miracle of her pregnancy after so many years of thwarted hopes. The birth of her son, Jason, was a turning point, a joyous event that also symbolized for Nancy her own potential for renewal after years of stress and suffering.

The bonds among our participants are strengthened as they learn about the mind-body connection and the practical ways it can be applied. Over the course of ten weekly sessions, we cover a great deal of ground. (The regular sessions last two and a half hours, but we also have one half-day and one all-day session, the latter including husbands.) First, I leave a half hour to forty-five minutes before the session starts for the participants to talk among themselves. Initially, they use the time to get acquainted. As the program progresses, they use the time to discuss recent experiences relating to their infertility, or any other issues they wish to explore. It becomes a kind of mini–support group that creates and strengthens connections among the members.

Following this initial time for sharing, I start each session by teaching a different method for eliciting the relaxation response. Then I discuss a particular mind-body method that is to be the theme for the week (eventually covering all those explained in chapters 4 to 8 of this book). I don't talk for too long, because I want the members to break into small groups for an experiential exercise in that method. For instance, I explain the journaling exercise (see chapter 8), and they go off to practice this approach and share their experiences and insights in small groupings.

These exercises give the women a chance to know each other in the positive context of learning and practicing new ways of coping with emotional and medical hardships. They forge connections based on more than just sharing the worst, most painful aspects of infertility. While they have opportunities to express negative feelings openly, the exercises are constructive efforts toward growth and acceptance, efforts carried out collectively with a sense of adventure and camaraderie. This approach differentiates our program from standard support groups, which can be superb but which don't teach practical mind-body methods.

I also give brief educational talks on various topics related to fertility, such as assisted reproductive technologies and adoption procedures. My colleague Margaret Ennis, M.A., comes in to teach yoga, demonstrating gentle postures and positions women can do on their own. We also make time for snacks and informal discussion.

The program I've just described can be followed on an individual basis. Indeed, I often teach the same approaches to individual patients in one-on-one sessions. I will now show how you can apply mind-body methods for the specific purpose of coping with infertility and reclaiming your life. The only missing element is the group connections, which you can cultivate on your own by joining a support group, reaching out to other women with infertility, or at least opening up to empathetic friends or family members.

Relaxation: "Now I Have My Life Back"

*W*omen with infertility take to relaxation like the proverbial ducks to water. Many have felt so out of control for so long that they have forgotten how to breathe, how to take in simple pleasures, how to laugh, how to sit quietly. As they learn to elicit the relaxation response, all of these capacities gradually return.

When you start this practice after years of struggle, you may notice what my patient Vera observed: "I've been so stressed out for so many years that I stopped realizing how stressed out I was." At first, your relaxation practice—sitting quietly and focusing within—may alert you to tensions present in mind and body. Try not to be alarmed. Accept this reality with compassion, recognizing that you've been through a great deal of emotional and often physical turmoil. Know that the more you continue this practice, recognizing and accepting your tensions, the closer you come to melting those tensions. Over time, they do melt.

Do your best to shelve any notion that you are doing relaxation in order to get pregnant. If your focus is on pregnancy, you may unwittingly rob yourself of the opportunity to truly relax. Keep reminding yourself that your purpose is to get your life back, which means finding time to put aside thoughts of infertility treatment, and pregnancy. What relaxation methods work best? Every method can be useful for women with infertility; you can use your own body sense and emotional intuition as guides as you select ways to elicit the relaxation response while coping with the peculiar trials of infertility.

The body scan is especially helpful to ease bodily tensions that build up over years of riding the infertility roller coaster. (The analogy works: think of what your body feels like when you're on an *actual* roller coaster—every muscle is tense.) The pelvic exams, blood tests, and medical procedures alone are invasive and stressful, but the emotional vicissitudes leave their mark on your musculature as well as your mind. If your mind wanders and you need a more concrete exercise, progressive muscle relaxation (PMR) takes the body scan a step further, instructing you to tense and relax muscle groups from head to toe.

Meditation is useful for many infertility patients, though it requires the discipline of regular practice. One of my infertility patients, Yolanda, whom I described earlier, chose the focus phrase "calm perseverance." It's exactly what most infertile women need, as they endure rounds of treatment and cycles of hope and disappointment. Among the most powerful focus phrases for women trapped in the tensions of trying to achieve pregnancy is also one of the simplest: "Let go." In this context, "Let go" does not necessarily mean "give up." It means, "For now, I am going to leave behind all thoughts and feelings about infertility."

Meditation can nourish the calm centeredness that allows women to progress consciously toward a healing resolution, whatever that may mean to the individual. One such patient was Maria, who entered our program after five years of unsuccessful efforts to conceive a biological child. After countless hormone injections, six intrauterine insemination procedures, and four cycles of in vitro fertilization, Maria was running on empty. On the surface, her stance was one of indomitability. She would keep doing high-tech treatments until one succeeded. Just below the surface, she was scared, hurting, and nearly hopeless.

When Maria first entered our group, she only let us see the surface. "I was definitely in denial," she remarked. "I said to people, 'I'm going to beat this thing. I know I'll have twins.' But really there was a lot of anguish and a lot of tears. My husband was worried to death about me."

As Maria grew comfortable with the other group participants, her defenses lowered. She began to acknowledge her despair; she opened up to other women and became receptive to their support. "Suddenly," said Maria, "I was waking up to the reality of what was happening to me."

Meditation helped Maria to wake up. She used a Sanskrit mantra in her daily meditations, which both comforted and centered her. Maria's commitment was strong. "I made absolutely sure to tell my husband to protect my time and space to meditate," she said. "He had to deal with the phone, so I could get some quality time." For Maria, meditation was an exercise in both relaxation and letting go. Her newfound inner calm enabled her to confront her fertility situation without blinking. She and her husband, Gregory, finally sat down and discussed their options with a level of clarity they never had before. After completing our program, Maria and Gregory decided to adopt. Meditation helped her let go of her tensions; it also helped her to let go of her hopes for a biological baby. She knew it was the right decision for her, because it wasn't imposed by any outside person or influence. Rather, it stemmed from an inner awareness achieved in stillness. Maria and Gregory adopted over a year ago, and their daughter is the great joy of their lives.

To cultivate tranquility and spiritual connectedness, some of my infertile patients turn to prayer, using words or phrases that are meaningful based on their religion or belief system. Whatever practice you choose, try to focus on a prayer that helps you to achieve peace of mind.

Mindfulness is extraordinarily helpful to many infertile women who've lost their ability to be in the present, to enjoy the life of the body and senses. One patient, Faith, had been dealing with infertility for three years. She had had four intrauterine inseminations and three GIFT procedures, a laparoscopic procedure in which eggs and sperm are placed directly into the fallopian tubes. After all these difficult medical encounters, not to mention the emotional upset of remaining infertile, Faith used mindfulness to rediscover the present moment.

"I was finally able to be aware of what was around me, rather than always being preoccupied with what was coming up next week or next month, or what happened three months ago that was still impacting me," she said. "Using mindfulness, I could be in the here and now. I began to see things more clearly, and my whole situation began to seem less horrific."

Mindfulness and other aspects of our group helped Faith rediscover the essentials of living. "The group opened up my vision. I could enjoy golf without thinking about infertility, enjoy my husband without thinking about infertility."

Mindfulness also helped Faith continue medical treatment, because the distress of the past and fear of the future did not direct all her actions. She took each medical step one moment at a time, and eventually—a year and a half after completing our program—a so-called natural IVF procedure helped Faith to conceive her first child. Her daughter is now two years old.

Guided imagery can take you on a trip far different from the unnerving roller-coaster ride of infertility. You can use audiotapes as a guide as you take an imaginary walk on a beautiful beach, or a stroll by a mountain stream. (See Appendix B for information on how to order these tapes.) If tapes don't work for you, or if they stop working, create your own self-styled imagery for relaxation and peace of mind.

Selena, a five-year veteran of infertility who'd had surgery and several high-tech procedures, used imagery to relax. She recruited her husband to join with her in creating relaxing images. He'd walk her through memories of a vacation they once took on a tropical island. "He had me waking up in the morning, opening the blinds to an ocean view, the sunlight pouring into our room. I slipped on my bathing suit and strolled down to the sea, passing the cabana and the pool until I reached the beach. I'd feel the sand under my feet as I walked along, my eyes darting from shell to shell, noticing shapes and colors, bending from time to time to grasp one for my growing collection."

Selena then started using these vacation images to relax on her own. She also created imagery about fertility that gave her peace of mind. Selena imagined that she was pregnant. "I visualized the planting of a seed, the pregnancy, the birth, holding the baby, taking care of the baby, the whole scenario," she said. "It made me feel wonderful, because I was continuing to undergo IUIs and other procedures. The imagery gave me a positive attitude, like there was a purpose for doing all this."

Selena did eventually become pregnant after an IUI procedure. Did the relaxation she gained through imagery help her conceive? Did it somehow make her more physiologically "receptive"? Or did it just keep her motivated to continue treatments? We can't know the answer, but we do know that Selena's imagery was profoundly calming and reassuring.

I can't recommend Selena's approach to everyone. Indeed, if you try imagining pregnancy, pay attention to whether this worsens or relieves the cycle of hope and hopelessness. Forgo this method if it makes you more anxious and rely strictly on relaxation techniques that do not focus on fertility. But Selena responded to her own inner call, and her visualization helped her with ongoing medical treatments. When it comes to the creation and use of imagery, listen only to guidance from your own instincts and emotions.

Mini-relaxations are extremely helpful for daily stressors, as well as for stressful medical encounters: pelvic exams, blood tests, IUIs, and every phase of assisted reproductive technologies. Waiting for results of hormone evaluations, hysterosalpingograms, pregnancy tests, and other crucial exams can be excruciating. Use minis to alleviate your inner distress. Take deep abdominal breaths whenever you feel overwhelmed by the medical treatments and emotional fallout of infertility.

Set aside time every day for the relaxation response, using whatever methods work best. Remember that your regular efforts—about twenty minutes once or twice each day—have enduringly positive effects. Over time, you will regain your healthy sense of control. Mind and body will become more flexible, less reactive to stress, and more able to ride the roller coaster without succumbing to anger, despair, or exhaustion.

As Faith once said, referring to the results of regular relaxation: "Now I have my life back."

Cognitive Restructuring: "I Could Have a Baby"

*T*he nasty mind of the infertile woman can be terribly active. Punishing thoughts abound. "I'll never be a mom" and its close cousin "I'll never have a baby" are most common. Here are a few other typical negative tape loops of patients I have treated over the years:

> "I can't do anything right."
> "Infertility is my fault."
> "God is punishing me for _____." (The blank is filled with a variety of supposed "bad" behaviors, including abortions, sexual behavior, and mistreatment of husbands or parents.)
> "I'm infertile because I don't deserve to be a mother."
> "If only I had tried when I was younger."

Use the skills of cognitive restructuring to question and replace these thoughts, each of which can be harmful to your health and well-being. (Refer to chapter 5 for the four questions to catch the nasty mind.) Think of these beliefs as viruses to be vanquished by an imaginary "immune system" of the mind: your restructuring skills can eliminate destructive thoughts just as surely as your white blood cells can eliminate destructive microbes from the body.

Certainly, you may find bits of truth in thoughts such as, "If only I had tried when I was younger." But that thought can take over your consciousness, twisting truth into a punishing tirade against the self. Women who blame themselves for waiting too long are innocent of all charges they level against themselves. Life circumstances, including the commitment of time needed to jump-start a career, tight finances, and the hard work of establishing a healthy relationship, are common reasons for late starts, and none of them are reasons for self-condemnation.

Many of these negative thoughts are outright falsehoods. The blame that infertile women heap on themselves has no rational basis. Laurie, a thirty-eight-year-old woman who felt that infertility was somehow her fault, had one constant negative tape loop: "I can't do anything right." She used the four questions to come to the following realizations: (1) this negative thought contributed to her stress; (2) it came from her mother, who used those very words many times when she was an impressionable, dependent child; (3) the thought was not logical, because she was a successful social worker, admired by her coworkers, and she had a good marriage to a man who also admired her; and (4) the thought was not true, because it was a gross generalization based on her inability to conceive a biological child. Some factor(s) beyond her immediate control caused her infertility, which was therefore not her fault. Laurie had, in fact, been doing everything in her power to achieve pregnancy.

Once Laurie recognized what she'd been doing, she wanted to stop hurting herself. She came up with a perfect restructuring: "I can't do *everything* right." And she stopped lumping infertility in the category "Laurie's failure."

If you believe that infertility is a punishment, whether your sin is birth control, an abortion, or some other religious or interpersonal transgression, you must question these ideas. You can remain true to your spiritual beliefs without flagellating yourself. In addition to cognitive restructuring, reach out to friends and loved ones. If your guilt is rooted in your religious background, talk to a therapist, counselor, or a member of the clergy who you trust. None of us should keep punishing ourselves for decisions or mistakes of the past, especially when our current circumstances are hard enough. I also strongly recommend group support with other infertile women.

The thought I hear most often, "I'll never have a baby," seems pretty logical to women who've tried unsuccessfully to have a child for three, four, five years or longer. But I ask them to make a tougher examination of this thought. Here is a dialogue I've had with women about "I'll never have a baby."

Q: Is this thought contributing to your stress?
A: Absolutely.
Q: Where did you learn this thought?

A: I'm not sure.

Q: Did your doctor say you could not have a biological child?

A: No, he never said that. He thinks I could have one.

Q: Is this a logical thought?

A: I guess not. To my knowledge, I am still biologically able to have a baby.

Q: Is the thought true?

A: I can't say it is absolutely true. It may be true, it may be false. No one can predict the future.

Q: Why are you continuing to pursue medical treatment for infertility?

A: In the hopes that I can have that baby!

Q: Then part of you must believe it is possible, or why would you continue to expend so much time and energy?

A: Part of me does think it is possible.

You can see that this dialogue is not an exercise in Pollyanna thinking. The proper challenge to "I'll never have a baby" is not "Of course you'll have a baby!" Who could believe that? But "I'll never have a baby" is as illogical in its *extremity* as "Of course you'll have a baby." For infertile women who do not have a medically irreversible obstacle to giving birth, the truth lies somewhere in between. The honest restructuring is, "I *could* have a baby," which is often enough to keep women's spirits afloat as they pursue medical and psychological treatments for infertility.

Emotional Self-Care

Ella lived with her husband, Jim, in a country house with one of those long porches, replete with wooden chairs and a rocker. There was also a swinging bench that hung from the porch ceiling by chains and had comfortable seat cushions. In recent years, the couple had been shuttling back and forth to the specialist's office, mired in the month-to-month disappointments of infertility. Saddled with work pressures as well, Ella always felt as though she had no time to breathe or think. Stressed and fatigued, Ella would sometimes glance at the swinging bench as she rushed into or out of the house, momentarily wishing she had time to sit there and daydream.

Ella joined the Mind-Body Program for Infertility, and during the session on self-nurturance, she realized that she'd stopped taking time for herself. That week's assignment was to engage in strictly pleasurable and relaxing activities. As Ella later told me, she did not know what to do. Two days later, she noticed the swinging bench and remembered how often she thought about sitting there, whiling away an hour with her thoughts. For the rest of the week, she did her homework—lolling in that bench by herself every day when she got home from work. It became a time for Ella to collect her thoughts, to settle down from all the anxiety and confusion. Ella noticed that the swinging bench had an almost magical effect on her spirit. Parking herself there became synonymous with letting go, relaxing, finding herself again.

The teachings on self-nurturance are critically important for women dealing with infertility and multiple miscarriages. One of the reasons these women tend to be so depressed and anxious is that they feel unentitled to basic pleasures. Time is short, marriages are strained, medical encounters are tough, and a sense of hopelessness lurks beneath the surface of daily events.

If you see yourself in this description, follow the guidelines in chapter 6, taking at least a half hour each day for activities with no other purpose than to nourish mind, body, and soul. Get a regular massage. Buy flowers for yourself. Select foods that you enjoy. Take yourself out for a meal. Read a trashy novel. Take a luxuriant warm bath. Ask yourself what kind of music is relaxing or soul-satisfying, being sure to listen to a selection or song every day. Substitute quiet reflection or good literature for excessive TV watching. Such activities are not wastes of time. Worrying, squabbling, overworking, overeating, and substitute relaxations like excessive TV *are* wastes of time. Borrow from these blocks of wasted time in order to nurture yourself with genuinely pleasurable activities that strengthen your self-esteem.

Emotional expression is also central to our program. Few infertile women I have met are not, on some level, responding to their situation with anger and sadness. But many are not aware of these feelings, which swim below the surface of consciousness. Why do women with infertility repress these emotions? Because they are painful and feared as potentially disruptive, and because the ultimate outcome of the fertility struggle remains a mystery. There is an aspect of the mind that says, "Wait. Maybe you'll get pregnant, and you won't have to feel so angry and sad." Although anger and sadness can be suspended, they can't be banished from the mind.

In truth, women can feel and function better by acknowledging and sharing difficult emotions, even if the outcome of their effort to give birth is unknown. Certainly, a day may come when a biological or adopted child will wash away the bitter disappointments. But until that time comes, many women suffer by bottling up their distress. Here's the paradox: women with a constructive outlet for anger and grief tend to be more hopeful and energetic. Because they can confront the unhappy possibilities, they are less frightened by the prospect of an unsuccessful attempt in any given month. Releasing anger and sadness can smooth out the roller coaster, so the dips and sways are less drastic. Women who work through difficult feelings are better able to maintain a genuine positive attitude.

Faith, the patient who used mindfulness to regain her footing in everyday life, also found a way to accept the sadness below the surface. "You can't negate the hopelessness or depression that comes up once in a while," said Faith. "That does not mean you're clinically depressed. You can have these emotions when you know that you're not going to feel that way forever. You can call a friend who understands. You talk it out with her, and you come out of it feeling better."

After completing our program, Faith continued to move forward with medical treatments. With her new coping skills, including emotional aware-ness, she could handle whatever challenges arose, which included high-tech surgical procedures. Faith also became a peer counselor who joined our groups and spent time with new infertility patients, offering her experience, wisdom, and support. Helping others buoyed her own spirits, and now, two and a half years later, Faith has six-month-old Marissa to nurture.

Women with infertility are often angry at their bodies for supposedly betraying them. They're angry at husbands for being unable to understand. They're angry at doctors for putting them through so much, all for naught, and at medical personnel who don't always show compassion. Expressing and managing anger in a constructive way is essential for these women.

If you need to work with anger, start by writing in a journal. Spill out your fury toward doctors, insensitive family members, your husband, friends with kids, friends who are pregnant, your body, yourself. Let it rip, but don't stop after one session. If you do, you may feel worse. Focus on the most upsetting events regarding your infertility, and take several days to peel away the emotional layers of anger and hurt. You may start by writing about early events you've never come to terms with. (One patient wrote about her first failed IVF cycle two years earlier.) Continue by writing about ongoing events, the month-to-month cycle of hope and hopelessness. Over time, you'll be better able to cope because you have integrated a part of yourself that may be wounded but is also fierce and powerful.

Writing helped one of my infertility patients, Maryann, to uncover a hidden source of emotional trouble. She had tried to get pregnant for three years, with many failed medical treatments along the way. When she first joined our mind-body group, Maryann was downright depressed. The thought of never having a biological child was unbearable, and she would not even consider adoption.

During the group session in which I teach the writing exercise, Maryann had an emotional catharsis. She wrote about her infertility, and in one sitting she recognized why the entire experience had been so painful. At the age of twenty, Maryann, who came from a religious family, had had an abortion. Immediately after the abortion, she felt both searing guilt and profound loss. But she shelved these feelings, and they gripped her unconscious for over a decade. She wanted a biological child for the same obvious reasons that so many couples want a biological child. But unconsciously, she also wanted to overcome the guilt and grief associated with her abortion. In her mind, having a biological child would somehow vanquish the old pain.

As Maryann wrote, she explored these emotions and issues without flinching. She wept over the child never born, and she recognized how her guilt and grief caused so much of her suffering over infertility. As Maryann continued to write, she developed an entirely fresh perspective on her struggle. She finally let herself off the hook, realizing that she was young and in trouble when she had her abortion. And she was no longer trying to escape a lingering, unacknowledged sense of loss. Soon thereafter, Maryann and her husband decided to adopt a child. Ever since, she has been unambivalently joyous about her decision.

Use journaling to write out all your feelings, not just guilt or anger. Let your notebook be a repository for anxiety, grief, exhaustion, disgust, despair, hope, humor, and self-discovery. This process can also help you make sound decisions: which treatments to pursue and which to avoid; when to move forward and when to rest; when to give up on medicine and when to adopt; whether to adopt or whether to find peace and happiness without children. Decision making is an affair of the head and the heart. Be sure to engage both as you search for the right turns toward parenthood and personal growth.

Healing the Strain on Couples

The effects of infertility on couples is often striking, and strikingly common. When women get together in our groups, they are both amazed and relieved when they hear stories of marital difficulties so similar to their own. The relief comes when they realize they are not odd ducks with peculiar weaknesses in their relationships, weaknesses that speak poorly of them and their partners.

It is hard for men to understand what women go through with infertility—the medical workups, the side effects of powerful hormones, the sense of embarrassment and failure. It is also hard for women to understand what their male partners go through—the helplessness to bring about conception, the insecurities when they contribute to the biological problem, the power-lessness to make it all better for their wives. It is hard for both members to grapple with the effects of infertility on their sex lives, their social lives, their ability to enjoy simple pleasures together.

It's even harder to bridge communication gaps when men and women speak a different language, as Deborah Tannen has pointed out. The solu-tion for infertile couples is not to try to change the other person's commu-nication style. The solution is to sit down and translate your partner's language into one you can fully understand. (See chapter 7 for detailed guidance on couples' communication.)

Most often, if you listen to your husband or male partner, you will hear themes of helplessness, confusion, or shame. (The latter is more common when there is a male factor involved in infertility.) If you recognize how he is feeling—even when you think he's not doing a good job expressing himself—let him know that you get it. A more fruitful dialogue will begin.

A typical trap among women is to wish silently that he would meet your needs regarding infertility, offering more practical help, empathy, and emo-tional openness. It's another example of the mental pitfall that we should be able to read each other's minds. It is your responsibility to state your needs clearly, as requests rather than demands, and to assert yourself when he is distant or unresponsive.

In our program, we get husbands involved by inviting them to three sessions, the first, seventh, and ninth ones, the ninth being an all-day affair on a Sunday. When I designed the program, I decided that it had to meet women's needs first, bringing women together with other women to heal the wounds of infertility and reclaim their lives. I therefore believed that it should not be a mind-body program for couples, because women are gener-ally more affected by infertility than men (which is not to minimize men's suffering one iota).

On the other hand, I also knew it would be wrong to exclude male partners, given the profound effect of infertility on couples. The changes I encouraged women to make in their daily lives are far tougher when their partners have no knowledge of or exposure to mind-body medicine. These partners may be alienated when their wives go off for twenty minutes to relax, or threatened when their wives assert their needs and start to take better care of themselves.

When men come to our groups, they're exposed to our methods and they learn firsthand what to expect. We briefly teach them to elicit the relaxation response, and they experience the positive benefits for themselves and their wives. They discover that our purpose is not to create an all-female enclave of complaint. On the contrary, they see that their wives are working to strengthen themselves *and* their marriages. Once these goals are clarified, the men can become even more supportive of their wives' participation. Sometimes they practice relaxation or minis or cognitive restructuring along with their wives. Instead of joining together for one more nail-biting attempt to get pregnant, they finally join together to recover from months and years of tension, to revive the relaxed sense of fun that got lost in the fertility shuffle.

During the seventh session, the men spend time with a male psychologist, to air feelings and get support from other men who understand their side of the infertility experience. The all-day Sunday session has a marvelous effect. First we do an hour and a half of gentle yoga stretching. Then we watch a hilarious tape of Lorretta Laroche's routine on using humor to reduce stress in daily life. The couples then take a mindful walk along the river that runs behind our hospital. They walk together wordlessly, feeding the ducks mindfully. Doing something so simple together, with full awareness in the moment, is like returning to the ABCs of relatedness.

In an exercise I learned from Steven Maurer, M.A., I have each couple go into a room together, where each partner takes turns speaking while the other listens. As mentioned in chapter 7, they speak about three subjects. First, something you like about your spouse you have never told him/her. Second, something you like about yourself that you've never told him/her. Third, something you like about your relationship you've never told him/her. The couples return to the group with a rosy glow about them. After years of focusing on struggle and failure, often with a buildup of resentment, this exercise reminds partners what they love and admire about each other and themselves.

"My husband, Sam, is kind of resistant to groups," said Gail, a recent member of our program. "He is a computer analyst and I am a social worker. I like groups, I believe in them, and I believe in therapy. His attitude is more, 'No, I don't want to get on the floor and do yoga. And I don't like groups!' But he came, and he took to the yoga. He even liked meeting with the other guys. He got into the whole day, and it turned out to be a beautiful one for both of us."

Gail and Sam walked and fed the ducks by the river without a word spoken, yet a new understanding grew between them. When one of them did speak, during the communication exercise, the other did not say a word.

"That helped us not only to say, 'I love you,' but to explain why we still admire each other," she said. "It brought back a real closeness."

Such communication exercises are especially helpful for healing rifts that can evolve over years of struggle with infertility. In my experience, it is rare for women and their male partners to share an exact perspective about where they are heading; one member of the couple may wish to move to the next level of high-tech treatments, while the other may wish to continue at the current level, or abandon the effort for a biological child altogether. One may embrace adoption while the other does not. Only a concerted effort to understand each other can preserve the couple's closeness.

You don't need our program to practice these exercises. To take a mindful walk with your partner, all you need is your legs and your partner. To sit and say what you like about yourself and your mate, you only need yourself, your mate, and a willingness to be open. While the structure and support of our program help, you can provide your own structure and procure your own support.

If your marriage is strained by infertility, I recommend that you take these steps:

- Take care of your own well-being with mind-body medicine, including relaxation techniques.
- Share your efforts toward self-care with your partner, but avoid accusations and defensiveness.
- Encourage your partner to join with you in self-care (e.g., relaxation, cognitive restructuring, self-nurturance), but only if he seems interested.
- Practice healthy communication skills, including the exercises above, and resuscitate the positive in your relationship (see chapter 7).
- Get support from other women with infertility, as well as family members and friends. Consider a support group such as those sponsored by RESOLVE.
- If infertility is causing severe anxiety or depression, seek professional psychological help.
- If infertility causes ongoing, severe problems in your marriage or relationship, consider joint therapy with a trained counselor or psychotherapist who specializes in treating infertile couples. Call RESOLVE for referrals to mental health professionals who regularly work with infertile couples.

One of the issues you can address in couples counseling is the loss of spontaneity in your sex life. But a few commonsense suggestions also help. Try not to be tyrannized by scheduled sex. If need be, take a few months off your schedule to have sex only when you want to. One option for couples who have yet to begin high-tech treatments is unassisted IUIs, which don't involve drugs and are exactly timed to deliver your husband's sperm during ovulation. This eliminates the need for obligatory sex every other day around the time of ovulation.

The focus of all these suggestions is the recovery of normalcy. Infertility can throw off your normal rhythms and behaviors as a couple. Faith summed it up when she said, "We had been married for six years before the hellishness started. We had a lot of fun together, until infertility hit us like a ton of bricks."

The program helped restore their capacity for fun, and it reminded them how it got lost in the first place. "When the program was over, we said to each other, 'If we could get through infertility, we could get through anything.'"

Group Support: "Now I Have
Sixteen New Friends"

*H*ow important is the support of other women in the group? Here's what Rena had to say: "I was looking for support but I couldn't find it. My family didn't have a clue. I remember going home for holidays, and I'd bring articles and newsletters on infertility. I hoped someone would look at them or ask about them, but they never did. It was hard for me to talk about, and hard for them to know what I was going through.

"I felt totally alone until the group," Rena added. "These women opened up a whole new world, one that was so comforting. Now I have sixteen new friends."

There was never any question about whether they understood. Their talks during the pregroup gatherings helped them exorcise feelings of isolation, loneliness, and frustration. Rena's experience exemplifies those of most of our participants.

Humor bonds them together, too. For Rena, the first few meetings included an outpouring of laughter as well as tears. "One time we covered the absurd stuff that goes on with infertile couples," she said. "Like people standing on their heads after intercourse to get the sperm in there. Or husbands who wear ridiculous boxer shorts because someone told them briefs were bad for sperm counts. Sometimes there was break-out laughter. Other times it was just outward grins—or inward ones."

Most groups continue to meet after the ten-week program finishes. They typically convene once every four to six weeks to schmooze, catch up on fertility treatments or adoptions, and offer the ongoing support everyone needs to keep on keeping on.

Rena continues to meet with her group members, and they have especially strong ties with one another. She recently told me that one of her compatriots, Jenna, had a dream that crystallized Rena's own feelings about the group. In reality, Jenna had gotten pregnant a few months after completing our program. But her pregnancy had been rocky, and the night her water broke she was terrified. When she fell asleep that evening, she had a dream in which every single one of the women entered her room and joined together in a circle around her bed. She instantly felt her fear subside, because these women—who knew her so intimately—had surrounded her with warmth and care. Jenna awoke with that feeling, and it helped her through a difficult birth two days later.

As with any groups, some "click" better than others, but the vast majority of women feel warmed and accepted by their fellow members. One of the groups that clicked especially well keeps meeting to this day, three years later. Dubbed the "CBS group" (because they all joined after seeing a report about our program on the *CBS Evening News* with Dan Rather), these thirteen women formed unusual bonds. In terms of motherhood, they also had remarkable successes within a short time span. Today, twelve of the thirteen are mothers: seven with biological children and five with adopted children. With several second births and adoptions, these thirteen women now have seventeen children among them!

The mind-body program appears to spur women toward biological or adoptive birth, since the majority of participants become parents within a year of completing the program. Sometimes the results astonish me, as with a recent group in which twelve of fifteen women (80 percent) had biological babies within two years. But usually there is a roughly equal mix of biological births and adoptions.

Can you get the support you need without a group? Yes, by networking to forge connections with other women struggling with infertility. You can also procure empathic support from friends and family by letting them know what you're going through. Formal groups do offer something unique, however. Support groups are widely available through RESOLVE. (Consult Appendix B, page 404, for RESOLVE's phone number, to locate the group nearest you.) If you join an infertility support group, and commit yourself to the mind-body approaches recommended here, you will be creating your own comprehensive program for infertility!

High-Tech: Hanging Tough, Moving On

*I*n today's world, coping with infertility means more than coping with infertility. It can mean coping with high-tech medicine, which creates its own unique set of stressors.

Since this is not a book about fertility medicine, I refer you to other books for information about the choices available and the complex procedures involved. (Two good ones are *How to Get Pregnant with the New Technology* by S. J. Silber [Warner Books, 1991] and *Getting Pregnant When You Thought You Couldn't* by H. S. Rosenberg and Y. M. Epstein [Warner Books, 1993].) I can tell you that hormonal drugs such as Clomid, Pergonal, and Humegon; intrauterine inseminations with or without drugs; and assisted reproductive technologies such as IVF, GIFT, and ZIFT are all becoming standard approaches of fertility clinics across the land. These methods can involve administration of injected drugs by yourself or your partner, minor surgical procedures, repeated blood tests and ultrasounds, and ongoing visits to clinics or hospitals.

I don't mean to frighten you, because many women cope well with these circumstances, and the best fertility clinics are well designed to keep your stress and discomfort to a relative minimum. If you are fortunate enough to become pregnant within a reasonable time frame, you may not be unduly stressed by your experiences. But when you must continue treatment over several years, the effects can be cumulative, leading you to feel chronically stressed and dispirited.

Use the relaxation response and mini-relaxations to vastly improve your ability to cope with the stress of medical encounters and procedures. Elicit the relaxation response daily to reduce cumulative tensions, and to approach each day with greater calm and balance. You may also elicit the relaxation response at these times:

- In the waiting room of your doctor or fertility clinic.
- Before and after any surgical procedure. Prior to surgery, it will help reduce anxiety; afterward, it will reduce muscle tension and pain.
- During procedures such as intrauterine inseminations and "tubograms," in which dye is injected into your fallopian tubes. Consider the body scan, or any other method that likewise relaxes abdominal

and pelvic muscles. This should make the procedure more comfortable and less anxiety-provoking.

During these procedures, you may not always have the fifteen minutes or so needed to elicit the relaxation response fully. If this is the case, try using mini-relaxations. You may also wish to practice minis:

- Before and during a blood test.
- Before and during injections, whether administered by your doctor, husband, or self.
- Before and during ultrasounds.
- Before and during the insertion of an intravenous needle (IV) prior to surgery.
- Before and during the egg retrieval phase of IVF.
- Before and during the transfer phase of IVF.
- Before and after the laparoscopy for GIFT or ZIFT.
- Before using the toilet on day 28 of your cycle.
- While waiting for the results of a pregnancy test.

Most of my patients feel that minis are among the most important tools they've learned for coping with high-tech fertility medicine.

If you are taking hormonal drugs, discuss all potential side effects with your doctor. They can cause psychological effects such as mood swings. If you're constantly upset with yourself, your partner, or your coworkers, consider the contribution of hormonal medications. Being aware of these side effects will reduce your perception that you are completely out of control. You will also be able to ask loved ones for more understanding, letting them know that you are "under the influence" of fertility drugs.

If stress and depression can influence fertility, can stress and depression influence the success of high-tech methods such as IVF? Two recent studies conclude that the answer is yes. One group of investigators followed 330 IVF patients, one third of whom were undergoing their first IVF cycle, two thirds of whom were "veterans" who'd been through it before. Patients who were depressed before starting IVF had significantly lower rates of success. This was particularly apparent among the veterans: only 13 percent of the depressed patients became pregnant, while 29 percent of the non-depressed patients conceived—more than double the success rate of the others. In a recent Canadian study of forty women undergoing IVF, the twenty-three who did not become pregnant reported significantly more stress during various stages of the IVF process. They also had a poorer biological response to the treatment, such as fewer eggs and embryos.

Such findings lead inevitably to this question: Could mind-body medicine raise the success rate for women undergoing high-tech methods such as IVF? Preliminary data indicate that it does. In a pilot study of IVF patients in our Mind-Body Program for Infertility, we found that 37 percent of them got pregnant during their first IVF or GIFT attempt after going through our program. (Many of them had had multiple failures of IVF and GIFT *before* entering our program.) By comparison, the nationwide success rate for women doing IVF on any given cycle is between 15 and 20 percent. Our current clinical trial will provide more certain answers, but it does seem that mind-body medicine improves outcomes for women undergoing in vitro fertilization.

Yet the reality remains that many women, with or without mind-body medicine, undergo numerous cycles of IVF, GIFT, or ZIFT without success. These women continually confront the question, When do I stop?

If you are one of these women, then you know that head and heart constantly bat this question back and forth like a tennis ball. Your head says stop, your heart says keep going. There is no prescription for when to stop; you must let the tennis match play itself out. But be aware of signs of emotional exhaustion—don't let your heart overrule your head to the point of collapse. Nor should you let your head overrule your heart, leaving you with a sense that you've acted preemptively. Keep open the lines of communication with your partner and your doctor, and they will help you make an informed decision that honors both head and heart.

For many women, the adoption option keeps hope alive. They can go through several cycles of high-tech treatment knowing that a lack of success will not prevent them from becoming mothers. Should they decide to cease treatment, they benefit by acknowledging and sharing their sadness over the loss of a biological child, a passage that enables them to move on.

Indeed, after they have grieved their loss, moving on to adoption becomes a more joyous process. They aren't harboring a disappointment so profound that it prevents them from wholeheartedly embracing adoption and the child they are fortunate to adopt.

Hillary's story illustrates how the adoption decision can be made. At age forty, she and her husband, Max, had been riding the infertility roller coaster for four years. When she entered our program, she felt isolated, confused, and raw. "I'd been living my life in menstrual cycles," she said. "And I needed to get back my sense of perspective."

Hillary's perspective began to return when she connected with fourteen other women "who spoke the same language." A dedicated practice of body scan and yoga helped, too. Exploring the emotional issues associated with infertility was hard but fruitful. "Sometimes I felt so vulnerable," she said, "as if I had been stripped down to my soul."

But Hillary was received in a caring atmosphere, and confronting raw emotions enabled her to move forward with strength and self-awareness. She wrote out her anger toward the medical community, whom she felt had failed her. "They did not do a good job monitoring our case," she said. "They had me do ten IUIs when, given my age, I should have had more aggressive treatment sooner. I was so angry. By writing, I got it all out of my system. I put the resentment behind me."

Before coming to our group, Hillary had started to grieve the loss of her capacity for a biological child. Adoption had always been in the back of her and Max's minds, but Hillary knew that she could not move forward with an open heart until she accepted her loss. Her grieving process resolved itself with the group's loving support.

Toward the end of our program, Hillary and her husband began the paperwork for adoption of a child in China. They also prepared for an IVF cycle a month later. The day they went to the IVF clinic to get their medications, they came home to a phone message: they had a referral for a Chinese baby. Hillary and Max canceled the IVF cycle and went for the adoption. Given Hillary's age and everything they'd been through, their hearts and minds told them it was the right decision at the right time.

Ever since they went to China to adopt their daughter, Lola, the couple has never looked back. "I know this will sound weird," says Hillary. "But I am so glad I did not have a biological child. Because I have the child I was supposed to have. Lola is the person who was supposed to be in our home."

A fair number of my patients who remain unable to conceive decide not to adopt. Frequently, these are women who've gained self-esteem and a capacity to live in the moment. Along with their partners, they feel that they're enjoying life too much to take on parenthood right away, if at all. With their new perspective, they set aside the adoption decision. Others rethink their whole concept of parenthood, while still others were never drawn to adoption for a variety of reasons. Of course, this is a uniquely personal decision for every woman and every couple. But the decision not to have children, I have found, can be made consciously—not as a default or defeat but as an assertion of what feels right for that couple at that time.

Maggie's six-year struggle with infertility was rough, and joining our program initiated an emotional healing process that led her to put off parenthood. Maggie had blamed herself for the couple's problem, based on her tubal scarring. (Surgery to remove the scarring had been a success; the couple's doctors are not sure why she has not been able to conceive.) Her work in our group revealed to Maggie just how much blame she had heaped on herself.

"During the yoga session, I spent the entire time crying," she recalled. "I was crying for myself, because I had been beating up on myself so badly. Then I cried because I was just so tired of having my body manipulated by people."

Self-nurturance was the most important teaching for Maggie. She began to rent "stupid funny movies," she gave herself permission for pleasurable activities, and she protected herself from the pain of other people's insensitivities, including members of her own family.

At a neighborhood meeting of women, a discussion arose among a group of pregnant women in which they talked excitedly of their pregnancies. Maggie was upset, but she was coping so much more effectively that she was not devastated. "I had a bad day," she said. "But that's a lot better than having a bad year."

Maggie was able to grieve the loss of biological parenthood *once she forgave herself for the problem*. The group's compassion helped with that, but so did Maggie's courage in confronting her pain and finding self-forgiveness. "I learned that it was real pain I needed to own," she said. "Then I could move on and forgive myself. But part of forgiveness is realizing that you're not this isolated sufferer. You are one among many."

She adopted a "one day at a time" attitude that brought more pleasure into her life. Maggie gradually accepted that she probably would not be a biological parent, and with the grief came a sense of liberation. "The relaxation and group support helped me to accept the path I was traveling. I learned to be comfortable inside my own skin, whatever was going to happen. I began to see this process as one of spiritual growth." Maggie and her husband, Michael, used meditation and prayer to enhance that growth process. Their mutual work of acceptance and forgiveness brought them closer than they'd been since the beginning of their fertility ordeal.

Maggie and Michael have decided, for the time being, to stop all fertility treatments and put off adoption. They leave the door open to the possibility, within the next few years, of adoption or an egg donor procedure. But their newfound spirituality and their revitalized marriage are more than enough for today.

There is a potentially positive outcome for every woman dealing with infertility. While we celebrate pregnancies in our groups, we do not elevate pregnancy above any other outcome or option. We celebrate adoptions with equal fervor, and we celebrate women who choose to stay childless. I hope you will find value and meaning and reason for celebration in your outcome, whatever it may be.

Molly's Story: The World in Color

Molly, an accomplished pediatric oncologist working at a major hospital, described herself as "a pretty upbeat person, by nature." But at age thirty-seven, three years of infertility had cast a dark shadow that gradually eclipsed her sunny side. After five IUI procedures with Pergonal, two unsuccessful IVFs, and one complicated ectopic pregnancy, Molly and her husband, Peter, seemed to be handling it all with aplomb. But it wasn't until Molly joined our program that she realized just how devastated she was.

"After three years of this, I thought, 'Oh boy, I'm so tough, I'm so great.' But I had already crashed," she told me. "When I took [Dr. Domar's] test for clinical depression, my score was sky high. I'd been thinking, 'I am not depressed, I am not.' I didn't realize that I'd been walking around like a zombie. What helped was [Dr. Domar] saying that it was normal to be so depressed. All of a sudden it wasn't my fault anymore. It wasn't my fault that I had dust bunnies under the bed, that I couldn't smile, that I didn't want to talk to my husband."

Once Molly realized that her zombielike state was normal and not her fault, she could finally admit just how bad she felt. She also realized that job stress was making things worse (what I call "infertility plus one"). The head of her department was an extremely difficult man to work with, competitive and mean-spirited. He was also threatened by Molly, a gifted clinician and a strong presence in the department. Over time, it became clear to Molly that her superior wanted to force her out of the hospital.

These pressures at work combined with her fertility woes to overwhelm Molly. When I first met her, I asked her about her diet, sleep, and exercise. She'd been eating too much sugar, getting too little rest, and exercising too much. I told her that some infertile women who overexercise get pregnant when they stop. She immediately quit her daily practice of an hour on the StairMaster with a twenty-five-pound backpack. We talked about her depression, and I suggested she do something exceptionally self-nurturing. She bought herself a basset hound.

Inspired by the group, Molly decided to revive a past practice of Tibetan meditation, a discipline of clearing the mind through contemplation and visualization. Years earlier Molly had trekked in the Himalayas, meeting monks and learning about Tibetan Buddhism. (One of the things that drew her to our program was her knowledge that Dr. Benson had collaborated with the Tibetan Dalai Lama on workshops and scientific endeavors.) While her meditation practice was more rigorous than most of the ones I teach, it was basically similar in its elicitation of the relaxation response.

"Meditation was for my mind what exercise had been for my body," said Molly, referring to the discipline and the resulting sense of well-being. She also loved to take mindful walks in the woods with her new puppy. Communing with this lively little creature did wonders for her mood. "Ten-week-old puppies just follow you. You don't have to worry about them at all. Everything for them is a new discovery."

Molly was making new discoveries of her own. When I asked the group to write out their feelings about the most traumatic event of their infertility, Molly chose the lengthy surgery she had to resolve her ectopic pregnancy. Here's how she described the experience, and her catharsis during the writing exercise:

> I'm pretty brave, I'm a mountaineer, I've endured plenty of physical pain. I trekked the Himalayas in minus fifty degree temperatures. But when they wheeled me into the operating room during my ectopic pregnancy, I was terrified. The horror of infertility was somehow crystallized by the image of me lying on the stretcher, waving at my husband and being convinced I was going to die. I was under for six hours, a long time, and I was pretty sick when I came out. I had recurring nightmares about this whole experience. It sat in the pit of my stomach for years.
>
> For me, it became the image that captured the depression, the terror, the anger, the sadness. So I sat down and started to write and started to cry. One of my buddies happened to be sitting close to me, and both of us were writing about something pretty real. Both of us started to cry and sob and write and cry and sob. I realized I was into something important. When the class ended all of us were like bomb victims; we could barely walk out the door. Yet a few of us yelled at Ali [Domar], telling her it was the wrong timing. She felt bad, but she said that we should continue to write for the next two days. It seems you have to write for three days to exorcise the feelings.
>
> So I did, and I exorcised them. The surgery was an image that

had collected all the bad feelings. I wrote about waving goodbye to Peter as I was wheeled into the OR, and from there it became a stream-of-consciousness, James Joyce kind of thing. I wrote out my feelings about that incident, my fear of dying, my sadness about infertility. It was like a knot being dissolved.

The group's support helped Molly to work through her sadness. They also offered commonsense wisdom after she came to a session upset with herself over a screaming fight with her husband. "In years of marriage I've only had two fights like that," said Molly. Her fellow members instantly replied, "So what hormones are you taking?" Molly had been getting Pergonal injections in preparation for another IVF procedure, and emotional side effects were indeed the culprit. It was another time for Molly to let herself off the hook.

Her marriage, which had always been "excellent," was tested by infertility. Molly believed that "you can't work on the relationship until you work on yourself. When you do, the positive changes get transferred to the relationship."

Working on herself had positive ripple effects both on her marriage and her work. Molly used cognitive restructuring to explore her conflicts with the head of her department, and she realized that her helpless reactions to his angry competitiveness were throwbacks. "I saw aspects of my relationship with my dad in my difficulties with him." Her negative thought was "I am powerless." To restructure this thought, and the distress it caused, Molly asked tough questions. "Was I *feeling* powerless? Yes. Was I *really* powerless? No."

Molly realized that asserting her real power would not work with this superior, since there was no room for communication. Asserting her real power meant removing herself from the hostile work environment. During the time in our program, Molly found a position as head of a department of pediatric oncology at another hospital. It seemed too good to be true. She grabbed the opportunity, which offered greater prestige, salary, and autonomy.

All these changes had a healing effect on Molly's spirit. "It was fascinating to me, because one Sunday, in the middle of the program, I woke up and the change was undeniable. Remember the scene in *The Wizard of Oz* when Dorothy steps out of the black-and-white house into a world lit up with color? Well, that's what happened to me. I woke up and my depression was gone. Boom, like that. My whole life turned from gray to being as good as it gets."

Adding to the color, Molly showed up at the last group session with an announcement: her third IVF cycle, which took place toward the end of our program, had been successful. Molly was pregnant, and though she later had a tough delivery, her son, Greg, was perfectly healthy. Now two years old, Greg is a happy, energetic boy, and the couple could not be more grateful for his arrival.

Did the program help Molly get pregnant? As a physician, Molly can't say. But her gut tells her that her body changed with her emotional state. Was it the meditation? The dog? The writing process? The new job? She's not sure, though she suspects these elements combined to relieve her depression. Molly believes that her emotional improvement "really did change my chemistry." Whether that change helped her to conceive remains, for Molly, an enticing possibility. What is certain to her is that she woke up one Sunday morning, and her world was in color.

Twelve

◆ ◆ ◆ ◆ ◆

CALMING THE WOMB:
MISCARRIAGE AND
DIFFICULT PREGNANCY

*T*he woman whose pregnancy is uneventful, who sails smoothly from the first telltale signs to the first cry of her newborn, is fortunate indeed. She's also something of a rarity. Whether it's just morning sickness and cravings, or the more serious prospect of miscarriage or premature delivery, pregnancy can be a time of anxiety as well as a time of momentous joy. Expectant women can reduce the anxiety and optimize the joy by turning within, empowering themselves with behavioral approaches that calm the mind, and the womb.

Multiple miscarriage is common, and women with this problem experience similar feelings of loss and frustration as do those with infertility, but they must deal with another layer of fear and grief. One of my patients, Leah, was at the end of her tether after three miscarriages. The negative tape running through her head was "I can't go through this again. I just can't handle it." Even though she had no children and desperately wanted one, it got to the point where she feared getting pregnant again.

With Leah, and patients like her, I use cognitive restructuring to put the logic behind their thoughts to a rigorous test. "Do you really think that having another miscarriage will send you over the edge?" The question is not meant to minimize their fears but rather to get them to look more deeply behind them. When they do, they discover that they're stronger than they tend to believe. Often, they can handle another miscarriage, if they take the time to grieve, rest, and procure the support of loved ones. Of course, every woman has her limits, and I respect and support anyone's decision to stop trying at any point along the way. But I encourage women to make this decision after sustained reflection, not sudden reaction.

Leah came to feel that another miscarriage would not break her spirit. I helped her explore three possible paths. She could give up trying to get pregnant; try to get pregnant again right away; or wait six months before trying again. Leah chose the last of these. She wasn't ready to give up on biological parenthood, but she also wasn't ready to face the possibility of another miscarriage so soon. I would have supported any choice she made, but waiting made the most sense to her.

But Leah was still concerned about how she'd feel the moment she began trying again. I offered her this perspective: "Which would be more likely to break your spirit—worrying for six months, or nurturing yourself for six months?" Leah realized that she could focus on her own well-being for six months, and that another miscarriage, were it to occur, would not destroy her. It would be painful, but she now realized she had the strength to handle it.

As Leah waited, she got stronger. Six months later, soon after she started trying again, she became pregnant. Her fear of miscarriage returned, and she intensified her commitment to body scan relaxation and mini-relaxations. She used cognitive restructuring to remind herself that she could endure, no matter the outcome. She took each day of her first trimester one at a time, with as much calm and equanimity as she could muster. Today, Leah has a vivacious three-year-old daughter, Elizabeth.

I see many women undergoing difficult pregnancies, and women who've experienced multiple miscarriages. In my clinical experience, when women like Leah practice mind-body medicine, they appear to have a lower than anticipated rate of repeat miscarriage. Moreover, women undergoing difficult or high-risk pregnancies have a vastly improved ability to cope with their condition.

Why would mind-body medicine help women with miscarriages or a high-risk pregnancies? We know a great deal about certain risks to the developing fetus, such as caffeine, drugs, smoking, alcohol, and too many vitamin A pills. Avoiding these risks is essential for a healthy pregnancy. But another dimension of healthy pregnancy is a healthy mind-set. A variety of animal and human studies have linked *extreme* stress and emotional upset to miscarriage. For instance:

- Since the stress hormones adrenalin and noradrenalin can decrease blood flow through the uterus, the fetal blood supply can be compromised when the mother is unduly stressed.

- In animal studies, sudden drops in blood pressure and heart rate have been documented in fetuses when the mothers are exposed to experimental stressors, such as loud noises or irritating interlopers in the animals' cages.
- Various studies carried out in the late 1960s and the 1970s appear to show a high level of psychological distress or certain personality factors common among women who experience multiple miscarriages.
- In one comparison of sixty-one repeat miscarriers and thirty-five controls, the women with miscarriages showed signs of "indirect hostility" and "tension about expressing it." They also showed tendencies toward "self-compromising compliance" and dependence, and were "preoccupied with 'helping' themes and guilt themes."

It is important to note that the human studies are not definitive, because we can't be sure whether the psychological states and traits identified were causes of multiple miscarriage, or aftereffects of the repeated traumas. Nevertheless, it seems likely that extreme stress and difficulty in coping may contribute to miscarriage in at least a small percentage of cases. It is also possible that stress combines with other factors to cause some miscarriages.

Given these facts, those of you concerned about miscarriage can benefit from stress reduction, but there's no need for blame over so-called reproductive failures (another term that should be dropped from medical parlance). If stress plays any part in miscarriage, it is never intentional, and the circumstances are invariably innocent. I simply suggest that you consider stress alongside other physical variables, such as smoking or drinking, as one factor to be managed during pregnancy. Do so not in a spirit of blame, but in a spirit of heightened awareness and a desire to do all you can for your own and your baby's health.

Pregnancy is as good a time as any to improve your stress management skills. Moments of anxiety are normal during pregnancy, just as moments of anxiety are normal through various phases of your baby's development. So are anger, melancholy, rapture, pleasure, and a host of other emotions that accompany the massive changes associated with ensuing motherhood. But some expectant mothers experience undue anxiety, a loss of control that can cause emotional and physical ills. Think about it: if you can't handle your anxieties when pregnant, how are you going to manage your anxieties about your son or daughter until the day he or she goes to college?

For this reason and many others, pregnancy is a wonderful time to heed the call of mind and body for greater tranquility, attunement, balance, and self-care. You can create a warm, loving environment for your child's entrance into and presence in your world by treating yourself with the utmost care. And that means learning to manage stress constructively—meeting your own fears with compassion, riding waves of hormonal and emotional change with equanimity, overturning inner voices of negativity and blame. One way to nourish your developing baby is to nourish yourself on physical, psychological, and spiritual levels. Your self-esteem as a parent, and thus your child's sense of security, is bolstered with every step you take to enhance your mind-body health.

In this chapter, I focus on mind-body medicine for women with multiple miscarriages and difficult or high-risk pregnancies. Most of my suggestions also apply to any pregnant woman wishing to ride the biological and emotional waves of change with greater balance and ease. Doing so enables you to experience those high crests of joy—the moments of connectedness with the baby inside, and the glowing expectations of future happiness with that child.

Miscarriages: The Rhythm of Recovery

Miscarriages are surprisingly common. By one estimate, 23 percent of all medically confirmed pregnancies are "spontaneously aborted," the formal term for miscarriage. Most occur during the first trimester, although some happen later. One of the problems faced by women who miscarry is the lack of credence given to their pain by others, and hence the lack of support they receive. Often, women who miscarry once are subtly pooh-poohed because their mishap is indeed so common ("Everyone's had one"). On the other hand, women who repeatedly miscarry also don't get enough support, because too few other women in their immediate circle are likely to understand their experience firsthand.

There is yet another overarching problem. While our culture and social institutions do too little to honor and assist people in the process of grieving loved ones, they do even less to honor and assist women grieving children lost in pregnancy. To the expectant mother and father, miscarriage represents the loss of a child who was to be; it's not only the loss of a fetus, it's the death of a highly developed dream. Putting aside political arguments about the origins of human life, the fact remains that any woman who experiences miscarriage has lost, at the very least, the child she hoped to welcome into the world. Whether perpetuated by culture, family, friends, or the woman herself, a dismissal of this grief robs her of a chance to move forward with hope and confidence.

I must emphasize that a first miscarriage, or even a few miscarriages, is no reason to despair. *Most women who miscarry go on to have healthy pregnancies.* But your emotional well-being is enhanced when you can feel the sadness that inevitably accompanies miscarriage. (I make a sharp distinction between felt sadness and chronic despair. The former is dynamic and healthy; the latter is static and debilitating.) You may feel numb at first; that's a natural defense we use to protect ourselves in the aftermath of loss. But in time you can recognize and experience the sadness. Certainly the grief becomes heavier if you continue to have miscarriages. Indeed, multiple miscarriages can stretch your grieving capacities to the limit. But mind-body methods can help you to uncover hidden strengths that enable you to handle circumstances you never thought you could bear.

Women who experience multiple miscarriages live with fear and sorrow. Developing healthy, life-affirming ways to cope with that fear and sorrow is obviously important for psychological well-being. It is also possible that effective coping may reduce the risks of continuing miscarriages in women who do not have an established medical obstacle to giving birth. Although I have conducted no formal studies on this question, the majority of miscarriage patients who've joined my mind-body programs have since come to term. This includes patients who've had more than four miscarriages.

If you've had one or more miscarriages, I recommend that you embark on the mind-body program I will shortly describe. At the same time, if you've had more than one, it is crucial to have a complete medical evaluation and follow-up with an obstetrician/gynecologist who specializes in pregnancy loss. A variety of biological problems—many of them solvable—have been implicated in repeat miscarriages. Hormonal imbalances, immune system irregularities, structural problems with the uterus, and an "incompetent cervix" are among the causes, and many of these problems can be corrected through medications and/or surgery.

Coping with miscarriages involves a focused mind-body approach, with a special emphasis on restructuring fearful and guilty thoughts; grieving and procuring social support; self-nurturance; and relaxation. As you will see, the approach differs somewhat depending on whether you've faced one or several miscarriages, and whether you also have trouble getting pregnant between miscarriages.

Managing Fear and Guilt

Fear is the emotional currency in the daily lives of women with multiple miscarriages. Signs of bleeding or "spotting" are the main sources of dread, and women who have had even one miscarriage are liable to be anxious every time they head to the bathroom. It helps to know that bleeding is common during pregnancy; many women bleed lightly during the first few months, and some bleed throughout pregnancy. But women who've had miscarriages need more help than simple reminders that bleeding is often benign, because they do have to pay attention to these signs. The question is, how can they monitor themselves while retaining their emotional equilibrium?

If you are one of these women, eliciting the relaxation response on a regular basis throughout pregnancy is one way to damp down the flames of fear. Another useful way is to do mini-relaxations whenever faced with anxiety-provoking situations. A good time is when you go to the bathroom worrying that you'll see a telltale red splotch. You may also want to do minis throughout the day, whenever your activities are strenuous or stressful and you feel anxious about your pregnancy.

Cognitive restructuring is essential to help you transform repetitive thoughts rooted in fear or guilt. As with Leah, whose story I told at the beginning of this chapter, you can replace these thoughts with an awareness of past circumstances—be they prior miscarriages or other traumas—that you have handled with strength and resilience. You can marshal your resources to deal with almost any event that comes your way.

Many women with multiple miscarriages experience a problem that astonishes women with infertility: they actually *fear* getting pregnant. Some women have both problems—after having had one or more miscarriages, they wait endlessly to get pregnant again. These "miscarriage/infertility" patients have the double whammy captured by one of them, Suzanne, who said, "I dread a positive pregnancy test as much as I dread not getting pregnant." Living in the present—helped along by cognitive work and mindfulness—is the best prescription for these women. I help them to focus on one goal at a time: first pregnancy, then going to term.

Whether women suffer repeated miscarriages with or without infertility, the focus on hidden strengths is central to healthy coping. One approach is to search for these strengths in other areas of their lives. Among the comments I've made to such patients are: "Look at how well you handled your grandmother's death." "Remember how you dealt with that horrible situation with your boss?" "When you think about it, you coped with the last miscarriage very well."

Finding hidden strengths is one way to reinforce your sense of control when you feel as if your body is betraying you. It's also critical to counter any blame you heap on yourself or your body. If your doctor has identified a medical reason for your miscarriages, you can often undergo treatment to resolve the problem, which certainly is not your fault, whether the problem is anatomical, hormonal, or immunological. If your doctor cannot explain your miscarriages, it is just as important for you to reject self-blame.

One of my multiple-miscarriage patients, Eleanor, was told by her doctor that he could not identify a specific medical cause. Her negative tape was: "But there must be something wrong with me." I helped her restructure this thought with facts. When a woman has no medical problem, the likely reason for miscarriage is a chromosomal abnormality of the fetus. In other words, there was nothing wrong with Eleanor's body, but there was something wrong with her fetus. I reminded her that miscarriage is usually nature's way of resolving conceptions that won't lead to healthy babies.

Other women blame miscarriages on their own behaviors. They think, "I shouldn't have been on my feet all day." "I shouldn't have had that fight with my mother-in-law." "Why did I have that glass of wine on day 29 of my cycle?" "I shouldn't have had sex once I knew I was pregnant." If you've had a miscarriage and are hounded by such thoughts, you can restructure them in two ways. First, such factors rarely if ever trigger miscarriage. Extreme, ongoing emotional or physical stress may be a factor in spontaneous abortion, but it is not usually identified as the sole cause. Women with such thoughts usually look back at their activities in the hours or days prior to the miscarriage in search of something they did wrong. One patient who climbed a flight of stairs the day before a miscarriage decided that she'd found the reason, and she punished herself over it.

Although minor physical, emotional, or chemical stressors (e.g., a glass of wine) are unlikely to cause miscarriage, we cannot offer such women a signed statement to the effect that nothing they did had any influence on their miscarriage. That leads to the second phase of restructuring—the realization that they have done the best they could with the information available at the time. I've known few pregnant women who engage in behaviors that their doctors explicitly warned them against. Most often, women skewer themselves over activities that no one ever told them could threaten their pregnancies.

Although I reassure these women that their behavior probably had nothing to do with their miscarriages, I encourage them to let themselves off the hook no matter the cause. Invariably, they are succumbing to specific cognitive distortions, what Dr. David Burns calls "all-or-nothing thinking" and "mental filter." They find some imperfect behavior and use it to punish themselves for the loss of a baby. Or they pick out a single negative detail and dwell on it exclusively. If you are subject to such distortions, you must label and reject them, for they cause so much undeserved suffering.

The Grieving Process

After four miscarriages, Suzanne was in a deep funk. She was depressed and scared, caught between wanting to give up and wanting to keep trying. After joining one of my mind-body groups, Suzanne realized that she'd skipped the grieving process. "I didn't have anyone to grieve with," she said. "The people I went to for support after the first few losses said, 'Oh, you'll get pregnant.' My aunt had had five miscarriages and now she has seven children. It was never acknowledged by my sisters and brother, and my parents just didn't know what to say."

Looking back, it was clear to Suzanne what she needed to do. "I needed to breathe," she said. "I needed to cry, I needed to hurt. I actually wanted to experience the suffering—to feel it and be done with it." With our support, Suzanne was able to do her grieving. She felt less alone with her pain because we validated her feelings.

Suzanne's whole way of coping had changed. Soon thereafter, she had another miscarriage on Thanksgiving. It was a very early miscarriage, and Suzanne did not rush right to the hospital. Friends were soon to arrive for dinner, and her husband, Jack, wanted to call and cancel. "I told him no," recalled Suzanne. "These are good friends, and I wanted to share this with them. I don't mean in a sick way, but they know what we've been through. So I drank some wine, which my doctor had suggested were this to happen again. I relaxed, we cried, our friends came in, and we toasted our lost pregnancy."

Suzanne opened up more to her husband, family, and friends. Her depression lifted, and her marriage to Jack was revitalized. After several more miscarriages, she and Jack decided to put their efforts to become parents on hold. They wanted more time to recover, relax, and enjoy each other again.

Women experiencing multiple miscarriage do need to grieve, and if others don't validate their feelings they can at least validate their own. From the moment couples discover they are pregnant, they imagine what the baby will look like, visualize the baby's room, discuss names with each other.

But, because our society considers a miscarriage at six or eight weeks to be "no big deal," there is barely any recognition that a loss has occurred.

I've had several miscarriage patients who wrote letters to babies they had lost. They wrote about their hopes and dreams for the child, and their disappointment at being unable to fulfill those dreams. Addressing the letters with names they had planned for their children, these women gave credence and concreteness to their own loss; they also felt connected to the being who never made it out into the world. I would not recommend this letter-writing process to everyone, but it did help these women. If you think it will aggravate a deep wound, don't try writing such a letter. But if you think it will help you resolve your grief, proceed with gentleness and care.

It concerns me that some obstetrician/gynecologists instruct miscarriage patients to try to conceive as soon as their periods start up again. I've had many patients who get pregnant within two months of their second or third miscarriage, and they have not had enough time to grieve and recover. The unresolved grief only accumulates if they have yet another miscarriage.

As a result of this phenomenon, I often counsel patients to wait longer. Most of these women are in their thirties and a few extra months won't make any difference. Phyllis, who was thirty-six, had had four miscarriages, and her negative thought was "I can't take it anymore." Yet she felt compelled to start trying immediately after her last miscarriage. I emphasized that this was *her* choice, that she could proceed or take time off. Phyllis was a successful artist and the mother of an eight-year-old from a previous marriage, and the notion of taking time to focus on her work, her marriage, and her child—without constant worry about pregnancy and its aftermath—was a revelation. During this time, she bounced back from her cumulative losses, grounding herself again in the pleasures and challenges of everyday life. Her native optimism and energy returned. One year later, she got pregnant again, and this time she came to term.

Few of us can mourn our losses alone. We need friends and loved ones to salve the sting of isolation, an isolation that makes grieving so much harder. I'm not suggesting that women who've had miscarriages ought never to mourn in solitude. But the grieving process over miscarriage is no different from the grieving process over any loss—it has its own rhythm, one that shifts back and forth from solitude to support-seeking.

Most women benefit by sharing their grief, at least occasionally, with select family members and friends. They often benefit by grieving with their husbands; if they don't, communication and connectedness may break down. But couples cannot always "carry the load" by themselves; it's too weighty and it can foster a feeling of separation from the world. Thus, I encourage both partners in the couple to seek support from each other, friends, and family members in a balanced fashion. However, not all family and friends will be able to be there for you. Find those who can, and turn to them when you most need support.

Suzanne found her needed support. Initially, she and Jack had to come together. Suzanne was a member of our Mind-Body Program for Infertility (she also had trouble getting pregnant between miscarriages), and on the Sunday when the husbands join us, she and Jack participated in all the activities for couples—walking and feeding the ducks mindfully, and taking time to simply listen to each other. "It enabled Jack to finally share with me," she said. "And I finally realized that he was as affected by all this as I was. I also understood how *I* would feel if it was *him* having all these miscarriages."

The day helped Suzanne rediscover "what a truly compassionate man Jack is. He actually wanted to stop doing Pergonal to get pregnant because he could not bear for me to go through this anymore. For the first time I didn't just hear him saying these things. I listened."

Suzanne knew that the couple's infertility and miscarriages could either bring them closer or create a wedge. "I saw how it could rip a marriage apart very easily," she said. But the day together marked a positive turning point in their marriage. Healing subtle rifts in their relationship also made it easier for Suzanne and Jack to accept their inability to have a biological baby: they knew, in a deeper way than before, that they truly had each other.

Suzanne also healed subtle rifts in her family, rifts that had developed—or been exposed—over her reproductive troubles. Her sisters, who "reproduce like rabbits," felt bad for Suzanne. And she had trouble talking with her mother, who she presumed to be profoundly disappointed. Suzanne envied her sisters' seemingly special connection with their mother. "I saw the relationship that my mom shared with my sisters because of their children," she said. "When they had their babies she went to live with them for two weeks to help out, and they had this incredible bond. I desperately wanted that."

When Suzanne finally broached this subject with her mother, she was reassured. "Mom said she didn't care, because there are so many other things she and I have together." And her sisters described a different scene with their mother than the one Suzanne had imagined. Yes, they had shared something special, but they also had run-of-the-mill mother-daughter disagreements about child rearing. "Both my sisters said that Momma was telling them how to bring up their kids." Now Suzanne feels good about her family relations. Her parents and siblings "are very protective of me," she said. Because Suzanne began to state her needs with clarity, these potential rifts turned into sources of renewal.

Your husband, family members, and friends may not know how to respond to your distress over miscarriages. And you can't expect them to. Do you want to talk about the baby you've lost? Would you rather avoid the subject with certain people? Some women resent the questions of loved ones as intrusive. Others feel that a lack of comment means a lack of care. It's up to you to let loved ones know what kind of support you need, and when you need it.

As with infertility, there comes a point when couples dealing with multiple miscarriage decide they've had enough. Every woman and every couple has a limit to the sheer number of losses they can endure. It helps many women to bear in mind the adoption option. They can hold in their heart the fact that parenthood is possible, that the love they've invested in a hoped-for child can be given to an adopted child, who can be received into their families with just as much gratitude and delight. When and if they decide to stop, they move on to make that dream a reality.

Other couples decide to stop, and set aside the adoption option. After seven miscarriages and a calm resolution to stop trying, Suzanne and Jack have come to terms with their childlessness. Right now, her top priorities are her own health and well-being, her relationship with Jack, and her relations with loved ones. She has "explored what it means not to have kids," and for now, she is entirely comfortable with that decision. She loves children, and she and Jack enjoy their relationships with other kids, including nieces and nephews. "There are countless ways you can be caring and nurturing to children when you don't have children of your own," she said. "And you don't have to be up every night at three A.M."

For miscarriage patients who go on to have biological children, the grieving process is more readily resolved. For women who don't, it takes longer, but the hurt does heal. Suzanne says that "the grieving has taken a long time. But I believe in life after death, and I have come to terms with the miscarriages. And I don't need a funeral to mourn the loss of a part of my life, because my life is continuing. I keep growing. To me, it's like piano lessons. I'll always remember what I've learned."

Quiet the Mind, Calm the Womb

Women who've had repeat miscarriages live in a peculiar state of fear. Many patients monitor every pregnancy symptom, and a woman whose nausea subsides may worry that she's losing the pregnancy. Such women are robbed of the joys of pregnancy; their pleasure is undercut by moment-to-moment anxieties.

Given this state of affairs, my multiple-miscarriage patients rely on both regular elicitation of the relaxation response and mini-relaxations. Certain methods tend to work best. If you've had one or more miscarriages, I recommend that you do minis whenever you are anxious or frightened, whether upon heading to the bathroom, going to your obstetrician for an examination or tests, or having any sensation that raises concerns about losing your baby. I also strongly suggest a regular relaxation practice. You may wish to try meditation or breath focus to calm yourself, and a variety of focus phrases are appropriate. Iris, who had five miscarriages, was pregnant again—and very nervous. She and her husband both meditated, and they used the focus phrase "We will" (on the in-breath) "get there" (on the out-breath). Iris added an image that worked beautifully with this focus phrase: her infant child lying in a crib in the room they had prepared for his or her arrival.

You don't have to limit such phrases to your meditation practice. You can repeat calming, reassuring phrases or sentences to yourself throughout the day; these are commonly known as affirmations. Among the affirmations used by miscarriage patients are "I can handle it," "I am going to be okay," "I'm doing the best I can," and "I'm doing the best I can for my baby."

If you are so anxious that you cannot sit still for quiet meditation, then go outside and take a mindful walk if your physician allows you to walk. Mindful walking is one of the best approaches when you feel paralyzed by fear, because you focus on simple sensations in the moment—your feet on the ground, the fresh air coming in through your nostrils, the sensations of your limbs moving, the sights of nature, buildings, or people. Your mind is taken off anxiety, your body is moving, and your spirit can be liberated from future-oriented fearfulness.

One miscarriage patient, Kelly, chose a different approach to mindfulness practice. She bought herself a fish-shaped kiddie pool, similar to one she had as a child. She set it up in her backyard, filled it with water, and lay there for an entire afternoon watching the wind and the birds in the trees. Kelly described this as one of the wonderful afternoons of her life, and she spent many summer afternoons lying mindfully in her kiddie pool.

Body-oriented relaxations like progressive muscle relaxation (PMR) and autogenic training might raise rather than lower anxiety levels for women worried about their pregnancies, because they are already so focused on their bodies that it may not be relaxing to engage in even more body focus. The body scan has a somewhat gentler bodily orientation; try it if your goal is to reduce physical (as well as mental) tensions. Yoga may be excellent for some pregnant women, but I would not recommend it for pregnant women who've had many miscarriages. However, yoga is a great form of gentle exercise and relaxation for multiple-miscarriage patients between pregnancies.

Guided imagery is a good choice for women who need an internal escape from their worries. Consider using audiotapes as guides as you take a mental walk on the beach or a stroll by a mountain stream, or develop your own imagery for relaxation. (These tapes can be ordered from our institute. See Appendix B.) You can also conjure reassuring images of your baby thriving, connected to your nourishment and oxygen.

For everyday fears based on physical twinges or other supposed signs of miscarriage, use the "goose in the bottle" exercise (chapter 5) to remind yourself that you habitually spin worst-case scenarios out of normal signs or sensations. That is not to say you should ignore real signs such as spotting, but rather that you question the basis of nonstop, irrational anxieties.

A sense of humor helps, too. One patient, Tina, had had four miscarriages after years of intensive infertility treatment. She discovered she was pregnant soon after joining our mind-body program. Her first trimester was horrible, replete with cramping and the dreaded spotting. But she used relaxation and minis to transform her state of fear and fatigue. Her sense of humor emerged in our relaxed group setting, and her stories and jokes were as beautifully timed and outrageous as any stand-up comedienne's.

Tina shared many stories with us, including her strategy for getting her unsympathetic husband, Harry, to change his tune. She made Harry go through bogus IVF cycles, injecting his buttock with distilled water—just like her hormone shots. One time they were at the local pizza parlor with his buddies when the appointed time came. Though chagrined, her husband joined her in the bathroom for his mock injection. Tina's tales lifted all our spirits. Her pregnancy continued without incident, and six months after the program's end, she gave birth to a healthy, strapping little boy.

High-Risk Pregnancy

*W*omen who have miscarriages only during the first trimester are not generally categorized as high-risk pregnancies. The term is confusing, because these multiple-miscarriage patients are certainly at risk to lose their fetuses during subsequent first trimesters. Nevertheless, the "high risk" designation is generally (though not always) reserved for women who either have had, or are expected to have, unstable or uncertain pregnancies *after* the first trimester.

The medical reasons for this designation are many. Women who've lost pregnancies during the second or third trimesters will be considered high-risk during any later pregnancy. Women in their forties and those with gestational diabetes, DES exposure, a small uterus, or other uterine abnormalities may be considered high-risk. In many of these instances, medical treatment and careful follow-up can mitigate the high-risk factors. (For instance, certain medications can forestall premature deliveries.) Depending on the medical variables involved, women with high-risk pregnancies will be told by their obstetrician/gynecologists to curtail their activities. The restrictions range from a simple admonition to "take it easy" to total bed rest for many months.

Such women live with a certain amount of dread throughout their pregnancies. Not only do they fear bleeding and spotting, they fear cramps or any sensations that could be premature contractions. Doctors and medical personnel unintentionally contribute to the problem when they tell these patients to be on constant alert for any such signs. Self-monitoring is indeed necessary, but unfortunately, these women can become anxiously preoccupied with signs and symptoms. Because they do need to be on the lookout, I recommend that they use minis constantly to offset anxieties throughout the high-risk pregnancy. Be aware of your body, I tell them, but don't let your body become a source of strictly negative inputs about yourself and your baby.

If you are coping with high-risk pregnancy now, or will be in the future, you might try an imagery exercise that several of my patients have found extremely helpful. You can do this during minis, breath focus, meditation, or just throughout the day as you breathe. On the in-breath, feel the oxygen entering through your nose into your lungs. Now feel your heart beating and pumping that oxygen to your baby. Every time you inhale, you breathe in life-giving oxygen for your baby. Visualize your baby flourishing from this oxygen. As you breathe out, imagine carbon dioxide and other toxins leaving your baby and your body. Continue this visualization with each inhalation and exhalation for as long as you wish. This imagery exercise will strengthen your sense of control, your connection to your child, and your capacity for nurturance.

If you've been told to maintain bed rest, consider quiet meditations including breath focus, mindfulness, and perhaps body scan. This is a time when audiotapes are particularly helpful. How can you get social support when you're lying in bed? I have heard of support networks of women with high-risk pregnancies who are on bed rest. Check with your local chapter of RESOLVE to find out if such a network exists nearby. If not, ask your obstetrician if he or she has other patients on bed rest who might be willing to chat over the phone. Of course, you can try leaning on your husband, family, and friends. In the best of all circumstances, some of them will be delighted to offer both practical and moral support. But if they will not or cannot, it is especially important to seek out support from those who know exactly what you are going through.

Be vigilant about rejecting inner or outer voices of self-blame. High-risk pregnancies are difficult, and it's nearly impossible to be perfect. One patient on bed rest, Emma, carried her infant nephew up a flight of stairs to be changed. Moments later she started having premature contractions. She had to rush to the hospital, where she received medication to forestall early labor. Having been in our group, Emma knew how to question mind-tapes of self-blame, and this prevented her from sliding into a mini-depression over this event. Emma realized that she couldn't be perfect, that her one lapse caused some trouble but it did not cause her to lose the pregnancy. Do the best you can, but don't castigate yourself for imperfections.

Don't blame yourself for medical problems related to your high-risk status, either. They are not your fault! Sometimes the medical lexicon contributes to self-blame. For instance, some high-risk women have cervixes that dilate too quickly, so the uterus cannot hold a pregnancy. This is known to doctors as an "incompetent cervix." It's the kind of terminology that makes some women feel responsible for their own suffering. If you've been given this diagnosis, try changing the term. Give yourself an equally truthful but far kinder diagnosis: "I have an overeager cervix." Who could blame themself for a cervix all too ready to discharge a baby that is so loved and desired?

Mind-body medicine will help you to cope with a high-risk pregnancy. In my experience with high-risk patients, quieting the mind may indeed calm the womb. Thus, you may enhance your prospects of a safe and healthy pregnancy. But there are many variables in high-risk pregnancy, and you can avoid guilt over any negative outcome with the knowledge that you can't control every medical factor via the mind. Become an active participant in your medical treatment, in partnership with your obstetrician. That, too, will contribute to a balanced, healthy sense of control over your circumstances. Let this affirmation become your mantra: "I'm doing the best I can for myself and my baby."

Thirteen

* * * * * *

MINDING THE CHANGE:
MENOPAUSE

Gradually, women's experience of menopause is being transformed. No longer a silent passage, it has become an expressive one—talked about, analyzed, alternately feared and embraced. This cultural transformation has not put an end to harmful myths about menopause. But the greater openness has made room for healthier perspectives, and this positive development may also have positive medical consequences for millions of women.

Why would a healthier attitude help women with the medical aspects of menopause? Because our emotions and perceptions influence the subtle interplay of hormones and brain chemicals, an interplay that may help determine whether we're beset with symptoms during this period of flux. A healthy attitude toward the so-called change of life can smooth the passage, enabling women to realize their vast potential for joy and meaning as they enter the postmenopausal years.

Much has been written about this passage, and the constructive tone of the media's more recent coverage is helping women accept menopause as a natural process rather than a disease process. But for those of you whose experience of menopause remains fraught with anxiety or depression, or who have physical symptoms that disrupt your quality of life, reading helpful books and magazine articles is only a first step. To realize the positive medical consequences of a healthier attitude, you may need more focused help. That is where mind-body medicine comes in.

You can benefit enormously from targeted methods for relaxation, cognitive reframing, and emotional expression that transform menopause from a perceived time of decline to one of vast possibilities for greater freedom, creativity, and pleasure. That is what I offer my menopause patients, and that is what I offer you in this chapter. Mind-body medicine can be a highly effective adjunct to mainstream medicine for the treatment of menopausal symptoms, be they physical or psychological.

In research on which I have collaborated with colleagues at Harvard Medical School's Division of Behavioral Medicine, we've shown that eliciting the relaxation response can significantly reduce anxiety and depression in women at menopause. We have also proven that the relaxation response can significantly lessen the intensity of hot flashes, the most common and often the most disturbing medical symptom, which effects at least 75 percent of postmenopausal women. Being able to control hot flashes is no trifling matter. A woman's quality of life can truly be hampered by them, and symptomatic relief often has a positive ripple effect on every aspect of her life.

Consider the case of Jessica, a schoolteacher who was vexed by hot flashes every few hours, day and night. The worst episodes occurred in the classroom, when her preteen students would frequently act up. When they noticed her unraveling—often at the onset of a hot flash—they'd become even more rowdy. Her hot flash would instantly worsen, disrupting her poise and concentration. At the end of such days, which were all too common, Jessica would be reeling with frustration and fatigue. When she joined my mind-body group for menopause, Jessica learned to practice relaxation on a regular basis, and over several weeks the frequency and intensity of her hot flashes began to abate.

But I also taught Jessica to recognize certain "triggers," stressful incidents that precipitated her hot flashes. She realized that her students' acting out was her most common trigger. From then on, as soon as they began to behave badly she would practice a mini-relaxation. (Her students wouldn't even know she was doing them.) Jessica found that by doing minis in the midst of these stressful events, she could either shorten or completely prevent incipient hot flashes. Overall, she experienced a 70 percent reduction in both the frequency and intensity of hot flashes. A combined practice of regular relaxation and minis during "trigger" events allowed Jessica to regain control of herself and her classroom. In a few months' time, her relationships with her students and her self-image as a teacher—and a woman— were markedly improved.

Although we've shown scientifically that the relaxation response reduces both hot flashes and the psychological symptoms associated with menopause, I have found clinically that combining relaxation with other mind-body techniques is even more effective. In our mind-body group for menopause, patients have used cognitive restructuring to transform negative ideas about menopause—many of them cultural "implants"—into positive ones they could genuinely embrace. They developed constructive new ways to express their emotions and creativity. For these patients, mind-body methods sparked an exciting revelation: that the post-menopausal years could be among the best years of their lives.

These women discovered firsthand what Margaret Mead once called PMZ—"post-menopausal zest"—a time of renewed energy and meaning. Again, it is one thing for women to read about PMZ in a magazine article; it's another thing to experience it. For many, cultivating PMZ requires the development of strong coping skills. Specifically, they need skills that empower them to overcome obstacles—both internal (psychological) and external (cultural)—that block self-esteem, creativity, and restfulness. We teach our patients these coping skills, and their commitment to our program, which also includes a healthy diet and exercise, leads to greater post-menopausal zest.

Mainstream medicine can also contribute to PMZ, as well as to better physical health in the postmenopausal years. Physical symptoms such as hot flashes and vaginal dryness are caused by the inevitable loss of estrogen that takes place during the menopausal transition. This loss may also play a minor role in psychological symptoms such as depression. Thus, hormone replacement therapy (HRT), which involves supplements of both estrogen and progesterone, can offer significant relief for the physical symptoms, and sometimes the psychological symptoms. We also know that the loss of estrogen during menopause heralds an increased risk of heart disease and osteoporosis, and that HRT cuts down these risks for postmenopausal women.

But HRT is not a panacea, and it carries its own potential risks. The older treatment, ERT (estrogen replacement therapy), which involved supplements of estrogen alone, was found to increase the risk of uterine cancers, and possibly breast cancer. HRT, which adds progestins to the regimen, does not increase the risks of endometrial or cervical cancers, and it may even reduce them. But the jury is still out regarding HRT's influence on breast cancer. For every study that exonerates HRT, another study shows at least a modest increase in the risk of breast cancer among long-term users. Most recently, results from the largest study yet of HRT's safety were published in the *New England Journal of Medicine*. Women using HRT for five or more years after menopause were 30 to 40 percent more likely to develop breast cancer than those who did not use hormones.

What does all this mean? Here's the general consensus among doctors: if you have reasons to be concerned about breast cancer—particularly a family history of the disease—you should be cautious about commencing with HRT. It's best to balance your breast cancer risks against the potential benefits of HRT, namely, symptomatic relief and a reduced risk of heart disease and osteoporosis. Every woman at menopause should discuss the risks versus the benefits with her physician. But until we have definitive answers about HRT and breast cancer, your decision to move forward with HRT may be difficult, particularly when you have reasons to be concerned about breast cancer.

Thus, if you are suffering with menopausal symptoms but also worried about the risks of HRT, you may find yourself in a tough bind. Based on our data, and findings from several other studies, we can now offer a proven way to *reduce your hot flashes and distress without HRT*. At the very least, you can elicit the relaxation response and apply other mind-body techniques *before* turning to supplemental hormones. Your chances of gaining relief are high, but if you do not experience sufficient improvement, you can always proceed with HRT.

Mind-body methods are also invaluable as complementary medicine, applied alongside medical treatments such as HRT. Some of my menopausal patients are on HRT, but it does not provide sufficient relief from their immediate symptoms. Yet they choose to stick with their regimen because it offers some relief, or because they're worried about future heart disease and osteoporosis. So they combine HRT with mind-body techniques that reliably reduce their hot flashes and improve their state of mind. A new day is dawning, one in which mind-body approaches are being used along *with* mainstream medicine to produce the best possible results for women.

I certainly do not issue blanket warnings against HRT, which offers tremendous benefits to great numbers of women during or after menopause. Indeed, I have often facilitated a decision-making process that leads patients to choose HRT. I remind them that, overall, the risk of dying from heart disease is likely to be far greater than the risk of dying from breast cancer. But I do respond to the real dilemma of equally large numbers of women who are deeply concerned about risks, and whose doctors are concerned about risks, with mind-body medicine as a viable option to alleviate their suffering.

One of the myths of menopause is that some women's emotional troubles during this transition stem strictly from the loss of ovarian function and resultant drop in estrogen levels. They do not. Studies have *not* shown clear relationships between drops in estrogen and psychological distress in menopausal women. Much of the emotional upheaval attributed to estrogen loss may be due to events in women's lives, the turning points that occur in their forties and fifties. Their careers may be shifting, their husbands may be facing job changes, their children may be leaving home, and their parents may need caretaking. Physical symptoms such as hot flashes can cause insomnia, and the loss of sleep itself can trigger mood changes. These issues must be sorted out before estrogen loss is blamed for everything and HRT is embraced as a cure-all.

As Dr. Sadja Greenwood writes, "During the menopausal years the body goes through a major transition which is experienced differently by every woman, depending on her general health, her body awareness, and the rapidity of her hormone drop. Her psychological reaction to this transitional phase will be determined by both her biochemistry and her outer circumstances. Each affects the other—inner and outer worlds are inseparable, and in constant interaction."

In her fine book *Menopause Naturally*, Dr. Greenwood goes on to question the old scientific axiom that "biology is destiny." This conventional wisdom implies that we are helpless in the face of our own physiological transitions. "A more balanced viewpoint is that biology is only part of destiny, along with the social environment in which we live. Moreover, as we understand this riddle we can direct at least some of our destiny by choosing to enhance our health and self-esteem."

The mind-body techniques I teach women at menopause are tailored for just this purpose—enabling them to direct their destiny by choosing to enhance their health and self-esteem. Remember, feeling out of control may be women's least recognized risk factor for a vast variety of symptoms. A concerted effort to regain healthy control can be extraordinarily powerful medicine for women during this sometimes tumultuous passage.

Menopause: Facts, Myths, and Choices

Though menopause refers literally to the cessation of menses, the term encompasses the entire stage of a woman's life during which her ovarian function declines. For most women, this transitional phase, which usually occurs between the ages of forty-five and fifty-five, stretches from a few years before their last period to a year or two afterward. During this time, estrogen levels decline and menstrual periods become irregular until they eventually cease altogether. About 80 percent of women experience physical symptoms including hot flashes, night sweats, and vaginal dryness.

Though less common, headaches, weight gain, dizzy spells, and "fuzzy thinking"—an intermittent loss of mental acuity—also affect significant numbers of women.

During the menopausal transition, some women do become anxious and depressed. But again, the link between these states and the physical aspects of menopause—namely, the loss of estrogen—is tenuous. Scientific surveys show no peak of emotional illness during the menopausal years. Surely, if there was a direct cause-and-effect relationship between estrogen loss and emotional instability, psychiatrists would be besieged by women at midlife, and this simply does not happen. Women predisposed to depression (i.e., those with a previous history) are more susceptible during this period of hormonal flux, but life events and coping challenges remain the primary factors in the onset of their emotional distress.

It's important to recognize, however, that most women do *not* suffer through menopause. The old, bleak view of menopause stems partly from doctors and scientists who see self-selected populations of women with symptoms. The vast majority who aren't having trouble don't consult their doctors! Our youth-obsessed culture recycles the myth of menopause as an inevitable time of despair, and women therefore *expect* a plunge into melancholia. Indeed, as women's health specialist Christiane Northrup, M.D., has pointed out, "expectations of problems in menopause *lead* to problems." Though a cultural shift is evident, it has yet to fully detoxify the poisonous messages women have received for decades.

Although negative messages about menopause cause more trouble for women than perhaps any other factor, the physical symptoms are real and they can be aggravating. So, too, are the psychological symptoms, even if they aren't caused by estrogen loss. We must acknowledge and validate women's suffering at menopause without reinforcing its inevitability or holding false, harmful views about biological destiny and the loss of beauty and importance in society. Women are *affected* by their hormones, but they are *not at the mercy* of their hormones.

Today, about forty million U.S. women have reached menopause or are in their premenopausal years. By the year 2000, the number will verge on fifty million. Approximately thirty-five million of them will experience hot flashes. Effective treatments for hot flashes certainly are needed. When severe and left untreated, these episodes can sometimes lead to a spiral of insomnia, fatigue, and depression.

Vaginal dryness, irritation, and thinning can disrupt women's sex lives, which in itself can cause a case of the blues. (Vaginal atrophy is the medical term for this thinning of tissues, but don't let this label frighten you into thinking that the process is irreversible.) A variety of medical treatments, including HRT, can alleviate this problem and allow women to regain their sexual vitality, a point to which I will return. Though some women report a loss of libido unrelated to vaginal atrophy, others report heightened sexual desire and activity. Certainly every woman is different in this regard, but some patients' loss of desire has more to do with stress and relationship difficulties than with estrogen loss or vaginal changes.

The HRT Decision

Many menopause patients consult with me because of their physical symptoms, and because they're anxious about the HRT decision. But as soon as we begin talking, it becomes evident that they've come to me for reasons that go deeper. They dread the aging process. They worry that they are no longer needed by family members and friends. They feel that they've gained weight and are unattractive. Some are regretful that they've never pursued careers. Others are regretful that they've never started families. Still others are shaken when their children finally leave home. The multiple turning points for women in their late forties and early fifties can leave them spinning. When we first meet, they are dizzy with apprehension and the perception of loss of control.

In my groups and individual sessions with menopausal women, I offer mind-body methods that help women regain control over their bodies and lives, but even more is needed. Regardless of whether they go on HRT, women face certain health risks, and a healthy diet and exercise are key components of a comprehensive, "whole woman" approach to menopause. In my view, combining conventional and mind-body medicine with sound nutrition and exercise addresses every major health concern of midlife women: hot flashes, vaginal atrophy, "fuzzy thinking," depression, mood swings, and reducing the risks of cancer, heart disease, and osteoporosis.

Education is part of this "whole woman" approach, because the only way we're motivated to stick with behavioral changes—especially relaxation, diet, and exercise—is by understanding why they are so necessary. For instance, it's important to know that estrogen can protect our hearts. As estrogen levels fall during menopause, our cholesterol levels rise—including LDL, the "bad" cholesterol—and we become more susceptible to the development of plaque in our arteries. (Plaque causes atherosclerosis, the hardening of the arteries that causes most heart attacks.) For these and other physiologic reasons, our risk of heart disease increases during and after the climacteric. In studies comparing postmenopausal women taking estrogen to those who do not, the estrogen users have a 40 to 50 percent lower risk of fatal heart attacks. When progestins are added, as they are in today's standard HRT regimens, the heart risks are not lowered quite so much. (Most women and their doctors try to avoid estrogen alone, since without progestins it can increase the risk of uterine cancers.) Though we await final studies of how much HRT (estrogens *and* progestins) lowers our risk of heart disease, most doctors believe that the benefits are substantial.

Therefore, if family history and other factors lead you to be deeply concerned about heart disease, but hardly concerned about breast cancer, HRT might be a good choice. If your concerns are just the opposite—cancer but not heart disease—you may put off HRT. In any event, a low-fat diet and exercise are essential, because they certainly help prevent heart disease and may help prevent breast cancer! Moreover, since HRT is no guarantee against heart disease, those of you on HRT whose major concern is heart health should still follow a low-fat diet and exercise plan.

Let's not forget that stress, chronic anxiety, and depression may increase women's risks of heart disease, immune dysfunction, and, according to some studies, cancer. By helping you to manage stress, regain a sense of control, and realize your full potential, mind-body medicine makes its own vital contribution to preventing these dreaded diseases.

Another major health concern of women at menopause is osteoporosis, the progressive loss of bone mass and strength that occurs during the perimenopausal period—those few years when your periods become irregular and eventually stop. Estrogen deficiency is a contributor to osteoporosis, and HRT during perimenopause can indeed prevent progressive bone loss. But here again, estrogen loss is far from the only factor in osteoporosis, and estrogen replacement is not a cure-all. Lack of exercise, a high-fat diet, insufficient calcium and magnesium in the diet, smoking, excessive alcohol intake, and too much caffeine can all contribute to the loss of bone mass, strength, and quality. Whether or not you are taking replacement hormones, those of you concerned about osteoporosis should consider the low-fat, high-calcium diet and other lifestyle suggestions toward the end of this chapter.

Put simply, not every menopausal woman will choose estrogen pills or patches. And for those who do, pills and patches are just not enough. As helpful as these medications can be, we must not rely upon them solely, lest we ignore the deeper needs of mind and body for nurturance and nourishment.

Stress is a clear culprit in the mood swings and "fuzzy thinking" apparent in some menopausal women, and it exacerbates physical symptoms such as hot flashes. The fear of hot flashes can itself become a stressor—women start worrying about entering warm rooms, fearful of being embarrassed without a comfortable exit. A sensible medical program must therefore include stress management. For women at menopause, this means relaxation techniques and a restructured view of the transition, one in which doors to creativity and joy appear to be opening rather than closing.

Mind-Body Medicine for Hot Flashes

One of my earliest menopause patients, Edith, ambled into my office one day for her first consultation. She sat down in the chair across from me, appearing quite fatigued. I noticed that she was carrying a gargantuan pocketbook. It was so large that I uncharacteristically blurted out, "Wow, you certainly carry a big handbag!" "There's a reason," she promptly replied, reaching into the bag to remove a jumbo roll of paper towels. "This is what I need at all times," said Edith. Her hot flashes were so intense that tissues were as useless to mop off her sweat as they would be to blot up a spilled bucket of water.

Among the most disturbing aspects of hot flashes is the accompanying embarrassment, as Edith clearly exemplified. In public situations—especially in warm rooms—she feared the humiliation she'd feel if people noticed her profusion of sweat. If she had no ready access to a bathroom where she could pull out her paper towels, Edith would feel trapped.

Hot flashes cause many other problems, as well. When they are prolonged, they can be especially unnerving, causing women to lose their focus in work or social situations. And hot flashes are a major cause of insomnia, a frequent complaint of menopausal women who are kept awake at night by roiling sensations of heat in their face, chest, and neck. When I carefully question menopausal patients who are depressed, I often discover that sleeplessness is a root cause of their depression. Because they are up half the night, they're wiped out the next day, and they lose the ability to function at a high level. Eventually, this fatigue causes them to feel out of control. Like falling dominoes, hot flashes can trigger exhaustion, helplessness, and ultimately, depression.

As mentioned, relaxation and other mind-body techniques can alleviate hot flashes and hence break this vicious cycle. You may ask, Why and how does relaxation stem the tide of hot flashes? Simply stated, stress may not cause hot flashes, but it can definitely exacerbate them. Indeed, the hot flash itself involves physiologic changes similar to those of the fight-or-flight response, including a rise in stress hormones. Add actual stress to the equation, and a woman's hot flash will intensify because her sympathetic nervous system is that much more hyperactive. It would seem logical, then, that eliciting the relaxation response, which naturally offsets our fight-or-flight response, would help to alleviate hot flashes. And that is just what happens.

I collaborated with one of my graduate students in Harvard Medical School's Division of Behavioral Medicine, Judy Irvin, Ph.D., whose thesis project was a controlled study of relaxation for the treatment of menopausal women suffering with hot flashes. We recruited thirty-three women, ranging from forty-four to sixty-six years old, all in good health, whose periods had ceased for at least six months. All of them had at least five hot flashes per day. Each participant carefully recorded the frequency and intensity of her hot flashes, and we had each of them complete several psychological tests of mood states at the start and finish of the study.

Dr. Irvin randomly placed each woman into one of three groups. The first group was taught how to elicit the relaxation response, given a twenty-minute audiotape for home use, and asked not only to practice this method every day for seven weeks but to record their practice on a diary form. The second group was instructed to read leisure material every day for seven weeks and to record their practice as well. A third control group received no training or instructions whatsoever other than to record their hot flashes.

Here are the results of our study:

- Women practicing relaxation experienced a statistically significant decrease in the intensity of their hot flashes (a 28 percent drop in intensity). This did not occur among women who simply read for twenty minutes each day, or who were members of the control group.
- Women practicing relaxation experienced a significant decrease in tension and anxiety. Women in the other two groups did not.
- Women practicing relaxation experienced a significant decrease in depression and feelings of dejection. Women in the other two groups did not. (The women in the reading group actually showed a slight increase in depression.)

These findings demonstrated that *daily elicitation of the relaxation response markedly reduces the intensity of hot flashes, and it eases feelings of anxiety and depression among menopausal women.*

Women practicing relaxation did have fewer hot flashes, but not to the statistical level scientists use as a yardstick. (Dr. Irvin suspects that a significant decrease would show up in a larger study.) In my groups and individual practice, menopausal women usually experience reductions in hot flash intensity *and* frequency. In my view, the support from other group members or myself, the regular follow-ups, and the other mind-body methods—including mini-relaxations, cognitive restructuring, and emotional expression—work together with regular relaxation to create a powerful mind-body treatment for hot flashes, not to mention anxiety and depression.

No less than three studies by other scientists confirm our conclusion that relaxation techniques are effective against hot flashes:

- Researchers at Wayne State University divided fourteen menopausal women experiencing hot flashes into two groups. Members of one group were taught progressive muscle relaxation and the others were not. After six months, the women regularly practicing relaxation experienced a significant reduction in the frequency of hot flashes, while the control subjects did not. Overall, women in the relaxation group showed a 60 percent reduction in hot flash frequency.
- Psychologists at Eastern Michigan State University followed four women experiencing regular hot flashes. They administered a ten-session training program (over ten weeks) involving mind-body techniques, including relaxation, self-suggestions of cool thoughts and images, methods for marital stress reduction, and temperature biofeedback. After this training, the subjects averaged a 70 percent reduction in the frequency of their hot flashes—an improvement that held up after six months.
- Robert R. Freedman and Suzanne Woodward of the Lafayette Clinic in Detroit placed thirty-three women experiencing hot flashes in one of three groups. The first practiced paced respiration (a breath focus relaxation); the second practiced muscle relaxation; and a control group used alpha-wave biofeedback, which was not expected to have any benefit for hot flashes. The women doing paced respiration experienced a 40 percent reduction in hot flashes, a statistically significant finding that was measured with ambulatory monitors.

It's not hard for most of my patients to believe that relaxation can alleviate their hot flashes, because they are fully aware of how stress exacerbates them. Ursula, sixty, had hot flashes she described as "waves of heat." She had had a hard life, losing her husband at a young age and raising four daughters as a single parent. When I met her, Ursula had just remarried, and she described a series of tumultuous changes. "Being single for so long was stressful," she said. "But so was getting remarried, because the change was enormous. I went from being a single woman to a married woman, a working woman to a home-based woman, a mother with kids in the home to a mother with grown children and grandchildren. Not only that, I had moved from Missouri to Boston. All these changes added up to a lot of stress."

Ursula noticed her hot flashes worsening during stress, and they got so bad she decided to go on HRT. But, as sometimes happens, the HRT was not sufficiently effective. She joined our mind-body group for menopause, and began a regular practice of meditation, prayer, and mindful walking. She also learned to identify triggers, including bodily tensions that presaged her "waves of heat." "I could practically feel the adrenalin flowing," she said. As soon as she experienced these sensations, Ursula would immediately do a mini-relaxation. "I learned to get myself out of a hot flash very quickly."

Being able to control her hot flashes was a meaningful victory for Ursula. Her adjustments to a new marriage, home, and family role were difficult enough. Overcoming hot flashes eased these transitions, and reminded her that she had more control over her body and her life than she ever believed possible.

For relief of hot flashes, most relaxation methods can be effective. I recommend that you field-test several to determine which one or ones work best for you. However, autogenic training, which includes certain self-suggestions such as "My arm is warm" may not be indicated. You could actually bring on a hot flash this way. (You might also avoid my guided imagery of taking a hot bath.) The opposite may be true, as shown in the Eastern Michigan State University study, where cool thoughts and images helped to relieve hot flashes. Consider the mountain stream imagery (see Appendix B to order audiotapes) or other forms of guided imagery involving cool water as you elicit the relaxation response. (Cool baths, showers, or swims in crystal-clear lakes are among the possible choices.) Since physical activity is essential for menopausal women, a good choice is yoga, an active form of relaxation that also keeps the body limber. Susan M. Lark, M.D., author of *The Menopause Self-Help Book*, suggests that yoga can help to alleviate both hot flashes and vaginal dryness.

Mini-relaxations can help you to stave off hot flashes as they occur, or even before. As with Jessica, the schoolteacher who had worsening hot flashes when her students acted up, you can recognize certain external or internal triggers. As soon as you sense a trigger, you can practice a mini, right then and there. Many of my patients find that minis, used in this fashion, can either prevent or arrest hot flashes.

One of my postmenopausal patients, Rhonda, told me, "I'm too old to do these relaxation techniques. I just can't focus and concentrate like I used to." I gently told Rhonda that I believed that we are never too old to learn something new, but that we must find our own unique path to learning. To help her find her way, I asked, "What is the most wonderful activity you can think of?" Rhonda's answer was instantaneous: time spent with her baby granddaughter, Katya. Her visage lit up as she described a recent day in the park with Katya. "And you know what was the best part?" she said. "When Katya spontaneously came over and hugged me."

I asked Rhonda to sit back in her chair, close her eyes, and imagine Katya coming over and hugging her. "How did that feel?" I asked a few moments later. "So great, so calming," she replied. "Why don't you let that be your relaxation?" I said. "Take ten minutes each day to relax and imagine your granddaughter hugging you." That became her daily ritual, one Rhonda relied upon to ease her tensions and arouse a deep sense of well-being.

Eliciting the relaxation response can relieve other symptoms that afflict women at menopause, including headaches, palpitations, forgetfulness, "fuzzy thinking," fatigue, insomnia, and weight gain. Relaxation techniques do not appear to reverse vaginal dryness, but thankfully other treatments are quite effective. A variety of lubricants, including K-Y jelly, vitamin E oil, Astro-glide, and cold-pressed castor oils, are useful. HRT usually works well, restoring the estrogen that naturally prevents the thinning of vaginal tissues. For women who wish to avoid oral HRT, which has systemic effects, estrogen creams are available that can be applied locally and that generally provide good results. However, if you have a health condition or medical history—such as breast cancer—be sure to discuss this with your physician, since some estrogen may be absorbed through the vaginal wall.

Some women with chronic vaginal dryness have pain upon intercourse, and eventually the prospect of sex becomes fraught with anxiety. In some cases, women develop vaginismus—painful spasms of the vaginal muscles that preclude intercourse. Women with vaginismus can benefit from relaxation, especially body scan and guided imagery that enables them to relax the entire pelvic region. I have had patients who've overcome vaginismus with focused relaxation.

One of the most effective treatments for vaginal dryness may actually be quite enjoyable: sex. If you are able to maintain an active sex life with your spouse or partner, your ongoing activity will slow or prevent vaginal atrophy. Consider using a lubricant or estrogen cream initially; in time, you may no longer need it. Even if you do still need lubricants, having sex regularly will help to stop or slow this often aggravating symptom.

Changing Your Mind About the Change

Menopause has finally left the backstage of our collective consciousness to make a front-and-center appearance. But we still have a way to go before the vast majority of women accept menopause for what it is: a natural life passage that carries its share of loss and gain, sorrow and pleasure, new limits and new freedoms.

In America, where the premium placed on youth and beauty is so high, women report many psychological and physical symptoms of menopause. In Japan, where people view the aging process respectfully and the aged with reverence, symptoms of menopause are far fewer than in this country. This disparity is more proof that how women perceive menopause will affect how healthfully they endure the passage.

I believe that pernicious words, ideas, and images can be as dangerous to the health of menopausal women as genetic risks and hormonal shifts. When we adopt cultural notions that our attractiveness and worth to our families and communities are profoundly diminished as we age, we suffer in mind and body. These thoughts damage our self-esteem and increase our stress on a daily basis. We therefore need cognitive restructuring as a tool for personal liberation *and* health promotion, because this technique empowers us to question and replace such harmful thought patterns.

Here again, I do not use the cognitive method to create an unreal world in which aging is a strictly wondrous affair. For some women, the climacteric will be tumultuous, even *without* negative thoughts and stubborn symptoms. We all have to face what author Judith Viorst called "necessary losses," and many of them occur in our forties and fifties. Common examples are the death of parents, the loss of children from the home, the surrender of dreams that may be unattainable. And yes, our bodies age in ways that won't always delight us, even if we reject the media's absurd idealization of youthful physicality. But when we view every midlife event through dark-colored glasses, our perceptions are just as distorted as when we view every event through rose-colored glasses.

I encourage my menopausal patients to reframe their negative perspectives as ones that are nonjudgmental—accepting necessary losses while embracing newfound possibilities. They use cognitive restructuring to resist

external and internal voices of shame and demoralization, replacing them
with voices of self-acceptance.

Here is a sampling of the negative thoughts I have heard repeatedly from
my menopause patients:

- I'll never feel attractive again.
- My husband does not want me anymore.
- In terms of my career, it's all downhill from here.
- It's too late for me to realize my creative self.
- My sex drive has declined, and it will only decline further.
- My children don't need me anymore.
- I've gained weight, and I can't get it off.
- I'm useless to my family and society.

Any woman taking such destructive thoughts to heart is bound to become depressed! Every one of them is rooted in our ageist culture, which
assumes that aging is an inevitable decline into incapacity, fatigue, and de-
spondency. Yes, certain changes typically occur at midlife: it can be harder
to lose weight; libido fluctuates; and social and family roles shift. But none
of these transitions should ever be interpreted to suggest that menopausal
women cannot feel attractive, be fully sexual, come into their creativity,
develop careers, or redefine relations with loved ones in ways that are profoundly gratifying.

I encourage you to apply the four questions of cognitive restructuring to
all your negative tape loops about aging and menopause. Be systematic and
tough-minded—don't let false cultural and social assumptions make you
suffer, and don't accept viewpoints that reinforce helplessness and low self-
esteem. Find role models among women in their fourth, fifth, sixth, seventh, eighth, or ninth decades who live with zest, sexuality, creativity, guts,
and sharp intelligence. Take your pick: Elisabeth Kübler-Ross, Betty
Friedan, Julie Andrews, Nancy Kassebaum, Gloria Steinem, Vanessa
Redgrave, Margaret Thatcher, Coretta Scott King, Elizabeth Taylor, Jessica
Lange, and Candice Bergen, to name just a few candidates. Perhaps your
mother, aunt, or grandmother lives or has lived that way. It's not hard to
find women in the world who've resisted conventional nonsense about postmenopausal decline.

One of my menopausal patients, Rose, had been married for thirty-two
years with two sons and a daughter. When her children were young, Rose
spent all her time and energies raising them while her husband, William,

built his mail-order business. As the children grew up, Rose began working with William, and later, their two sons got involved in the business. "William was very successful," she said. "But our family's entire life began to revolve around the business."

At fifty-two, Rose began having severe hot flashes, as well as vaginal thinning and irritation that made her reluctant to have sex. Adding to her distress was a weight gain of twenty pounds, which made her feel ungainly and unattractive. Rose's low self-esteem as a woman and a sexual being led her to worry incessantly that her husband would be attracted to other women. She feared that if she left her job in his business—which she wanted to do—he might become involved with another woman.

Rose was also depressed because she felt that her life revolved totally around William and his business. She felt that her chances for her own creative life were slipping away, and so were her children, who she thought no longer needed her. Rose believed she'd given three decades of life to her children and husband, supporting and nurturing them—and what was there for her?

In our cognitive work together, I helped Rose question all her negative thoughts. Was she really unattractive? Couldn't she reduce her hot flashes and treat her vaginal dryness? Did her husband and children really no longer need her? Could she leave her husband's business, or find a better way to work with him?

This process yielded surprising new answers to questions she had never before put to the test. She could go on a healthy diet to lose weight and find effective treatments for her vaginal symptoms. She was invaluable to her husband in his mail-order business. All three of Rose's children still relied on her for emotional support. In fact, she had helped all three through recent troubles with spouses or partners. She could devote time to her own creative pursuits, including painting. Finally, she could negotiate with her husband about leaving his business or find another alternative.

Rose was able to follow through on every single one of these restructured thoughts. She lost weight; her sex life began to improve; she became more assertive with her family; she found time and a space for painting; and she and her husband embarked on a whole new business together, one that drew them closer together. But Rose would never have made any of these difficult transformations had she not first made revolutionary changes in her mind-set.

Women at menopause won't be motivated to achieve "post-menopausal zest," as Rose did, unless they dig out deeply embedded negative thoughts, expose them to the light of day, and allow them to shrivel and fade from consciousness. Once this happens, the road ahead is cleared, and the problem no longer is one of motivation but one of choices: as careers change, marriages mature, and children leave, there are open-ended new possibilities for work, love, and play.

You *can* change your mind about "the change." Yes, menopause is a major psychological and physical transition. Obviously you have no choice in such biological matters, but you do have choice with regard to your cognitive and emotional responses. You can say to yourself, "I feel terrible physically, I feel terrible mentally, I'm totally out of control." Or you can say to yourself, "This is a difficult time for me. What can I do to help myself through this transition? How can I make myself feel better physically? What can I do to reduce my distress, today and tomorrow? What can I do to improve my physical health? How can I follow this passage to higher ground, where I will have more energy, hope, connectedness, and creativity?"

Emotion and Creativity in PMZ

*M*any women have compared their experience of menopause to that of adolescence. Both can be stormy passages, when sudden fluctuations occur in our hormones, feelings, energy, and sexuality. We may not be prepared for these changes, and thus we feel out of control, particularly of our bodies. But menopause, like adolescence, can also mark a turning point of individualization, a time when we struggle to achieve a healthy separateness from those upon whom we've been dependent. (In adolescence the separation is from parents; at menopause, it's often from children.) Twisting our way through the pains of separation, we can refashion these relationships to achieve a more mature connectedness, in which our worth and autonomy are respected. In so doing, we also gain a greater maturity in our relations to everyone we care about. We find more of ourselves, including a richer capacity for self-expression in work and at leisure.

When menopause is viewed this way, the necessary losses are easily matched by the unexpected gains. Yes, we will be sad that our children have left home; that our parents are sick or gone; that our partners have not been able to fulfill all our needs; or that certain dreams have never been realized. And women who have not started families may feel regretful during the climacteric. Menopause can be a time to grieve over unfinished business of all sorts. However, when we experience and move through the grief, getting the support we need from loved ones, it will be far easier to recognize the potential excitement of this time in our lives.

Just as in adolescence, sadness and struggle at menopause often give way to newfound freedoms. Children are out of the home, and we can pursue creative work with fewer obstacles. The disappearance of our menstrual periods—and our need for contraceptives—offers the prospect of sex with more abandon. Greater opportunities may arise for travel and uninterrupted leisure with spouses, partners, or lovers—or by ourselves. We can take time to redefine priorities, and seek new levels of emotional and spiritual growth that we never even had time to *think* about before.

Lotte, fifty-eight, had worked as a real estate saleswoman ever since her two children were in high school. Her daughter and son had moved to other cities, and when her daughter-in-law gave birth to her first grandchild, Lotte wanted to be near them. She gave up her job, and she and her husband, Carl, who had just retired, moved a thousand miles away to Boston. It was a tumultuous time for Lotte. She was thrilled to be near her son, daughter-in-law, and grandson, but she missed her work.

"I had been a success, and when I left my job and home to move here, I lost control," said Lotte. "I wondered if I still had a function." Feelings of dislocation gave way to a stark depression and stress-related physical symptoms common after menopause, including headaches and dizziness.

When I worked one on one with Lotte, I first encouraged her to use relaxation techniques such as body scan to tune into herself with heightened awareness. She soon realized that although she missed work, she also missed her familiar role as a people-pleaser with friends and coworkers. Her self-esteem had been shaky because of this dependence on other people's responses. Now, Lotte used this transitional period to uncover hidden sources of self-esteem, ones that stemmed from within rather than without.

"I always have a tendency not to listen to my body, either because I am too busy or don't have enough time. I'm also the kind of person who is very nurturing, always trying to be good. I do many things simply because it's so hard for me to say no. I'm learning that women of my age and generation have given so much of themselves for others, and rarely think about themselves and what they need."

Much of Lotte's void had to do with the loss of positive feedback she used to receive when selling homes and entertaining friends. She learned to fill that void by transferring her energies from nurturing others to nurturing herself. "Reading has become important," she said. "When my children were small it was like a carrot in front of the donkey's nose—all I could think about was getting time to sit down and read. Now I'm giving myself that time, whether it's for reading, puttering, or nonsensical activities. I'm learning how to take care of myself and it feels great."

The move to Boston became a metaphor for Lotte's passage—she'd left behind old patterns and connections for new ones, including a change in her marriage. While Lotte got kudos from others for her marvelous caretaking, she never got the open demonstrations of love from Carl that she quietly longed for. As part of her cognitive and emotional work, Lotte stopped subtly struggling for Carl's affection. It was a huge step, because, as she said, "one of my crazy fears was that he would walk out on me." Rather than soothing herself with affirmations that he'd never leave, Lotte took a more daring step: "I came to terms with the idea that if Carl did leave me, I would be okay. I could live without him."

It was a seeming paradox, but Lotte's revelation that she could live without Carl brought them closer. Once she let go of her rigid role as the selfless, devoted wife—always maintained to hold his love—Lotte came into her own. Now that she was no longer straining to please, their love blossomed on a bedrock of Lotte's self-worth rather than self-sacrifice. She also gained the gumption to assert her needs with Carl, in order "not to let him get away with his controlling stuff anymore." She expressed her desire for greater equality in the relationship, to make it more of a partnership. Carl responded with a surprising openness and equanimity.

"We've been married over thirty-three years, and we still adore each other," said Lotte. "But now there is more of a growth process. I see other married couples who never seem to put it together. Thank God we've been able to put it together."

Remarkable change occurred over a two-year period, during which time Lotte shifted the ground of her relationships with her husband and children from one of insecurity to one of assertiveness, honesty, and a hard-won trust. After the dust settled, Lotte wanted to get back to work, but this time her purpose was not to fill an aching emptiness. She'd already filled that void with self-nurturance. Her purpose was to enjoy herself and to exercise her skills as a saleswoman. Lotte developed a part-time arrangement with a real estate company in the Boston area, and today her work is a source of pleasure and pride. So is her grandson, whose proximity makes it possible for Lotte to enjoy him every day of her zestful life.

Lotte's story illustrates how mind-body approaches can be seamlessly woven together to help women with the stressful aspects of menopause. Relaxation helped her tune in to her needs and her body; cognitive work changed her bleak view of midlife; emotional expression brought her out of her shell; and assertiveness transformed her marriage. In a matter of months, her depression and physical symptoms abated.

Anger can be a particularly liberating emotion for women who've spent most of their lives pleasing others. Donna, a sixty-year-old patient, spoke graphically about her repressive tendencies. "I don't show anger. I hold things in, I don't let them out. With my husband, instead of getting mad we simply wouldn't talk to each other. But it's changing. Now, when I'm angry with my husband, he knows it. We get it out and get on with our lives. Over and out."

Donna did the anger visualization I teach (see chapter 8), in which she imagined a dialogue with anger in the form of an animal. She took anger by the hand. "What surprised me most was the feeling that anger was my friend." The exercise helped validate Donna's healthy anger as it surfaced in her close relationships.

Her transformation took her family by surprise, but like Donna's recognition of anger as a friend, the surprise was actually welcome. One Mother's Day, Donna was talking to her eldest daughter, Kathy, on the phone. She made an offhand critical remark about Kathy's parenting of her young son, and Kathy exploded, upping the ante considerably. Although Donna knew she'd probably stepped over a line, her daughter's furious retort cut deeply. Donna burst into tears and told her daughter, right then and there, that she did not wish to be spoken to in such a hurtful way. The whole tenor of the conversation instantly changed.

"She loved that I had asserted myself," recalled Donna. "She thought it was great. Before we got off the phone we told each other how much we loved each other. I hung up, tears were streaming down my face, then I began to laugh. I was thinking, if someone asked me how I felt on Mother's Day, I'd say that I had the first big blowup with my adult daughter and it was so liberating. I was able to say these things and still feel loved, still feel that she would always be there."

Post-menopausal zest often heralds a surging of emotion and creativity. For women who've spent decades constraining both, whether in the service of career, family, or some combination, the fifth decade and beyond offer the prospect of freedoms never before tasted. But the potentialities can be either grasped or bypassed. Sybil was one of my patients who seized the opportunities offered in her early sixties. Her two daughters grown and married, Sybil had time to return to a great joy of her late teens and twenties: sculpture. She set up shop in a bedroom left vacant by one of her daughters, filling it with her tools and materials. The room became Sybil's artistic refuge, a place where for an hour each day she let her creative impulses bubble up, her mind fully focused as she chiseled, cut, and molded forms to her delight.

During and after menopause, find a room, even if only a metaphorical one, where you can let your creative sides bloom. At such times the medium is not the message. Any medium is message enough, to yourself and others, that it's your time to blossom. Whether the form is music, painting, sculpture, film, video, pottery making, basket weaving, acting, writing, or dancing, the process is what matters most. It can yield the highest satisfactions, and there's no doubt in my mind that creative expression is a boon to every woman's mind-body health.

Lifestyle Changes: Diet and Exercise

There are four salient reasons for a sound low-fat diet and consistent exercise during the menopausal transition and beyond: prevention of heart disease, prevention of osteoporosis, possible reduced risks of breast and colon cancers, and the general enhancement of mind-body health and energy during this time of psychobiological flux.

Heart Disease

You may be surprised to learn that heart disease is the number one cause of mortality in women over fifty. In fact, it is responsible for ten times as many deaths in postmenopausal women as breast cancer. One reason has become clear: estrogen helps protect against heart disease, and its depletion at menopause is therefore associated with an increased risk. Specifically, estrogen lowers the total cholesterol count while increasing blood levels of HDL, the so-called good cholesterol that appears to protect blood vessels.

Here is the key point: whether or not you choose to go on hormone replacement, a key strategy in lowering cholesterol and increasing HDL—and hence, preventing heart disease—is a low-fat diet. If you decide to go on HRT you will reduce your risks of heart disease. But don't be fooled into thinking that your daily dose of hormones is your only ticket to heart health. Heart disease is "multifactoral"—several variables are involved, and you take control of your well-being by addressing each one.

If, with your doctor's counsel, you decide *not* to go on HRT, a low-fat, high-complex-carbohydrate diet is obviously essential. A diet with a low percentage of fat (especially of the saturated variety) and generous amounts of complex carbohydrates—grains, fruits, and vegetables—is a safe, natural way to lower your cholesterol and your risk of heart disease.

Whether or not you choose HRT, you reduce your risk of heart disease when you:

- Adopt the low-fat, high-complex-carbohydrate diet described in chapter 9.
- Use a healthy diet to keep your weight down, though not through obsessive dieting and fear about a few extra pounds. Obesity is a risk factor for many diseases, including heart disease.
- Moderate your alcohol intake. Though several studies indicate that a modest intake of alcohol—say, a glass or two of wine per day—might reduce heart disease risk by raising HDL, other studies demonstrate that excess alcohol can increase blood pressure. (It may also contribute to breast cancer and osteoporosis.) My motto here, as with other life-style changes, is meant to cut through the thicket of contradictory media messages: Don't be confused, be sensible. An occasional drink, or even a regular glass of wine, beer, or spirits, is not a problem. More than two glasses per day may be considered excessive and potentially harmful in terms of heart disease risk, breast cancer risk, and addiction.
- Quit smoking. Smoking is a factor in high blood pressure and a known risk for heart disease. Use relaxation, behavior therapy, or any other technique that helps you through the withdrawal symptoms, including hypnosis and group support.
- Moderate salt intake. Excessive salt contributes to high blood pressure in some people, a key risk factor in the development of heart disease.
- Get regular exercise. The data on regular exercise and prevention of atherosclerosis and heart disease are unequivocal. As per the advice in chapter 9, there is no need to undertake a strenuous regimen. Daily walking is sufficient to reduce cholesterol levels and heart disease risk.

Every woman should have a regular "lipid profile" to determine her levels of cholesterol, HDL and LDL, and triglycerides. Ideally, you would like to have a cholesterol level below 200, an HDL over 35, an LDL below 130, and a triglyceride count under 250. Don't let test numbers be your only guide; you should also take into account other risks, including family history of heart disease, past or present smoking, high blood pressure, obesity, and a behavior pattern of hostility and cynicism. (Mind-body medicine, including relaxation, offers enormous help for modifying unhealthy behavior patterns.) Lifestyle changes will go a long way to reduce risk and bolster heart health, but you should monitor yourself on a regular basis and discuss all your options with your doctor. These options include both HRT and cholesterol-lowering drugs.

In a landmark study, Dean Ornish, M.D., the renowned cardiologist, has shown that an extremely low-fat vegetarian diet, along with regular exercise, stress management, and group support, can actually *reverse* existing heart disease. If you have heart disease, you may wish to follow Dr. Ornish's program, which has recently gained backing from a major health insurance company. (See his book *Dr. Dean Ornish's Program for Reversing Heart Disease*.) Consider his guidelines if you have heart disease or you are concerned about your risks and highly motivated to alter your lifestyle. But don't punish yourself with guilt if you have trouble maintaining such a low-fat diet; more modest changes are absolutely worthwhile.

Osteoporosis

Approximately one half of all postmenopausal women will develop osteoporosis, a progressive loss of bone mass and strength. Osteoporosis is a cause of low back pain, curvature of the spine, diminished height, and the all-too-common fractures of the hip, back, and wrist. As with heart disease, estrogen is a factor in osteoporosis: it appears to protect the bones from excessive calcium loss; to stimulate recalcification of bone; and to enhance calcium absorption. The loss of estrogen at menopause, along with other age-associated factors, contributes to a decline in the availability and balance of calcium. And calcium is the mineral that helps us maintain strong, healthy, flexible bones.

It's our job, then, to optimize our levels and absorption of calcium, and again, hormone replacement is not the only strategy. With or without HRT, we should combine diet and supplements in order to get sufficient calcium. The Recommended Daily Allowance (RDA) for calcium is 800 milligrams, but most nutritionists suggest between 1,000 and 1,500 mg to prevent bone loss. You will likely need both food sources and calcium supplements to achieve this goal.

Contrary to long-held popular opinion, dairy foods are not the only good sources of calcium. Many dark green leafy vegetables are also good sources. Make sure to include these calcium-rich foods in your diet on a regular or rotating basis:

- Low-fat dairy products: Dairy is indeed an excellent source of calcium, but you still want to avoid high-fat versions. Enjoy nonfat or low-fat varieties of milk, yogurt, cheese, and other milk-based foods.
- Fish: Salmon with bones (the canned variety has even more calcium than fresh), shrimp, canned sardines
- Fruit: Figs, rhubarb
- Vegetables, beans, and seeds: Collard greens, broccoli, kale, soybeans, mustard greens, turnip greens, tofu, sesame seed paste (tahini)

Calcium from food is likely to be absorbed better than calcium pills, although supplements are still considered useful to shore up our overall dosages. It is simply too hard for many women to eat enough of the above-listed foods to get optimal amounts. Calcium supplements can be taken as 500 mg tablets; a sensible dose is two of these per day for a 1,000 mg total. Not every calcium supplement is as good as the next; some are absorbed more readily than others. According to many nutritionists, the best choices are calcium carbonate or calcium citrate, both of which should be taken with food for optimal absorption. Antacids such as Tums are also good sources of calcium. Avoid antacid varieties that include aluminum; their calcium is less well absorbed.

Vitamin D is needed for the body to absorb calcium from the intestines. Sun exposure is needed for the formation of vitamin D, but we can't always get enough sun, and in any event we should limit our sun exposure due to the risks of skin cancer and premature aging. Fortified milk products or a daily multivitamin pill with vitamin D included are more than sufficient. Vitamin D in doses higher than 400 IU should be avoided due to its potential side effects.

Magnesium, an essential component of bone, is also helpful in prevention of osteoporosis. (Some studies point to its role in heart health.) It also helps to regulate absorption of calcium, prompting many nutritionists to suggest that magnesium supplements be considered, especially when one is also taking calcium supplements, in a roughly one-to-two ratio with calcium. In other words, 400–500 mg of magnesium may be taken with 1,000 mg of calcium. Food sources of magnesium, such as whole grains and green vegetables, are also important, and they contain an array of other essential nutrients.

Exercise is a critical component in any program for prevention of osteoporosis. The key here is weight-bearing exercise—any activity that puts weight on your bones. This includes exercises in which you carry your own weight, such as walking, jogging, and NordicTrack. Low-impact aerobics in the form of race-walking or dancing are superb. Biking is good but not great as a weight-bearing activity. Swimming won't do the trick for this purpose. Weight lifting is an excellent way to help maintain your bone density. But don't be daunted by these choices. If you're not likely to join a health club for its fancy equipment, or you're not inclined to lift weights, remember that walking or light jogging is a wonderful and undemanding way to meet your requirements for weight-bearing exercise for your lower body. For upper-body strength—elbows, shoulders, and wrists—use small weights or carry balls to squeeze as you walk.

Diet and Exercise for Symptoms

Healthy diet and exercise are also helpful in the management and prevention of menopausal symptoms, including hot flashes, insomnia, mood swings, and depression.

Huge meals, spicy foods, caffeine, and alcohol can worsen or trigger hot flashes and night sweats. Avoid all of these, but don't eat so little food that you are malnourished or overly thin. A normal distribution of fat is actually needed, since natural estrogen is stored in body fat.

Certain foods have estrogenic activity that may help with menopausal symptoms. Soybeans and soybean products such as tofu and miso contain phytoestrogens, which are weak estrogenlike compounds. One study published in the British medical journal The Lancet showed that Japanese women who had a high intake of soy products had fewer hot flashes and other symptoms of menopause. Other foods containing phytoestrogens include peanuts, cashews, apples, almonds, oats, corn, and wheat. Whether or not they reduce your hot flashes, most of these foods are worth introducing into your diet, although nuts are high in fat and should be consumed only in moderate amounts. Soy products are also excellent sources of protein and other vital nutrients.

A fair number of women report that vitamin E helps to relieve their hot flashes. There is little scientific evidence to support this claim, so I cannot make hard-and-fast recommendations. But vitamin E, a powerful antioxidant, has shown benefits for the health of our hearts and immune systems, and moderate supplementation carries no known risks. Taking 400 IU per day of vitamin E is considered completely safe, and you may give it a trial run for hot flashes. Avoid any dosages above 1,000 IU.

Exercise helps some women with hot flashes, though there is little data indicating what kinds of exercise are best. I recommend that you follow the same exercise guidelines offered for prevention of heart disease and osteoporosis, and you may also experience a reduction of hot flashes and other menopausal symptoms.

There is no doubt, as mentioned in chapter 9, that exercise can help women to manage both anxiety and depression. To the extent that you experience anxiety or depression during the menopausal transition, you have yet another reason to embark on a nondemanding exercise program of walking or other enjoyable forms of physical activity. Low-impact aerobic activity may enable you to raise your levels of endorphins intermittently, which often lifts women's moods, energy, and even their sense of self-efficacy.

A number of commonsense strategies are recommended for hot flashes, night sweats, and the resultant insomnia. Use cotton sheets and bedding that "breathe." Keep your bedroom cool, either through open windows or air conditioning. Finally, in cool or cold weather, dress in layers that you can peel off during the advent of a hot flash.

The Mind-Body Approach:
Putting It All Together

*I*t is possible to facilitate your own growth process at and after menopause, cultivating PMZ despite the obstacles. Though I've stressed the growth opportunities, there is no doubt that menopause can be a time of inordinate stress, primarily due to converging life circumstances. If you find yourself dealing with unavoidable family pressures, caretaking responsibilities, financial hardships, or family illnesses, it will be hard to view midlife as a wondrous time of expanded opportunity. All the more reason to adopt mind-body techniques and coping skills to alleviate distress and enhance control. The hard times will come and go, but you can always turn to your mind-body "bag of tools" to find peace of mind. It's also easier to implement real-world solutions to tough problems when you are calm and confident, as opposed to anxious and depressed.

Carrie had had a total hysterectomy in her late thirties, which brings about an early surgical menopause. It took years for her to deal with the emotional and physical repercussions. The hysterectomy, done to relieve the pain of endometriosis, may or may not have been necessary, but the doctor who recommended and performed the surgery frightened Carrie into believing that hormone replacement therapy would certainly carry unacceptable cancer risks. (She had no family history of breast cancer, and his excessive warnings were based on ignorance.) As a result, she never availed herself of HRT's benefits, which would have been especially helpful given Carrie's unique emotional and physical symptoms. (The worst were depression, insomnia, and severe vaginal thinning.) Carrie also believes that her emotional suffering was intensified because, for so many years, she handled the trauma of early hysterectomy by repressing all the associated emotions: anger toward her doctor; grief over the loss of reproductive organs and capacity; fear that she would no longer be fully alive as a woman.

Carrie now feels that her denial and avoidance led to a variety of additional symptoms, including food allergies, anxiety attacks, phobias about HRT and other medications, chronic flu symptoms, and back pain. She was in her late fifties when she came to me, and I taught her relaxation and cognitive restructuring, and encouraged her to talk out her feelings about the hysterectomy and early menopause.

With courage and unwavering commitment, Carrie took the ball and ran with it. Here is a list of what she did to transform her life:

- Mindful walks on the beach
- Breath focus meditation
- Listening to mountain stream imagery tape
- Doing self-created guided imagery of pleasant memories with her family
- "The construction or creation of a 'safe place' where I can pull myself out of any stressful event"
- Identifying cognitive distortions related to her fears and phobias
- Questioning every self-blaming thought she had about letting down her husband and children
- Meditative prayer and Bible readings
- Recognizing and expressing her anger from the past (mainly about her hysterectomy) and in the present (toward her husband)
- Opening lines of communication with her husband and children in family sessions with me
- Conquering fears about reaching out to family and friends for support

So comprehensive were Carrie's efforts that her mood state improved in a short time span. Her fears of medication were overcome just enough for her to commence HRT with a patch. The estrogen relieved some of her symptoms, including partial improvement of the vaginal dryness. As she continued over a period of months, her insomnia was cured and her aches and pains alleviated. She still struggles with anxiety attacks, but they are less disabling than before.

Carrie had to work on many mind-body fronts to get relief, and she feels it has all been worthwhile. She reclaimed her sense of control, and the positive ripples have touched her marriage, family relationships, and self-esteem as well as her physical health. Although the above list may seem daunting, each step and technique was part of a process of self-discovery, one that Carrie ultimately found exhilarating.

For women at or after menopause, a combination of mind-body approaches has, in my clinical experience, been most effective. I make the following overall recommendations:

1. *Relaxation:* Elicit the relaxation response through any method detailed in chapter 3, with the possible exception of autogenic training and the hot bath imagery. This enables you to achieve stress reduction, enhanced control, and relief from insomnia, anxiety, and mild depression. The chances are very good that your hot flashes will become significantly less frequent and intense. Use mini-relaxations when you sense hot flashes coming on.

2. *Cognitive restructuring:* Use the four-question method of cognitive restructuring to label and replace distorted negative thoughts about menopause, the aging process, your worth, and your potential for greater meaning, zest, and energy.

3. *Self-nurturance:* Recognize new freedoms and time available during this life transition, and take these opportunities to engage in strictly pleasurable activities and creative pursuits.

4. *Reaching out:* Social support is associated with reduced health risks and greater longevity. Establish or reestablish open communication with your spouse or partner, children, family members, and friends. Use the skills of communication and assertiveness detailed in chapters 7 and 8, respectively. Join volunteer, charity, or other social organizations, because they offer opportunities for fun and meaningful activities, not to mention a sense of community that can be emotionally and physically healing.

5. *Emotional expression:* Uncover areas where you have stifled awareness and expression of emotion due to early upbringing, family constraints, marital tensions, or sheer force of habit. Through visualization, journaling, and if need be, group or individual psychotherapy, develop constructive outlets.

6. *Low-fat diet and regular exercise:* Include extra calcium and the other supplements mentioned, namely magnesium and vitamin D, to prevent osteoporosis. Weight-bearing exercise is essential, including walking, jogging, and, if possible, weight lifting.

As you embark on a mind-body approach to the menopausal transition, be careful to ferret out the true causes of your symptoms or distress. Some may be related to estrogen loss, others will not be. For instance, mood swings may not be caused by hormonal fluctuations but rather by insomnia due to late-night hot flashes. Depression may not be caused by low estrogen but by increased stress due to live-in children or ailing parents. As with conventional medicine, successful mind-body medicine depends on proper diagnosis. Learn to pinpoint the sources of your discomfort, and take proactive steps to heal yourself.

Most of all, reframe your experience of menopause from one of decline to one of newly realized freedoms. The burdens of child rearing recede, leaving more time for strictly pleasurable pursuits. The inconvenience of periods and contraception disappears, which can herald a freer sexuality. The maturity gained through self-realization leads to deepening relationships and expanded potential for creative work. All of these possibilities are made more achievable with mind-body techniques. Post-menopausal zest is quite real for women who take control of their well-being.

Fourteen

• • • • • •

FAT IS A MIND-BODY ISSUE:
EATING DISORDERS

The tyranny of thinness is everywhere: in print ads showing models with sunken cheeks, flat stomachs, and spindly legs; in movies and TV shows whose stars have invariably perfect figures (read, ultra-skinny); in the flurry of self-help books and articles that promise a new formula with which to crack the code of the weight loss mystery. Every month we read about a new "zone," "factor," or miracle medication that will either squash our appetites, jazz our sluggish metabolism, or melt away extra pounds. In this atmosphere, even exercise can become an addiction, with some women overdoing their health club routine to the point of physical collapse.

The tyranny largely affects young women, who internalize these standards of beauty and never shake them, even into middle age. This mind-set can even affect children. We often carry the image of an impossible ideal with us through every phase of our life cycle. We don't feel adequate in our teens and twenties if we think we aren't thin or shapely enough, or our breasts are too small or too big. But we continue to feel inadequate in our late thirties and beyond, because we are no longer in our teens or twenties—the only time our culture says we can fulfill ideals of youthful beauty.

Our culture presents us with images that make it nearly impossible for us to maintain a robust sense of ourselves as attractive and worthy. It is a wonder we don't all have eating disorders. The only reason we don't is that toxic cultural messages can't get under our skin if we have strong inner resources, a family background that bred self-love and self-respect, and a social support system that offers validation. But many of us don't have these resources, or we have vulnerabilities (sometimes extreme) in our backgrounds and are therefore susceptible to the eating disorders of binge eating, bulimia, and anorexia.

These disorders represent only the extreme end of a long continuum of problems with food and weight. I would say that a majority of women have conflicts and pain about eating and body image, difficulties they live and struggle with on a daily basis. Only some of them develop full-blown eating disorders that require not one but a variety of psychological and medical therapies to resolve. This chapter offers mind-body treatments for diagnosed eating disorders, but the remedies apply just as surely to any woman who is troubled by food and weight.

The good news is that these treatments—especially the cognitive therapies—have become an effective first-line approach to eating disorders. In my clinical experience, combining these techniques with other mind-body methods improves the odds of success of medical treatments, should they become necessary.

A whopping 90 percent of diagnosed eating disorders occur among women. Given that society's edicts about thinness and beauty are aimed predominantly at women, this figure should come as no surprise. Eating disorders have more than biological and medical dimensions; they have psychological, social, and cultural dimensions as well.

As if to underscore the creeping effects of family dysfunction and cultural distortions on eating patterns, the actual incidence of medically diagnosed eating disorders is much higher than experts have long estimated. Daniel Goleman, Ph.D., the behavioral sciences writer for the *New York Times*, recently highlighted studies suggesting that anorexia and bulimia are twice as frequent as previously thought, and that "the incidence is increasing steadily." A prime culprit in this rise? The spread of dieting. For women suffering with anorexia, diets can be the first foray into extreme self-denial. For compulsive overeaters, an impossibly restrictive diet can stoke feelings of deprivation that in turn lead to binging. The same phenomenon occurs among bulimics, who then feel so much fear about weight gain that they regurgitate the food they have just ingested.

Women inculcated into the diet mentality live in a state of shame: in their own eyes, they are either "good" or "bad," depending on what they have or have not eaten. This "good/bad" dichotomy is part of the cultural climate of shame, a climate many of them internalized in dysfunctional families where every behavior and physical attribute was fodder for judgment and criticism.

Another reason for this spotlight on eating disorders is that they are a

For Susan-

Some inspiration for you, Always remember, You are a survivor.

The spiritual dimension is your core, your center, your commitment to your value system. It's a very private area of life and a supremely important one. It draws upon the sources that inspire you, uplift you, and tie you to the timeless truths of all humanity, and people do it very differently.

Thoughts are energy. And you can make your world or break your world by your thinking.

Our mind is just like every other part of us; it gets stronger when we challenge it. Happiness must be cultivated. It is like character. It is not a thing to be safely let alone for a moment, or it will run to weeds.

Memories are restatements of our experience. They can't show us anything new or move us beyond where we have been. Imagination, in contrast, expands on experience. It's a creative process, a tool for exploring our potential.

I stop struggling and fighting with my thoughts. I acknowledge them and give myself permission to go beyond them. Thoughts can always be changed.

Habit 1. Be Proactive, means being responsible for your life. You are not a victim of circumstance; you are exactly what you choose to be.

I am in charge of my thoughts. My power comes through the use of my mind. I choose thoughts that are loving and courageous.

We have unlimited choices about what we can think. I notice my thoughts, weeding out those that hurt me and nurturing those that help me.

Changes can begin in this moment. I am willing to change.

I stop all criticism of myself. I am always doing the best I can. I love and protect myself at all times.

I let go of the past and become a "now" person. This moment is a new beginning for me right here and right now.

Every good thought you think is contributing its share to the ultimate result of your life.

When one door closes, another opens; but we often look so long and so regretfully upon the closed door that we do not see the one which has opened for us.

serious threat to women's health. Women with anorexia are at greatest risk; when weight loss is severe, it can compromise every bodily system. (Many people first heard about anorexia after singer Karen Carpenter's untimely death due to complications of her anorectic weight loss.) The mortality rate among women with anorexia is 5 to 8 percent over ten years, primarily from the effects of severe weight loss or suicide. The purging of bulimics can cause life-threatening electrolyte imbalances, dehydration, heart arrhythmias, and a damaged esophagus and throat from vomit acids. Obesity from overeating is a risk factor for diabetes, high blood pressure, heart disease, and certain cancers.

But eating disorders threaten our health in other ways that are less immediately apparent but equally insidious. Stress and self-loathing around food and weight take their toll on both psyche and spirit. In turn, stress and self-loathing can harm our physical health, dragging down our energy, damping down our resilience and our resistance to illness.

In other words, fat is a mind-body issue. Women's self-esteem—a key factor in physical health, as we've seen—is often intertwined with body images that are shaped by families and culture. The constant guilt over weight gain leads many women to feel helpless, angry, and out of control. These states of mind can weaken the immune system and overtax the cardiovascular system.

There is a high incidence of depression, anxiety, and other psychiatric conditions among women with eating disorders. Whether these conditions are a cause or a result remains a contested issue. But many experts believe that depression is probably a cause *and* an effect of eating disorders. Women with low self-esteem and unresolved grief, anger, or sadness—factors that typically add up to depression—are more susceptible to eating disorders. And once a disorder develops, the painful cycle of addictive behavior, shame, and secrecy, not to mention the distressing medical symptoms, puts women at high risk for worsening depression.

The result is extreme emotional suffering and physical wear and tear. Fat is a mind-body issue, food is a health issue, and eating disorders are medical conditions with potentially dire consequences. One-dimensional approaches will not resolve eating disorders, because their causes run deep. Psychiatric drugs can be effective, but as a sole therapy they are usually insufficient. Mind-body medicine offers potential adjunct treatments for eating disorders because it addresses root causes: anxiety, the feeling of being out of control, internalized negative myths about beauty, an aching sense of emptiness, and damaged self-worth.

Mind-Body Treatment for Eating Disorders

Sandra was going through a difficult time in her marriage. Her husband, Gerald, was having to work late hours at his corporate job, and she was alone a great deal in the evenings. Gerald even brought work home on weekends, and she was often left to fend for herself. Sandra's health habits were generally good; she tended to eat low-fat, high-complex-carbohydrate meals. But Gerald's long absences led her to feel bored and frustrated, so she began to fall back on old habits of binging in front of the TV. Sandra would scarf down a whole bag of potato chips or an entire coffee cake in one evening. Her husband liked to nosh when he was home, so there was always junk food in the cupboards. Sandra lost control of her eating habits during this period, until she was eighty pounds heavier than her "ideal" weight on body charts.

As Sandra gained weight, her self-esteem, plummeted and she began to feel even more socially isolated. The couple had no children, and many of her friends were busy with their young babies. When she came to see me, she was immensely frustrated, unable to lose weight, and out of control.

The crux of Sandra's problem was diminishing self-esteem, centering around her weight. To make matters worse, every time she binged she berated herself, which drove down her self-regard even further. I taught Sandra to elicit the relaxation response, and she uses this practice to ease her anxieties. And rather than focusing relentlessly on weight loss, I targeted Sandra's key cognitive distortion: that her weight and body shape were the sole measures of her worth as a human being.

Using cognitive restructuring, Sandra was able to shift her focus away from weight. What made her feel worthwhile? What brought meaning into her life? Wasn't there more to her existence than her body image? Sandra saw that emptiness, loneliness, and fears about her marriage were root causes of her overeating, and she began to let herself off the hook about the addictive nature of her binging. But she had to find better ways to fill her void than with bags of chips and cookies.

Moving from insight to action, Sandra decided to do something that reminded her of her worth on other levels. She joined a local Big Sisters organization, and was paired with a twelve-year-old teenager, Felice. They got along famously. The young girl looked up to Sandra, and the relationship helped to heal Sandra's loneliness. It was a bond that called upon Sandra's compassion, wisdom, and humor—qualities she'd practically forgotten she possessed during the previous months of boredom and obsession about food and weight. Her self-esteem improved, and so did her marriage to Gerald. He was still not sufficiently present, but Sandra no longer spent those evenings and weekend afternoons feeling miserable and overeating.

Having rediscovered her sense of self, Sandra gradually gained control of her eating patterns. Using the "eating transitions" approach described in chapter 9, Sandra started to lose weight. (Once in a while she binged, but the frequency of these episodes declined markedly.) By the time we finished working together, Sandra had lost half of the weight she hoped to lose and was continuing to take off pounds.

Sandra's story exemplifies a mind-body approach to an eating disorder, in this case, binge eating (the current medical term for severe overeating). Relaxation and cognitive techniques helped Sandra gain awareness of her behavior and its causes, and to take proactive steps to address them. Perhaps antidepressants would have helped Sandra, but what if she had been given a prescription and no other therapeutic help? Would she have developed new coping skills? Would she have found out why she binged? Would she have joined Big Sisters and developed a relationship with a young girl who needed her help? I am in favor of medical treatment for eating disorders when deemed appropriate, but recent studies confirm the effectiveness of various forms of psychological therapy alone or in combination with anti-depressant medication.

CBT and Other Psychological Therapies

Cognitive-behavioral therapy (CBT, for short) is now considered a first-line treatment of choice for eating disorders, especially bulimia. Therapists who practice CBT for eating disorders teach their patients cognitive restructuring, an awareness of eating "triggers," and practical skills they can use to cope more effectively with stress. Dr. Stewart Agras, director of the Eating Disorders Program at Stanford University Medical School, has found that CBT helps about 65 percent of bulimics to stop binging and purging. (This figure is reflected in study after study.) In controlled trials, CBT has also been found to be more effective than antidepressant drugs, though recent evidence suggests that CBT combined with drugs may be slightly better than CBT alone.

Research has revealed that other psychological treatments can be as effective as CBT in the treatment of bulimia. So-called interpersonal therapy focuses on a patient's relationships and helps her identify difficulties—such as fears of rejection, social isolation, and relationship conflicts—that underlie eating disorders. Unlike CBT, interpersonal therapy does not focus directly on issues of eating and body image, but rather helps women to explore feelings that drive their disorders and to develop workable strategies for positive change in their relationships. Though its effectiveness in treating bulimia is less well studied, leading experts have noted that both cognitive and interpersonal therapies show effectiveness in the treatment of binge eating and anorexia.

Cognitive-behavioral therapy for eating disorders involves several key components:

- Self-monitoring helps patients recognize physical and emotional triggers of binging or refusal to eat. To better pinpoint these triggers, patients often keep a diary of eating disorder episodes.
- By developing effective coping strategies, patients learn better ways to manage frustration, anger, and powerlessness.
- Assertiveness skills help patients change or resolve unhappy relationships.
- Cognitive restructuring helps patients deal with distorted thoughts about food, eating, weight, and body image, and other negative "tapes" that fuel stress and helplessness in everyday life.

Typically, a course of cognitive-behavioral therapy will run for twenty sessions. For patients who suffer from deep-seated emotional problems or clinical depression, dysfunctional families, or abusive relationships, individual or group psychotherapy may be considered as a longer-term treatment, perhaps in addition to CBT. If you are experiencing any of these symptoms or conditions, consult a mental health professional, since they require proper diagnosis, treatment, and follow-up.

An Integrated Mind-Body Approach to Eating Disorders

In my own work with women with eating disorders, I have applied principles of CBT and interpersonal psychotherapy, along with other mind-body techniques. I first used this approach during my postdoctoral fellowship at Children's Hospital in Boston, where I worked with young women hospitalized for anorexia. These were patients who, due to a host of psychological factors, dreaded every meal. Often, the only way they knew how to maintain some sense of control—albeit an unhealthy one—was to refuse to eat enough food, or even to eat at all. In the hospital, they were obliged to eat scheduled meals. Given their rising anxiety levels as the time for meals approached, I taught them to elicit the relaxation response about twenty minutes before each meal. Frequently, this practice calmed them down sufficiently to make eating a far less upsetting experience. Relaxation timed in this manner became an extremely useful part of their therapy.

Though it remains largely untested, an integrated mind-body approach to eating disorders makes common sense, since many of its features come from the two methods that *have* been proven to work—CBT and interpersonal therapy. In addition, I use relaxation in a targeted fashion to help women cultivate healthy control, the loss of which is a key factor and feature in eating disorders.

Most relaxation techniques can be used by those of you with eating disorders, although some may prefer to bypass body-focused methods such as progressive muscle relaxation (PMR), autogenic training, or body scan. Paying too much attention to your body parts may exacerbate your tendency to judge yourself. If so, rely on meditation, mindfulness, or guided imagery. However, trust your intuition. Some women in the process of healing their eating disorder may use body scan, for example, to tune in to their bodies with gentleness and compassion.

Eating disorders are often associated with shallow breathing. The cultural bugaboo about weight can cause you to chronically contract your abdominal muscles, which makes it nearly impossible to breathe correctly! If you can't breathe, you can't relax—your brain receives messages that you are oxygen-starved, and your anxiety levels rise even if you don't know it. *The solution is to shift from shallow chest breathing to deep abdominal breathing whenever you practice relaxation.* Use the breath focus (chapter 3) and the mini-relaxations (chapter 4) on a regular basis. In the privacy of your own room, allow your stomach to rise and fall, knowing that life-giving oxygen is reaching into the bottom of your lungs.

My philosophy is simple: eating disorders are multileveled problems that require multileveled solutions. Each method I employ deals, in some fashion, with common precipitating factors: an aching emptiness, unmet needs for love and support, and a loss of control that patients desperately try to rectify with large quantities of food or dangerous forms of self-restraint.

Recognizing the emotional triggers for binging or self-denial is a pivotal aspect of my work with these women. Sometimes I observe very consistent patterns, which I point out to patients, encouraging them to become aware themselves. Take, for example, the woman who binges every time her mother calls. Or the woman who binges and then purges after arguments with her husband. Or the woman who stops eating every time she is neglected or hurt by an abusive boyfriend. Awareness of these triggers is often the first phase of a healing process.

The next, proactive phase is to make outer changes in relationships, and inner changes toward healthy control, self-acceptance, and peace of mind. The woman who finally realizes that she binges every time her mother calls can do it differently next time. After a stressful phone conversation, she can stop, take a deep breath, and realize what is happening to her. The urge to run to the fridge may pass when awareness intercedes in its place. Then, she can do a mini-relaxation to generate inner calm and control. Next, she can turn to her partner or call a friend and talk about why the phone call was unpleasant. Finally, with her own insights or with the help of a therapist, she can find out whether a different approach with her mother would reduce her own tensions. Does she need to be tougher with Mom? More assertive? Less reactive and furious? Kinder? Positive change in the mother-daughter relationship—which is often a particular problem for women with eating disorders—may alleviate the conditions that trigger episodes.

Finding a safe place to express positive and negative emotions—be it a journal, a therapist's office, or both—is also crucial. Women can stop using food to squelch emotion when they have healthier outlets. Once that happens, they can actually *enjoy* food without having to overindulge.

I also encourage women with eating disorders to nurture themselves in every way possible, since their eating patterns are unsuccessful attempts to fill their own emotional voids. They can care for themselves and give themselves pleasure in other, more genuinely satisfying ways.

In the following sections, I will show how these mind-body methods can be used to treat the three main eating disorders—overeating, bulimia, and anorexia. What if you can't tell whether you have a full-blown disorder or a less threatening, more typical problem with over- or undereating? In each of these upcoming sections, I present guidelines for you to determine whether you should seek professional help. If you have any doubts, err on the side of caution and call your physician for a consultation and referral to a mental health professional. Often, when we are suffering with a serious condition, we are simply and innocently unaware of its severity.

Overeating and Binge-Eating Disorder

Many women struggle with overeating and the obesity that often results. Those who regularly and repeatedly eat large amounts of food within fairly short stretches of time (an hour or two), and who feel they lose control during these episodes, may have binge-eating disorder. The line between typical overeating and binge-eating disorder can be fuzzy, but look out for these additional signs of the actual disorder:

- Eating more rapidly than normal
- Eating large amounts when not physically hungry
- Eating until uncomfortably full
- Eating alone out of embarrassment
- Feeling disgusted, depressed, and guilty over one's eating
- Binging, on average, at least two days a week for six months

Use these signs as guidance regarding your status, but you don't have to fulfill all these criteria to have an eating disorder. Moreover, even if you don't "qualify" for this diagnosis, you may still have an eating problem that deserves early attention, lest it become worse and develop into a disorder.

Based on my own experience with patients, here is a brief overview of a mind-body program to embark upon if you overeat or binge regularly. Consider taking action in these seven areas:

1. Identify emotional triggers that precede binges, such as boredom, anxiety, and other emotional reactions to stress, pain, or difficult relationships.
2. Identify cognitive distortions—automatic negative thoughts that upset you, depress you, or drag you down. These thoughts can involve eating, weight, or other realms of everyday life, including frustrating relationships, work pressures, or creative blocks.
3. Devise assertive actions you can take to change conditions that trigger your eating episodes. Take a hard look at your relationships, and find out whether you need to communicate your needs and rights more clearly and forcefully.
4. Practice the relaxation response and mini-relaxations to calm feelings of anxiety, helplessness, or hostility that prompt you to overeat.
5. If grief, fear, or anger is at the root of your overeating, use journaling to explore and express these feelings.
6. Substitute pleasurable, self-nurturing activities for overeating or binging.
7. Use the "eating transitions" approach (chapter 9) to slowly change your diet to one that is healthier and more balanced. Don't fall into the trap of feeling guilty over supposed transgressions, because this

guilt will cause you to abandon all efforts to eat more healthfully. Remember, this is not a diet and you are not in food prison! Your goal should not be thinness, but rather healthy self-nourishment. If you approach overeating this way, your motivation to change will stem from self-love, not self-loathing. And most women who adopt this approach benefit from a fortuitous side effect—a gradual loss of pounds that tend to stay off.

One of my patients, Paula, suffered with chronic pain from fibromyalgia. She was also a binge eater. She had problems with overeating before, but they only got worse as her chronic pain condition dragged on, causing her to feel ever more powerless and miserable. Through cognitive work, Paula saw clearly how binging made matters worse. "I came to the realization that I was hurting myself with food," says Paula. "Chronic pain was hard enough. Eating over it, and gaining weight, only doubled my suffering."

Overeating exacerbates unhappiness for women in any stressful situation, be it chronic pain or other illnesses, divorce, the loss of a job, troubles in a marriage, children who act out, or financial problems. Paula turned a corner when she decided to change her eating patterns. "I felt like I had too little control over my pain," she commented. "But how I dealt with food *was* in my hands. I could do a lot more about that."

What Paula did was to elicit the relaxation response to calm herself down when her pain or other stressors got the best of her. Perhaps the most useful method I taught her was to substitute self-nurturing behaviors for overeating whenever anxiety would strike. "I wrote a list of good things I could do for myself and pasted it on my refrigerator," says Paula. "I made sure I did something on that list every day." A year later, Paula's list is still there, and she makes checks by the self-nurturing suggestions every time she carries one out. Here are a few examples from Paula's list:

- Cook a healthy home meal rather than going next door to the pizza place.
- Buy flowers for myself.
- Have lunch out with a good friend.
- Shop at a health food store for healthy goodies.
- Get a face mask and manicure at my favorite salon.
- Go to my health club for exercise.
- Take a bath mindfully.
- Treat myself to relaxing imagery tapes.

Paula recently told me that she and her husband were going on an overseas vacation as a treat for themselves on their fifth anniversary. After several years of chronic pain, Paula feels that she deserves this break, even though it will be rather costly. But the vacation is part of her strategy of self-nurturance, a strategy that not only keeps her spirits afloat, it prevents her from lapsing into overeating.

Over the course of several months, Paula took off fifteen pounds, and she continues slowly to lose weight. She feels lighter, more energetic, and better about herself. She also feels better able to manage the pain of fibromyalgia.

As in Paula's case, self-nurturance can be used as a behavioral technique. Why not do something nice for yourself instead of something—like binging—that only yields shame, self-doubt, and powerlessness?

If you overeat or have a binge-eating disorder, follow the seven suggestions listed on page 319. Find the relaxation technique that works best for you. Identify and practice your own list of self-nurturing behaviors. Find out what past events, family dynamics, and current relationships are at the root of your addictive behaviors. Use journaling to uncover these emotions, events, and relationships, but remember that writing should only be an adjunct to psychotherapy for serious eating disorders.

Studies have shown that women with eating disorders are, in fact, more likely to have a past history of emotional, physical, or sexual abuse. In the case of sexual abuse, many women overeat with the unconscious intent of making themselves as unattractive as possible to men. Their aversion to men's sexual interest is easily understood once the real history is unearthed. This pattern won't change unless or until a therapeutic process allows for exploration and healing. If you think that early or recent abuse is an underlying cause of your binging and overweight, consult a psychotherapist trained in the treatment of eating disorders.

Bulimia

*B*ulimia nervosa, as it is medically known, is the condition of binging followed by purging. As with binge eaters, bulimics ingest excessive amounts of food in short time periods (an hour or two), and experience a lack of control over their eating during these episodes. Such episodes are followed by purging (self-induced vomiting) that occurs at least twice a week for three months. In their desperate efforts to prevent even the slightest weight gain, bulimic individuals also misuse laxatives, diuretics, fasting regimens, or excessive exercise.

Bulimia has received a great deal of publicity since the early 1980s, and celebrity admissions—most notably Princess Diana's—have brought the disorder to the forefront of public consciousness. In Diana's case, the nature of bulimic suffering is all too clear: By her own acknowledgment, a profound despair about personal relations—characterized by a sense of betrayal and powerlessness—is at the core of her condition. Her self-destructive behavior, shrouded in shame and secrecy, has nevertheless barely concealed her cry for help. This is quite typical of bulimics, whose disorder is often invisible to the outside world until their cover is somehow blown. Though some have been shocked, Princess Diana appears to have done a great service with her recent admissions, and with her explanations of how and why women can become bulimic. Perhaps this will lead to greater empathy and support for women with eating disorders, and to more readily available treatments.

As I've emphasized, cognitive-behavioral therapies have a fine track record for treating bulimia, and so do interpersonal therapies. As I do with binge eaters, I treat bulimic patients by combining elements of CBT and interpersonal therapy with mind-body methods, most especially relaxation. For the most part, once they can stop binging they have less need to purge and their bulimic condition subsides. Thus, if you suffer with bulimia, I strongly recommend the same seven steps listed on page 319 for the treatment of binge eating. Taken together, these steps represent a comprehensive mind-body approach to bulimia.

Bulimics suffer with negative thoughts about body image. The obsessive need to binge to fill an inner emptiness is matched by an equally obsessive need to keep off weight, as though every additional pound were a symbol of worthlessness. A typical negative tape loop, "I'm fat," is often an outright distortion among bulimic women. If subject to such thoughts, you can be helped to recognize that you are not overweight, or not as overweight as you believe. Also, the deeper thought or feeling is generally "I'm disgusting" or "I'm worthless." These beliefs can be restructured once you accept, in your heart, that body shape cannot and should not be the sum and substance of your self-image.

Given today's cultural standards, if everyone's sense of self was entirely dependent on body shape, 95 percent of us would walk around filled with self-loathing. From a cognitive perspective, the solution is to focus intently on all our strengths as women. We can ask ourselves: Are we good partners? Wives? Mothers? Friends? Professionals? Workers? Artists? Are we wise? Compassionate? Creative? Helpful? Decisive? Courageous? We need to find areas in which we feel good about ourselves, or areas where we have the power to make changes that enable us to feel good about ourselves. Once we do, the issue of fat falls into proper perspective. Yes, our figure matters to us. But, as an aspect of self, it is only one aspect of a much larger whole. We often forget that our essence has more to do with soul than with size or shape.

In many cases, the inner voice of the bulimic—the one that screams invectives at her for eating too much and fears gaining those dreaded extra pounds—belongs to someone in the past or present. Often it is the woman's partner or mother.

One of my bulimic patients, Cynthia, thirty-three, was an attractive, successful, well-to-do professional. Yet she had binged and purged on and off since she was a teenager. Now her bulimia was getting worse, and her esophagus was becoming damaged from purging. When Cynthia came to see me, she was scared and out of control. But I also recognized that her meticulous and scrupulously honest personality could be a positive factor in her struggle to overcome bulimia.

I taught Cynthia a variety of relaxation techniques to quiet her anxieties, and then made her a deal. She would agree to sit down for a twenty-minute relaxation practice every time she had the urge to binge/purge. Then, after eliciting the relaxation response, she was free to decide whether or not she would binge. To seal the deal, we would both sign our names to an actual written contract. Cynthia agreed. I filed the original, and she took home a copy.

The contract worked. For the most part, Cynthia's relaxation practice would relieve her tensions enough to help her resist binging. The fact that the contract was not compulsory—that she had a choice in the matter— vastly reduced the elements of guilt and shame that only reinforce addictive behavior. Indeed, once in a while Cynthia did go ahead and binge. But her relaxation practice made it genuinely easier for her to choose to abstain. Over time, she built up an authentic mastery over her eating patterns. When she no longer binged, she had no reason to purge and her bulimia was finally under control.

But her treatment did not begin and end with our relaxation contract. To maintain her gains, Cynthia had to uncover factors that had caused and perpetuated her bulimia. In our cognitive work together, it became clear that her binging episodes were mostly triggered by conflicts with her five-year-old daughter. Whenever the daughter would act out or express anger, Cynthia took it to mean that she was a lousy mother. I helped her realize that children who *never* act out toward their parents will never gain their autonomy. Some misbehavior and anger is to be expected as part of the normal process of a child's growth and development.

With further exploration, it became clear that Cynthia had an exceedingly fraught relationship with her mother, in both the past and the present. Her readiness to believe she was a lousy mother was an outgrowth of her tremendous rage toward her own mother. Since she secretly harbored this anger toward her own mother, she unconsciously assumed that her daughter must also harbor such ill will. From then on, Cynthia kept a journal of her feelings, focusing on her troubled relationship with her mother. Her notebook became a cauldron into which she could pour her red-hot rage. She remembered her mother's comments on her "chubbiness" as a child and preteenager, and how deeply they wounded her. Her bulimia had originated with these early wounds. Cynthia's case demonstrates the efficacy of a comprehensive mind-body treatment for women with bulimia. Relaxation addresses the anxieties and cognitive restructuring opens the door to deeper levels of insight. Therapy is absolutely necessary to explore early or present-day familial sources of bulimia, but there is much you can do right now to promote your own healing process.

Anorexia

Certain telltale signs and symptoms are apparent in women—especially teenagers and young women—who suffer from anorexia nervosa.

- Refusal to maintain body weight at or above a minimal normal weight for your age and height
- Weight loss leading to maintenance of a body weight that is 85 percent or less of what would be expected
- A failure to make expected weight gain during a period of growth, again resulting in a body weight that is 85 percent or less of what would be expected
- Even when already underweight, an intense fear of weight gain or fat
- A disturbance in the way you experience your body weight or shape (e.g., you think you are fat when in fact you are too thin)
- Self-evaluation influenced far too much by body weight and shape

Certain physical and psychological factors are apparent in women suffering from anorexia: the absence of three or more consecutive periods in women who've started menstruating, intolerance of cold, complaints of feeling bloated after normal-sized meals, irritability or outright depression, fatigue, or a tendency to bruise easily. Of course, the most obvious physical factor is increasing skinniness, though some women hide their stick-thin figures under baggy, bulky clothing.

As mentioned, anorexia can have life-threatening medical consequences, including severe heart problems. Women who do not get relatively early treatment may end up in the hospital. A combination of inpatient and outpatient treatment is often required to turn around this disorder. In the hospital, doctors can control the environment and provide the nutrition, calories, and support needed for weight gain. Antidepressant medications can play an important role in the treatment of anorexia, because many patients are severely depressed. The "chicken or the egg" question about whether depression is a cause or a result of anorexia becomes irrelevant when a patient's distress is a factor in her refusal to nourish herself. In these instances, psychotherapy, medication, and caring support are all needed right away.

When I worked with young anorexic patients at Children's Hospital, one seventeen-year-old, Helene, exemplified many of the patterns one sees repeatedly among anorexic patients. She was a high-achieving student who ran the school newspaper and participated in every extracurricular committee in sight. A year or two earlier she had decided that she was vastly overweight and went on a diet that never stopped. She was actually proud of the fact that she weighed eighty pounds. Helene was finally admitted to the hospital because she was in denial regarding her condition and its threat to her health and well-being.

When I sat and talked with Helene, I realized that she did not seem terribly invested in getting better. She was gripped by her desire to be ultra-thin and by her distorted body image. As with most anorexics, the refusal to eat is a misguided attempt to exert control, and Helene certainly did not like feeling out of control. But she admitted that her intense anxiety before each meal *also* made her feel out of control, and I recognized this as a positive sign. I offered her several relaxation tapes, letting her know that she could reduce her own anxiety by practicing relaxation twenty minutes before each meal.

It wasn't an instant cure, but Helene gradually became able to eat without such intense anxiety. She remained an inpatient for over a month, then went home for weekends, a transitionary period until she was discharged completely. During this time, she took the relaxation tapes home with her, and she used them consistently. Over the next year, Helene was able to gain enough weight to get herself out of the danger zone. She stabilized her eating habits and her weight at a reasonable level, while continuing supportive therapy on an outpatient basis.

With Helene and anorexic patients like her, I have also used cognitive therapy to deal with thoughts and emotions that drive their behavior. Typical thought constructs among anorexics include "Fat makes me ugly," "Being thin gives me power and control," and "Boys will like me only if I am thin." We can find out together where these ideas come from. Typically, there is a confluence of messages from their families, peers, and the broader culture that leads them to fear an extra ounce of fat. We talk about what is "normal" and "healthy," how we need some fat on our bodies to survive and stay healthy.

Here again, this cognitive exploration can open doors to deeper awareness, since family issues often reside at the core of anorexia. Some patients get direct messages from parents that they must be perfect in every way, including the realm of the body, which requires that they maintain modelesque proportions. It is no wonder that fat becomes an enemy for these young women.

Many want to retain a "little girl" body. They often dread the growth of breasts, the appearance of curves, and the onset of menstruation, all of which represent the sexual maturation process—coming into womanhood. The reasons for these fears are unique to each individual, but a fair number of anorexic women have been sexually abused. These patients may associate sexuality with pain and suffering, and they wish, unconsciously, to forestall their own sexual development. Other girls fear growing up and taking on greater responsibilities, being more like the mothers toward whom they feel ambivalence or hostility, or having to live up to impossible standards of perfection laid down in their families or school environments.

Given the complex of causes, anorexic patients require psychotherapy in addition to mind-body techniques, coping skills, and medical treatment. Family therapy is also important for many women with anorexia. The entire family may suffer when one member is in trouble, and family treatment can be a positive educational process for both the patient and her parents and siblings. It also offers an opportunity to explore emotions and conflicts that have been shrouded in secrecy. Indeed, anorexia, and other eating disorders, can sometimes be a catalyst for families to confront their patterns, to open new lines of communication, and to heal wounds that have been festering for years or decades.

♦ ♦ ♦

Eating disorders may be psychiatric conditions, but it should not be forgotten that they are also cries for help. Medications should only be part of an overall treatment plan. The first step toward healing is to acknowledge your disorder and seek help, remembering that there is reason for optimism: various therapies have been proven effective, and mind-body medicine offers new ways to exert personal authority in your life. You don't need to binge, purge, or starve yourself to feel in control. You may need to change how you cope with stress, how you relate to your family, and how you think about beauty and sexual identity. Let your disorder be a spur to deeper transformations that elevate your quality of life and health.

Fifteen

✦ ✦ ✦ ✦

FROM TRAUMA TO TRANSFORMATION: BREAST AND GYNECOLOGIC CANCERS

Michael Lerner, head of the Commonweal Cancer Help Program in northern California, compares the experience of being diagnosed with cancer to being thrown out of a helicopter over a guerrilla war zone with a parachute, but with no compass, no weapons, no map, and no training in survival. A woman diagnosed with breast or gynecologic cancer is rarely prepared for this odyssey. Before she can fully comprehend the diagnosis, she may be scheduled for surgery, with chemotherapy, radiation, or hormone treatments soon to follow. Typically, she is an active, healthy person who suddenly faces an array of side effects. Without some kind of survival training—in the form of education, therapy, coping skills, or all three—this is no easy terrain.

One woman with breast cancer described the diagnosis and its aftermath as an emotional tidal wave, an image that captures what many patients experience. With that first wave comes shock, often followed by surges of fear and sadness. These stormy seas are hard to navigate, but through it all, she must stay levelheaded enough to make tough decisions. She must procure information from doctors, decipher complex medical concepts, and garner second opinions. She may have to choose among a variety of treatment options, knowing that her choices could influence her long-term health. Partners and children and parents are scared, too, and she must find a balance between their needs and her own. Rarely does the world of medicine ease this entire process, and women must often fight for information and support.

Given these hard realities, how can a woman diagnosed with cancer thrive and survive? How can she participate in her own recovery? Does her active involvement really make a difference?

In the past decade, we have learned that women with cancer can participate in their own recovery. They can thrive in the face of immensely trying circumstances, and their active involvement can make a difference in their recovery. When women with breast or gynecologic cancers are engaged in their own healing process, they not only cope better, they may strengthen their biological defense against cancer.

Mind-body medicine for cancer is not a cure, but it is an empowering approach that helps women with every aspect of healing—physical, emotional, and spiritual. It offers tools and skills that enable many women to navigate that perilous terrain known as cancer.

At the Deaconess Hospital, I see women with breast and gynecologic cancers. The latter category includes ovarian, uterine, vaginal, and cervical cancers. I usually treat them on an individual basis, although some cancer patients have participated in my general mind-body groups. (My colleague at the Deaconess Hospital, Ann Webster, Ph.D., runs groups specifically for cancer patients and for AIDS patients.) I teach these patients all of the mind-body methods at the core of this book, but I tailor them for the realities of cancer and its treatment.

Joyce had recently been divorced when her doctor broke the news: "You have breast cancer and it has spread to your lymph nodes." Joyce felt out of control before this diagnosis; afterward, she was spinning in all directions. Convinced she was going to die, she came to me for individual sessions. Initially, I taught her relaxation techniques and mini-relaxations to better manage the anxieties and side effects associated with surgery and chemotherapy. Then we addressed Joyce's desire to make comprehensive changes in her life. She was ready to jettison her unsatisfying relationships and sedentary lifestyle. Beneath her desperation, I sensed an ardent yearning to live. I encouraged Joyce to channel her fierce determination and energy into achievable goals.

Most of all, Joyce wanted to quit smoking. It was her most stubborn habit, one she felt could only compromise her efforts to get well. However, attempting such a major lifestyle modification and failing would probably reinforce her sense of helplessness. I encouraged her to master simple things first, such as taking a mindful walk each day. Then she moved on to the next behavioral or emotional challenge. With each new modification, Joyce's confidence grew, until she came to believe that she could influence her own recovery. She began asking for support from friends and family, accepting more than she'd been willing to in the past. She searched for and found joy in fleeting moments with friends, at work, in nature.

If quitting cigarettes had been her first task, Joyce might have failed and given up all efforts to change. But the other changes gradually strengthened her self-assurance, making it possible for her to take on the smoking challenge. (Over the long haul, addictive behaviors are impossible to change unless you find a better way to manage stress.) Eventually, she did quit smoking. Her triumph over tobacco was a turning point, but Joyce came to feel that her newfound capacity for pleasure and meaning—an unexpected victory—was even more significant. It helped her to endure the stress of cancer and the uncertainty of her future. Today, Joyce is a cancer survivor, five years after her doctor's grim prognosis.

Mind-body medicine can assist women through every stage of coping with cancer, from the shock of diagnosis to the decisions about treatment; through surgery and adjunct therapies such as chemotherapy and radiation; through the side effects of treatment and the aftermath—living life fully after cancer. There has been much controversy about whether mind-body therapies can promote cures or lengthen the life span of cancer patients, and I will address this controversy shortly. But the medical world and the general public hardly realize that mind-body medicine has been scientifically proven to enhance the quality of life of cancer patients, especially as they undergo medical treatments.

Some of the most impressive data involve the use of mind-body techniques to relieve pain and the side effects of treatment. William Redd, Ph.D., of Memorial Sloan-Kettering Cancer Center in New York, a leading expert in the field, points out that 25 to 65 percent of patients in chemotherapy report nausea in anticipation of treatment. Progressive relaxation, imagery, hypnosis, and cognitive approaches can relieve this anticipatory nausea and vomiting. In Dr. Redd's review of recent studies, he wrote, "The consistency of the positive results obtained in the group of studies just reviewed is remarkable, because clinically significant reductions in anticipatory nausea and vomiting were achieved despite wide variations in the type of cancer, stage of disease, and chemotherapy protocol." My colleague Ann Webster has also shown that relaxation and other mind-body techniques relieve anticipatory nausea and vomiting.

Although there are fewer studies on the use of mind-body methods for nausea and vomiting that occur after treatment, one team of researchers reports positive results. T. G. Burnish and his colleagues found that patients using relaxation and distraction techniques experienced significant reductions in nausea. Studies have also shown that mind-body methods can:

- Relieve pain associated with cancer and its treatment
- Promote normal food consumption and weight gain among cancer patients
- Reduce insomnia in people with cancer
- Alleviate anxiety in children undergoing cancer treatment
- Lessen fear and apprehension among patients undergoing painful diagnostic and treatment procedures

Women must often deal with particular adverse effects from their medical treatment. Some women with breast cancer will lose a breast to mastectomy, while others who have gynecologic cancer may lose their ovaries, uterus, or both. Mastectomies and hysterectomies may take a toll on women's sexual identity, libido, and self-esteem. In premenopausal women, the surgical loss of ovaries, or the loss of ovarian function due to chemotherapy, leads to instant artificial menopause. These women are suddenly subject to hot flashes, night sweats, vaginal drying, and other unnerving symptoms. Many of them cannot take hormone replacement pills for their symptoms because they may pose an additional risk for recurrent cancer. What are these women to do? Mind-body medicine offers a myriad of options.

Take the case of tamoxifen, a hormonal treatment for breast cancer. Tamoxifen is an estrogen blocker proven effective in the treatment of postmenopausal patients, and now being tested in premenopausal patients. Approximately half of the women taking tamoxifen experience hot flashes. Recently, my colleagues and I wanted to find out if women stuck in this bind could benefit from the relaxation response.

We recruited a group of breast cancer patients, all taking tamoxifen, who were experiencing significant hot flashes as a result of their treatment. Half of them were taught to elicit the relaxation response, while the other half continued to monitor their hot flashes but were not taught relaxation. After one month, the women doing relaxation experienced a 42 percent reduction in the frequency of tamoxifen-induced hot flashes, while there was no significant change among women in the control group. We also found that women doing relaxation had a decrease in the intensity of hot flashes, while women in the control group actually experienced an increase in hot flash intensity.

Our study offers evidence that mind-body medicine can help breast cancer patients with hot flashes, an aggravating symptom of hormone treatment that, for many patients, cannot be reliably relieved in any other fashion.

We are learning that mind-body medicine offers the most powerful tools currently available to help cancer patients with their symptoms, which include pain, the side effects of treatment, nagging fears, debilitating depression, and the feeling that their lives and bodies are somehow not in their own hands.

In Ann Webster's groups at the Deaconess Hospital, she empowers men and women with cancer to take control of their health through active involvement in every phase of treatment and recovery. Mind-body techniques are central to her work with cancer patients. Frequently, I will see patients with breast or gynecologic cancer soon after they are diagnosed, to help them get through the initial shock and to offer them hopeful options for coping with the struggle ahead. Soon thereafter, many of these patients enter Dr. Webster's group, ready to embark on a learning process that turns cancer from a nightmare into an opportunity for growth. It is a tremendous inspiration to observe the progress of cancer patients in my practice and in Dr. Webster's mind-body groups.

Both Dr. Webster and I have worked closely with oncologists and surgeons at the New England Deaconess Hospital and at several other Boston hospitals affiliated with Harvard Medical School. Until recently, Dixie Mills, M.D., was a breast surgeon at the Deaconess Hospital, where she collaborated closely with us. Dr. Mills would frequently walk one of her recently diagnosed breast cancer patients directly over to our offices down the corridor. Usually one of us was immediately available to meet with the patient, who, as you might imagine, was almost always distraught.

It was Dr. Mills's philosophy (and ours) that women just told that they had cancer should not be sent home reeling after a discussion of medical treatment plans. Either Dr. Webster or I would sit down with the patient and describe her options for self-care. We let her know that Dr. Mills and other cancer specialists would be providing the best possible medical treatment for her disease, and we would be providing mind-body methods she could use to strengthen her own resources for recovery. This message—delivered within hours of a startling diagnosis—laid the groundwork for hope and empowerment.

Though Dr. Mills has moved to a women's health practice in Yarmouth,

Maine (Women to Women, headed by Christiane Northrup, M.D.), we continue to collaborate with cancer specialists and to offer patients our methods and our message about self-care. In our meetings with each patient, we provide this framework only after we have listened to her, whether she wishes to express her fears and feelings or discuss her thoughts about treatment. We let her know that we respect her singular needs and responses. The vast majority of women respond warmly to this approach, because they appreciate the support we offer, they are grateful for the acknowledgment of their uniqueness, and they avidly want to be engaged in their own recovery process.

What does it mean to be engaged in the recovery process? It means that the patient informs herself about her treatment alternatives, and she makes conscious decisions along with her physician and cancer specialists. It means that she trusts and relies upon her doctors, but she *also* trusts and relies upon her own capacities for emotional and physical healing. It means that, despite her fears and doubts, she can find something meaningful in the crisis of cancer and her brush with mortality. She becomes emotionally and perhaps spiritually engaged in a process of self-awareness—discovering for herself what it means to be fully alive.

There is no question but that women who become engaged in their own recovery can improve their quality of life. However, another question is more difficult to answer: Can being engaged in your own recovery help you to live longer?

Cancer and the Mind-Body Link

*F*ifteen years ago, a psychiatrist at Stanford University School of Medicine, David Spiegel, M.D., had a mission. Dr. Spiegel believed that group therapy and other mind-body approaches could definitely enable cancer patients to cope more effectively with their illness. He just as surely believed that group therapy could *not* help cancer patients to recover physically or to live longer. He was extremely skeptical of the claims of some holistic practitioners who thought that psychological treatments could, in some instances, promote physical recovery in people with cancer. So Spiegel—a rigorous and respected researcher—decided to initiate a study that demonstrated the benefits *and* debunked the myths about mind-body treatment for cancer.

Dr. Spiegel recruited eighty-six women with advanced, metastatic breast cancer, all of whom received similar medical treatment. But half of them were randomly assigned to Spiegel's group therapy program, while the other half received only medical care. After ten years, Spiegel and his colleagues discovered that not only did the women in therapy cope more effectively, they also lived *twice* as long as those who did not participate in therapy. Metastatic breast cancer carries a grave prognosis, and only three women were alive after ten years. But all three had been in the therapy group.

"We were shocked at the magnitude of the effect," said Dr. Spiegel after the results were published. "We expected no biological effect from the psychological one." The findings caused Spiegel to change his attitude. Though he is careful not to recommend mind-body treatments as potential cures for cancer, he believes that his study revealed a mind-body link in cancer. When cancer patients join a group that provides support and healthy coping strategies, the benefits may extend to the body, strengthening their resistance and enhancing their recovery.

In 1989, Dr. Spiegel's results were published in the prestigious British medical journal *The Lancet*, which also published an editorial praising his scientific methods. Soon, leading critics in mainstream medicine acknowledged that Spiegel's study was something of a breakthrough.

What, exactly, went on in Dr. Spiegel's groups that may have helped women with advanced breast cancer to live longer? Here are the elements:

- Patients received the social support of other women with the same illness, women who could understand their unique suffering.
- The group offered a safe place in which to share emotions such as grief, fear, and anger. "One role of the group," wrote Spiegel in his *Lancet* paper, "might have been to provide a place to belong and to express feelings."
- Each patient was taught self-hypnosis and other relaxation techniques to control pain.
- The women were encouraged by the therapist (a psychiatrist or social worker) to be more assertive with doctors and oncologists.
- The therapist enabled women to openly discuss and master fears of dying. Women were able to explore existential and spiritual issues related to both living and dying.
- A therapeutic attitude encouraged women to cherish each day—to lessen social obligations, repair valuable relationships, and realize their creativity.

Although our style and emphasis may differ, in our programs at the Deaconess Hospital for cancer patients (and other conditions), we teach many of these same approaches: relaxation, coping skills, assertiveness, expressing emotions, group support, reaching out to friends and family. The effects on cancer patients cannot always be measured, although our clinical experience confirms that mind-body medicine yields significant psychological and physical benefits.

Was Dr. Spiegel's finding a fluke? Probably not, given his methodological rigor. But he is repeating his earlier study with a larger group of cancer patients, and he is searching for evidence of how a mind-body treatment could lengthen life for women with breast cancer. Specifically, he has included sophisticated tests of his subjects' immune systems to determine whether his therapy boosts their cellular defense against cancer cells, thus explaining how a psychological therapy could influence their physical recovery.

In 1993, another remarkable finding seemed to confirm that Spiegel's discovery was no fluke. A psychiatrist at UCLA, Fawzy I. Fawzy, M.D., had followed a group of patients—half of whom were women—with melanoma, a potentially lethal skin cancer. Half the patients received his group therapy, which included three primary components: supportive group interactions, cognitive therapy for the development of active coping, and relaxation techniques. The other half received the same medical treatment, but no group therapy. After six years, Dr. Fawzy discovered that patients in his groups were *three times less likely to suffer a recurrence, and three times less likely to have died.*

Dr. Fawzy also uncovered an important clue as he searched for reasons why patients in his groups were more likely to thrive and survive. He found that patients who were most distressed at the beginning, but who developed, over time, *an active way of coping with their stress,* were significantly more likely to remain free of disease. It was a powerful piece of evidence, suggesting that people with cancer can change their mind-set and behavior, and these changes can have a positive effect on the healing process.

In earlier research on these patients, Fawzy also found that individuals in his groups sustained significant increases in natural killer (NK) cells for six months after completing the program. Since NK cells have been shown to eliminate metastatic cancer cells, it is possible that these patients were better able to resist the spread of the disease. That would explain why they had a much lower rate of recurrence and death.

These findings are at the forefront of a new field—psychoneuroimmunology (PNI)—that explores the complex linkages between the mind, the nervous system, and the immune system. Although it is still early, PNI research on cancer has already produced tantalizing data. These data reveal that how we think, feel, and act can influence our immune system—our defense against viruses, bacteria, fungi, and cancer cells. Although thoughts and emotions are not simple determinants of our risk or recovery from cancer, they do appear to play a role for some individuals, a role that is worthy of further study.

Earlier studies in the 1970s and 1980s combine with the recent breakthroughs to create an intriguing puzzle about cancer and the mind, a puzzle with pieces still missing but nevertheless a discernible picture. For instance, a pioneering British investigator, Steven Greer, M.D., joined with colleagues Tina Morris and Keith W. Pettingale to track a group of sixty-nine women with early breast cancer. At the study's outset, they evaluated how each woman was coping with her cancer diagnosis. Five years later, they found that patients who exhibited fighting spirit were more than twice as likely to be alive than patients who were stoic or hopeless in their response to cancer. These remarkable findings held up over the course of fifteen years.

What is fighting spirit? As defined by Dr. Greer, it is exemplified by cancer patients who take charge of their medical care, and who are determined to beat their disease. But Dr. Greer admits that other factors may be involved, including the ability to express intense emotions such as anger, assertiveness, optimism, and a strong will to live. In his book *Freedom and Destiny,* the late psychiatrist Rollo May wrote, "Spirit is that which gives vivacity, energy, liveliness, courage, and ardor to life." His words could apply just as well to "fighting spirit."

One of my patients with ovarian cancer, Vera, appeared to lose her fighting spirit. Vera came from an impoverished family in the South, and she'd worked hard to become a physical therapist. A spunky, vivacious, intelligent thirty-year-old, Vera had been the first member of her family to attend college. To attain her success, she'd overcome many financial and emotional obstacles, with little support from her family. Only a few months before her diagnosis, Vera had married and was facing a bright future. In one fell swoop, her doctor described a grim prognosis and recommended a complete hysterectomy as her only hope for survival. Though it meant she would never have biological children, Vera felt she had little choice but to go through with the surgery. As if that weren't enough, she then had to endure painful side effects from both chemotherapy and radiation. It was too much to bear, even for someone as spunky as Vera. She became listless, depressed, even hopeless. Her negative tape was "What's the use? I'm going to die anyway." She barely had the interest or energy to fight.

I started by teaching Vera to elicit the relaxation response and to use mini-relaxations, which she utilized before, during, and after her rather grueling chemotherapy treatments. Her practice reduced her nausea, lessened her pain from IV needle insertions, and partly relieved her anxiety about the whole process. In our cognitive work, I helped her question her defeatist assumptions about her medical treatment. I made her put "What's the use?" to the test, reminding her that her oncologist believed that the combination of her surgery and adjunctive therapies offered her a real chance for survival. If she did nothing, her chances would dwindle. This realization seemed to stir Vera's fighting spirit.

We also talked at length about how far she'd come in life. I reminded her of how much energy and ingenuity and commitment it took for her to overcome her background, become successful, and find a wonderful man to marry. Our cognitive work progressed, and eventually Vera adopted a radically different position: "If I could beat poverty and ignorance, I sure as hell can beat cancer."

Both Vera and I knew there was no guarantee, but from that point on she began to fight, once again showing her customary pluck. To keep it up, however, she could not deny her emotional pain, for denial only sapped her energy. We talked about her many losses—of her feminine organs, and most especially her child-bearing capacity. She grieved these losses, and then we talked about what it meant to reproduce biologically. In time, she was able to accept this loss, realizing that she could still be a mother through adoption.

Happily, Vera's husband, Tony, was wonderfully supportive and loving throughout her ordeal. Her spirits remained afloat with his help, and together they began to pursue adoption. At the same time, she managed to continue her work as a physical therapist. She even joined a new and more lucrative group practice, becoming codirector within a year's time.

Five years after her diagnosis, Vera is alive, well, and according to second-look surgery and follow-up tests, completely free of cancer. She has two adopted children and her marriage to Tony remains strong. Not only had Vera's fighting spirit returned, it saw her through the darkest times of her life.

We see elements of Vera's fighting spirit in research that has identified positive factors in cancer patients whose immune systems tend to remain strong, and who either live longer or recover more readily. Chief among these factors are coping skills, emotional expression, assertiveness, and the presence of strong social support. Here are some of the key findings in recent years. Take note—most of these studies involve patients with breast cancer.

- While at the National Cancer Institute, Sandra M. Levy, Ph.D., and her colleagues studied patients with early breast cancer. Women who complained, had trouble adjusting, had more energy, and had stronger social support also had stronger natural killer (NK) cells, which are capable of destroying wayward cancer cells. These women also had fewer cancerous lymph nodes, signaling a more favorable prognosis. Dr. Levy viewed these patients' "difficulty adjusting" as a sign that they more openly expressed their negative emotions. In a later study, Dr. Levy showed that women who actively pursued social support, and who felt that they had strong support, had significantly livelier NK cells.

- At the University of California at San Francisco, Lydia Temoshok, Ph.D., evaluated psychological and medical factors in a group of patients with melanoma. Those who demonstrated what she calls the "Type C behavior pattern"—tending to repress negative emotions and trying to please others at all costs—had thicker lesions, which meant a less favorable prognosis. Using sophisticated tests of emotional expression, she found that patients who were more able to express both positive and negative feelings had a stronger immune response against their own tumors. (They literally had more cancer-fighting white blood cells at the site of the tumor.) These expressive patients also had less aggressive cancers.

- Mogens R. Jensen, Ph.D., of Yale University, followed a group of cancer patients for two years. Women who repressed emotions, felt helpless, and avoided thoughts and feelings by daydreaming had cancer that spread more rapidly. By contrast, women who did not fit these categories—who expressed their emotions and did not employ a strategy of avoidance—had a 46 percent higher rate of remission.

- A group of oncologists in New Zealand, led by Alan Coates, M.D., followed 243 women with advanced breast cancer while measuring their overall quality of life. They found that women with better physical well-being, less pain, and better mood—and whose physicians had given them higher quality-of-life ratings—lived significantly longer.

These studies add depth and richness to our understanding of factors that may, indeed, favorably affect cancer survival. Fighting spirit does appear to involve expressing both positive and negative emotions, active coping, maintaining a good quality of life, and establishing strong social support. With regard to breast cancer, I would add that the recent political activism of women with breast cancer is probably valuable both for the changes it will make in society, and for the positive changes it could make for the women themselves. By lobbying for more research to fight the disease, demanding better medical treatments, and changing the culture to get rid of the stigma associated with the diagnosis, such women stoke their own fighting spirit, which may well promote their recovery.

The will to live, once described by the late Norman Cousins as a "blazing determination," makes every day count for women with cancer. We still need more data to prove that blazing determination helps women to live longer, but we already know that it injects meaning and purpose and joy into their lives, whether that time is measured in weeks, months, years, or decades.

Mind-Body Medicine for Cancer Patients

*A*propos of political activism, I recently caught a local news story about a march of breast cancer patients, and one of the women was interviewed by a reporter. Her words stayed with me. "You have to understand," she said, "I was an extremely active, healthy person. I was absolutely fine. They discovered a lump in my breast, and all of a sudden, I became a patient. Before I knew it I was in surgery and getting chemotherapy that did make me feel sick. This disease can strike healthy young women who instantly lose their sense of what's normal."

Mind-body medicine helps women with cancer to retain their sense of what's normal. Although for many cancer patients it is best to confront rather than deny the reality of their illness, it's also best for them to stay in the stream of life, lest they begin to define themselves as a sick person, or even worse, "a cancer victim." I teach mind-body techniques for cancer patients with this goal in mind: to help them tap their inner resources in the face of so much stress and fear. Cancer psychotherapist Lawrence LeShan says that he works to help patients discover not what is wrong with them, but what is right with them, and I concur with his method. Cancer can remind women of their vulnerability, but it can just as surely awaken them to their strengths.

With women with breast and gynecologic cancers, I use the same methods described fully in the first half of this book, but I gear them to the specific stresses these women confront in the aftermath of their diagnosis. If you have been diagnosed with cancer, refer to chapters 1 to 9 for a complete explanation of mind-body techniques, but pay close attention to the following exploration of how you can tailor these methods to meet your own needs.

If you choose to embark on the program that follows, bear in mind that mind-body medicine is not a cure; nor should you judge your efforts on the basis of your disease outcome (e.g., "I had a recurrence so I must not have been committed enough to mind-body healing"). Mind-body factors in wellness should never become one more basis for self-blame. There are too many unknowns about the causes and progression of cancer for anyone to say that a person's mental state was the primary reason for her disease or decline. Know that your efforts are worthwhile on their own terms, not just because they could contribute to your physical recovery. Proceed with hope, but without illusions.

Relaxation and "Minis"

You can elicit the relaxation response in order to allay the immediate, sometimes overwhelming anxieties associated with your cancer diagnosis and treatment. A recent review in the *American Journal of Surgery* highlighted studies that show that relaxation, guided imagery, hypnosis, and other related techniques do more than lessen anxiety—they actually boost and balance various immune functions. Although we cannot yet say that improved immunity directly translates into better physical recovery, the data from doctors Fawzy, Levy, and Temoshok suggest that it can make a positive difference.

As mentioned, relaxation techniques can empower you to reduce anticipatory nausea and vomiting; relieve the pain associated with surgery, chemotherapy, radiation, or cancer itself; and lessen the discomfort and fear associated with medical procedures, including injections, intravenous administration of drugs, magnetic resonance imagery tests (which some patients experience as claustrophobic); and other invasive tests. I recommend to patients that they bring relaxation tapes with them to the doctor's office or hospital, and use them before or during the procedure, whenever possible. Mini-relaxations require no tapes and can be practiced instantly with the simple shift from chest to abdominal breathing, anytime, anywhere. Most of my cancer patients find minis to be invaluable tools for managing their anxiety and discomfort.

At least one study has shown that eliciting the relaxation response will reduce nausea and vomiting after your chemotherapy treatments. Try this method; if it doesn't work, don't continue. Practice relaxation when you are not actively nauseated, and when you are, rely on methods of distraction such as TV watching, or listening to relaxing music. As mentioned earlier, we already know from our own data at the Deaconess Hospital that women taking tamoxifen can elicit the relaxation response to reduce the hot flashes that occur as a result of this hormonal treatment. If you are taking tamoxifen, I suggest that you practice relaxation every day, and that you practice a mini as soon as you feel a hot flash coming on.

The technique that helps most under these circumstances is doing a regular relaxation practice of your choice every single day at a fairly regular time. Any method will do, unless you have had a mastectomy or hysterectomy and prefer not to focus on body parts, as in progressive muscle relaxation (PMR), autogenic training, and body scan. (Some women may wish to use these methods to reconnect with their bodies; others will be made more anxious. Absolutely trust your intuition.) When you take tapes with you to the doctor's office or hospital, breath focus, meditation, and guided imagery are especially recommended. You're not going to be able to do yoga postures in your doctor's waiting room, and you might get embarrassed if you started tensing all your muscles (as in PMR) as you lie on your doctor's examining table!

Guided Imagery

Although it is basically a relaxation technique, guided imagery may also have some special applications to cancer. You may have heard of the method advanced in the 1970s by radiotherapist O. Carl Simonton, M.D., and Stephanie Simonton, Ph.D., detailed in their book *Getting Well Again,* of cancer patients visualizing their chemotherapy drugs or white blood cells as heroic cancer fighters that vanquish malignant cells in the body, wiping them out with dispatch. The Simontons believed that their methods, combined with psychotherapy, could boost the immune system and help at least some patients to recover. Although their research at the time did not adequately answer this question, studies in recent years have supported at least some of their views, especially the value of supportive therapy. We still don't know if visualizing your white blood cells as strong and effective actually *makes* them strong and effective, although Dr. Stephanie Simonton recently revealed data from a study she led at the University of Arkansas showing a 47 percent increase in the responsiveness of key white blood cells—T-lymphocytes—in cancer patients who had practiced guided imagery.

Until we have more answers about this method, I recommend and teach guided imagery as a means to relax, and to reduce symptoms and side effects. I know that guided imagery is useful in these areas, and patients do not feel that they have been set up to expect miracles we cannot ensure. (Please note that Stephanie Simonton has been extremely careful not to set up her patients in this manner, but she stands by visualization as a method that can, in some cases, bolster anticancer defenses.) If you wish to use guided imagery as a healing approach, I suggest the Simontons' *Getting Well Again* and Martin Rossman's *Healing Yourself.*

What methods of imagery work best? The guided imagery tapes listed in Appendix B are highly effective for relaxation, and the tapes work well when you are going through anxious or painful times with chemotherapy, radiation, diagnostic or medical procedures, or the aftermath of surgery. (You can order them from our institute at the address given.) Included are exercises in which you see yourself taking a walk on a deserted beach, strolling down a path toward a mountain stream, or gradually immersing yourself in a luxurious hot bath.

You can also create your own guided imagery. Think of a place from your past or present that has always made you feel safe, and use your imagination to transport yourself there. One of my breast cancer patients, Victoria, always felt safe as a child at her aunt's country home. It had a sprawling backyard with a marvelous view of a valley. On a hill across from the valley stood a stately white mansion. When Victoria was undergoing some rather grueling chemotherapy treatments, she would close her eyes and see herself sitting back on a lawn chair in her aunt's yard, gazing over at the hill and the white mansion, which somehow represented to her the prospect of happiness. She also thought of her aunt, who was always warm and accepting.

You can also fashion images that help reduce your distress and side effects from treatment. Elizabeth Tyson, a breast cancer patient of Dixie Mills, M.D., went through thirty-three sessions of radiation therapy, imagining rays of warm sunlight entering her body. In other instances, it comforted Elizabeth to imagine scenarios of the radiation successfully doing its job of eliminating cancer cells. She'd visualize a benign healing light that would only zap cancer cells but no healthy cells. When asked how exactly the light would accomplish this end, she answered, "Deep frying!"

Cognitive Restructuring
As a reliable, time-tested treatment for depression, cognitive therapy—which includes the restructuring of negative thought patterns—can be in-

valuable for cancer patients. As part of a broader mind-body program, it is extremely effective in reducing distress and bolstering patients' fighting spirit. Indeed, Dr. Steven Greer, who has studied and defined fighting spirit, developed a mind-body program for cancer patients (called "Adjuvant Psychological Therapy") that features cognitive restructuring as a central component.

Cancer is such a frightening disease that it is easy for patients to get locked into a position of fear. Even if their prognosis is excellent—as in very early breast cancer—many patients are still plagued by anxieties. In these instances, cognitive restructuring can be used to reject baseless, "all or nothing" thoughts and "mental filter" that allow patients to ignore whatever good news they may receive regarding their prospects for recovery.

But all women with cancer, including those with a less favorable prognosis, can benefit by reframing their relentless negative thoughts about the future. I've asked patients, "Does your worrying help to stave off your worst-case scenarios?" The logical answer is always no. What could help to stave off worst-case scenarios is a clearheaded, assertive effort to get the best possible medical care.

But how can they short-circuit their anxious thinking? One approach is to focus on today, on life in the moment with all its potential for wonder and pleasure. I remind them that all we have is the moment, that each of us is mortal and vulnerable whether or not we have a life-threatening condition. Rather than allowing moment after moment, day after day, to become suffused with fear about what might happen five years into the future, why not live these days with zest and purpose?

I never use this method to deny women's legitimate fears, or to prompt them to deny their own fears. You can and should discuss your fears openly with a therapist, a friend, family members, or your physician. Sharing anxieties about death can be an enormously healing endeavor, as Dr. David Spiegel has shown. But cognitive restructuring is useful when you are *stuck* in fear, and your thought patterns have become distorted as a result. These thought distortions then contribute to a circular pattern of negative beliefs and anxious emotions. The chain must be broken, and one point of attack is relentlessly negative ideas such as "Cancer is going to get me."

Christina was diagnosed with endometrial cancer at a time in her life when a long-term relationship was dissolving and pressure at work was becoming hard to bear. After surgery, she began to worry about everything, most especially the return of her cancer. Christina was clearly overwhelmed, and it was affecting her judgment to the point that baseless negative thoughts were taking up all the space in her consciousness—space she could have used to devise solutions to some of her problems, as well as to enjoy the moment. After I worked with Christina, she was able to restructure her anxious preoccupations about cancer.

"We settled on the simple idea of me living for today," she remarked. "I try to make the most of it. The truth is that my doctor said the condition is not life-threatening. I am going to die like everybody else. In my everyday life, I feel that I handle stress very well now, and my career certainly is stressful. It helped to put the cancer in its proper perspective."

When stressed, some of us wallow in negative thoughts, others fend them off with great effort, while still others refuse to entertain a single negative thought. In the face of a life-threatening diagnosis, these patterns come to the fore with a vengeance. A balanced approach might be to acknowledge our negative thoughts, but then to put them to the test. Of course, many negative thoughts about cancer are not distortions. For instance, women with advanced breast cancer are not lying to themselves when they say, "I could die from this disease." The question is, what does a woman do with such thoughts? Does she let them destroy her hope for good quality of life? Or does she acknowledge them, work with them, and let them motivate her to fight for life—whether that means a longer life or a more joyous life, regardless of how much time may be left?

Women who've undergone mastectomies or hysterectomies may have the negative thought "I'm damaged goods." If you are one of these women, a support group of others who've been through it can help to restructure this distortion. You will see evidence firsthand of others who are not ashamed of their bodily changes, who are strong and energetic and attractive. If you are not feeling that way now, you can feel that way soon. You may have lost a sexual organ or organs, but you have not lost your womanhood.

Expressing Emotions

The data on emotional expression and cancer prognosis continue to build. As shown in a 1974 study by Dr. Steven Greer, and suggested by several other research findings, suppression of anger may contribute modestly to the risk of breast cancer for some individuals. (This controversial proposition still has not been nailed down.) But the work of Sandra Levy and David Spiegel provide clearer evidence that expressing emotions can be a positive factor in recovery from breast cancer.

Over many years, bottling up anger appears to drain our energy, sap our spirits, and possibly even suppress our natural defense against disease. I don't belong to the camp whose members say that we must express each one of our angry impulses, spewing venom in every direction. There is much to be said for managing and communicating anger in a manner that is socially responsible. But we all know the difference between placid people who are genuinely contented and those who keep an airtight lid on their discontent. The latter do not appear to benefit psychologically or physically from their stance; they'd be better off expressing hidden frustrations in constructive ways.

If constructive expression of anger can be good for the body, one can only imagine how important it is for cancer patients. As I have observed among my patients, a woman with breast cancer tends to harbor anger toward a range of targets. She may be angry at her body for its seeming betrayal; at society for not coming up with a cure; at her doctors for not offering a surefire treatment; at industry for allowing toxins into the environment that she suspects have contributed to her cancer; at drug companies for developing treatments that are not curative, yet have so many side effects; at her husband for not having to endure what she's going through; or at friends who don't have breast cancer and don't "get it."

What do women do with all this anger? The Pennebaker method of writing out emotions (see pages 161–64) can be used to drain off the excess, so to speak, through uncensored, uninhibited writing. You can experience a catharsis as often as needed by writing your deepest thoughts and feelings about your illness and its repercussions. If you wish, write letters to industries, the drug companies, doctors, health-care personnel, your husband, your body, your friends. Upon reflection, you probably won't wish to send them, though perhaps you will decide to put postage on one or two.

Anger can be an energizing emotion, especially for cancer patients who feel weighed down by fear and sadness. Anger is a part of the fuel for fighting spirit—the opposite of despair and hopelessness. Let your anger be a spur to getting the best possible treatment, to fighting for your rights as a medical consumer and a human being, and to getting the support you need and deserve during this difficult period. (See pages 172–76 in chapter 8 for information on assertiveness skills.) Remind yourself that your anger is normal and healthy. There is no reason for you to blame yourself for being angry, or for any spate of emotions in the aftermath of a cancer diagnosis. (Just try your best not to "dump" them on people you love or, for that matter, on unsuspecting health-care professionals.) These feelings are entirely normal and a sign of your aliveness.

When cancer patients use mind-body methods, I often see an orderly unfolding of their emotional states, as though the layers of the proverbial onion are peeling away before my eyes. They first come to me in a state of high anxiety, and relaxation techniques melt some of this anxiety. What emerges next is anger, followed by a deep sadness. The anger may protect them from sadness, but if they cannot access the anger (or get stuck in it) they often can't experience the sadness. Instead, they remain at a surface level of hopelessness, a state of mind and heart that may weaken their immune defenses. Following this progression of emotions—whether in the context of journaling or psychotherapy—can actually help *relieve* hopelessness or depression. Paradoxical though it may seem, feeling authentic anger and sadness over a cancer diagnosis is likely to *prevent* a lapse into despair.

The ultimate purpose of emotional expression is not to let yourself be ruled or terrorized by anger or sadness. Rather, you can use anger to protect yourself as you cope with the tribulations of cancer and its treatment. And you can let sadness be a gateway to honest acceptance of your illness, and ultimately, to a positive recognition of what is worth fighting and living for.

If you get stuck in anger, the result can be rage, hostility, or cynicism. If you get stuck in sadness, the result can be clinical depression, or crying jags that don't seem to stop. In either of these cases, you must not judge yourself as somehow a failure in your struggle with cancer. This "stuckness," too, is entirely normal and very common. It is a signal of one thing only: you may need specialized professional help, including the support of a therapist and/ or group, to move through difficult emotional states. As cancer patients across the country are learning, there is no shame in that.

Coping Skills

When you are living with cancer, perhaps the most important coping skill involves your ability to procure social support throughout the hard times associated with your illness. For some of you, a partner, husband, family member, or good friend is all you will need. But for others, it helps to weave a fabric of support among partners, family, friends, and fellow travelers—other women with breast or gynecologic cancers. Shortly, I will return to the crucial issue of social support.

On a practical level, certain strategies will help you to handle the treatment phase of your recovery. One patient with breast cancer, Winona, was about to undergo an arduous six-week regimen of chemotherapy. She was anxious and forlorn about the weeks ahead, worrying not only about side effects but about keeping up her commitments at work, obligations to her family, and so on. I suggested that she plan the six weeks ahead of time so that she could preserve her energies and protect herself. For Winona, that required a strong focus on self-nurturance and asking for help. I encouraged her to plan activities that she loved to do, and to forsake obligations that would drag her down. She did not have to give parties that strained her resources to the hilt. But she could schedule time with friends and relatives she most enjoyed. She could also decide ahead of time who she wanted to accompany her to the hospital for her chemotherapy treatments.

The plan helped Winona maintain her sense of control; she knew she could do things to make herself feel better, so the six-week course, though difficult, did not seem as bad as her fears dictated. I encourage all my cancer patients to adopt a similar strategy. I also recommend that you give yourself as much time and leeway as possible to recover from surgery, chemotherapy, and radiation. Work and family obligations will always intercede, but make a pact with yourself to honor your needs for rest, relaxation, and the quiet times that foster emotional and physical healing.

Self-nurturance, the subject of chapter 6, ought to be one of your central coping strategies. Feed your senses, your intellect, and your emotions with art, music, or film. If you can, take walks in nature, or find time by the ocean or any setting that stirs your spirit. Buying yourself flowers or new clothes or getting manicures or pedicures are ways to feel good about yourself when treatments and hospital visits get you down. If you've experienced hair loss from chemotherapy, get the loveliest bandanna or hat or wig you can find, unless you're one of those unusual souls who wishes to brandish a beautiful bald head for all the world to see. Remind yourself that your hair will grow back, though it may return with a somewhat different texture or color. Enlist a hairdresser who promises, in the event of any changes, to provide whatever touch-ups you need to get back your previous look and style, or to create a whole new style that reveals another side of you.

A good example of self-nurturance in the face of obstacles is Peggy, a woman with cervical cancer who had two preteen kids who loved loud rock music. Peggy complained to me that she never got a chance to listen to music she loved—jazz by artists like John Coltrane and Charlie Parker. I told her that as part of her treatment she should listen to John Coltrane and Charlie Parker every day for half an hour. She had to get assertive with her two children to wrest that time with the stereo, but she succeeded. (It helped when she thought of it as a medical necessity!) Peggy not only made a statement to her family—that her priorities were important—she got the soul nourishment she needed every day.

As Thomas Moore writes in *Care of the Soul*, such assertions may seem minuscule in the grand scheme of things, but they are not minuscule, especially when you are trying to transcend the aggravations and anxieties of cancer. When doctors and therapists talk about coping skills for cancer patients, they often mean getting the practical help and support you need, and that is crucial. But they rarely mention the need to fill a hunger for meaning and pleasure and fun, which is just as crucial.

Getting the Support You Need

Though I referred to them in chapter 7, I must reiterate the findings of a 1995 study conducted by researchers in Canada and published in the renowned medical journal *Cancer*. Led by epidemiologist Elizabeth Maunsell, Ph.D., the team followed 224 women with breast cancer that was either confined to the breast or had spread only to nearby lymph nodes. As a measure of social support, they asked the patients whether they confided in a person or people during the three months after surgery. The seven-year survival rate among women with no confidants was 56 percent. By contrast, the survival rate for those with one confidant was 66 percent, while the rate for those with two or more confidants went up to 76 percent. The researchers concluded that "social support appears to warrant serious consideration as a factor that may favorably affect breast cancer survival."

Consider the contrast between the survival rate of women who had no confidants—56 percent—with the survival rate of women who had two or more confidants—76 percent. If a chemotherapy study found that a new drug yielded a 20 percent increase in the survival rate of breast cancer patients, you would know it because of the hoopla in the media. Moreover, pharmaceutical companies would probably pour millions if not billions into further drug development for this agent. But what we are talking about here is social support—people to confide in during the crisis of cancer.

Formal groups for cancer patients provide such support, and the evidence from Dr. David Spiegel and Dr. Fawzy I. Fawzy provides confirmation that such groups can indeed extend life for some patients. But I cannot overemphasize that the most tangible and enduring benefits of such group programs are the improvements in quality of life. These improvements stem, in large part, from the warmth and connectedness that so often occurs among women facing the same life-altering condition.

There are many different kinds of groups available for women with breast or gynecologic cancers. If you endeavor to find a group, be aware that different groups have different emphases. Dr. Spiegel's initial groups were for patients with metastatic breast cancer, and he focused quite a bit on issues of death and dying. His patients, who did not have favorable prognoses, seemed ready to confront these realities, and doing so strengthened their bonds, brought their authentic emotions to the fore, and helped them to live in the moment. But such an approach might not be at all appropriate for patients with a different stage of disease—say, early breast cancer patients. These women may not wish to explore issues of death and dying, since their death is not an imminent likelihood and it could cause them unnecessary distress. They might do better in a different kind of group, one more focused on here-and-now coping strategies.

Some support groups are places where women can vent their feelings and share their experiences. With a good leader or therapist, these groups can be superb. But I have heard complaints from some women who feel that the emphasis becomes either too negative ("bitch and moan" sessions) or too positive (Pollyanna optimism, with no room for sadness or anger). A group with a strong, well-trained leader and a good chemistry among the participants can avoid these traps by providing a proper balance between opportunities to share distress and opportunities to develop strengths and optimism and the prospects for greater joy in life. For this balance to occur, a sense of humor on the part of the group leaders and participants is practically essential.

My colleague Ann Webster runs separate groups for cancer and AIDS patients with just such a balance, but they are not standard support groups. Though time is provided for sharing of feelings and experiences, her groups—like my own—are mind-body groups that focus participants on constructive coping skills and relaxation techniques. This brings people together not only to share but to create bonds around a collective effort to develop skills that are empowering and enlivening.

But therapy groups or support groups are far from the only avenue for women with cancer to get the support they need. I emphatically encourage my cancer patients to weave that fabric of support into their daily lives. If there is too little support in their own social fabric, it becomes harder for formal groups to fill in those gaps. Whether or not they have supportive family and friends available, they still must make efforts to procure support through their willingness to reach out.

In some instances, this means summoning up the courage to ask for practical support. If you are sitting home at three in the afternoon after returning from a chemotherapy session feeling so lousy that you don't know how you're going to cook dinner, call a friend and ask him or her to come over and help. Women with cancer don't always realize that truly good friends want an opportunity to offer assistance. In fact, it is typically a great relief for friends when they're asked for favors—it gives them an opportunity to express their care and to do something about their own distress on your behalf.

I often say that there are two skills cancer patients must acquire fast, and they may seem contradictory: asking for help and saying no. When you are anxious, sad, or just plain tired, self-nurturance requires you to do both. Your family members, in particular, may make demands you cannot meet, and it is up to you to let them know your limits clearly, firmly, and, to the greatest extent possible, without resentment. They have a right to ask; you have a right to remind them that you're too exhausted or preoccupied or in need of downtime—whatever the reason—to meet their needs as you might have in the past.

But it is also your responsibility to let your needs be known. Avoid the "mind-reading trap" in which you expect friends and family to have clairvoyant powers with regard to your needs. I have reminded cancer patients that I am a clinician who works with women with medical conditions, and I am no better able to read their minds than anyone else, since every person's needs are so utterly singular. Your husband, children, parents, and friends must know what you want—more or less contact; more or less practical help; to be accompanied to treatments or not to be accompanied; to plan more or fewer social events, and so forth.

My patients with cancer often complain that their husbands or partners are not sufficiently empathic and supportive. This can be a real problem, but if the relationship has a solid foundation of trust, it can be overcome. Patti, a breast cancer patient I saw several years ago, had this complaint about her husband, Lenny. I worked with them as a couple, and what began as an acrimonious discussion became an insightful exploration. Rather than spend so much time on charges and countercharges, I turned to Lenny and asked him to talk about his family background. He revealed just how uncommunicative his father had been. During family crises, his mother would get upset and his father would take to his room. He rarely showed affection and recoiled from any upsets or conflicts. The discussion helped Patti to understand that Lenny wasn't offering a certain kind of support because he never had a model for that behavior—never once had he witnessed his father providing it either for his mother or himself and his siblings. It was an enormous insight for Patti, who could better empathize with Lenny. Once the heavy-duty pressure was off, and he better understood his own difficulties, it became easier for Lenny to openly express his love and concern. The purpose was not to deny or push aside Patti's upset, but to derail the dynamics of blame, and to engender a deeper dimension of understanding.

Women with cancer may be unaware of the degree of their partners' fear and concern. Partners often try hard to mask that fear, believing that it will only cause their loved ones more distress. But this noble motivation can have unexpected and unfortunate consequences, when patients come to believe that their partners don't care enough. Frequently, husbands or companions care so much that they are frozen in their expression of love. They are simply terrified of losing their loved ones. The same can be said for parents, children, and friends. Women with cancer need communication skills to find out the truth, which may involve some risk-taking but is well worthwhile. I have seen many couples and families bridge what initially appeared to be unbridgeable gaps by speaking up and discovering what is beneath surface behavior. It is a surprisingly common though unexpected occurrence when, in the shadow of cancer, couples and families forge an emotional healing they never knew was possible.

Breast Cancer

Breast cancer may seem like an epidemic, but it is not. We often hear in the media that one in nine women will contract breast cancer during her lifetime, but the statistic is misleading. Many breast cancer cases occur among elderly women, and the possibility that a lump found at any given time in your life cycle will turn out to be cancerous is far, far less than one in nine. This is especially true for women under forty, which is why they are not told to have regular mammograms. (The current general recommendation is for a baseline mammogram at age thirty-five, and then one every year or two after forty.) Breast cancer is the most common malignancy among women, with about 180,000 new cases each year in the United States (though lung cancer causes more deaths each year among women than breast cancer). This certainly explains why breast cancer is a leading health concern of women, but I do see evidence of media-driven hysteria that only leads women to be even more stressed out than they need to be.

Which leads me to specific good news: early detection of cancer when it is still confined to the breast results in up to a 90 percent cure rate. I recommend that you practice regular breast self-examination and follow the guidelines for regular mammography—doing so can clearly save your life. Large-scale studies have shown a 30 percent decrease in cancer mortality among women over fifty who received regular mammograms. The details of a program for early detection and breast cancer prevention are beyond the purview of this book. For that purpose, I strongly recommend *Dr. Susan Love's Breast Book*.

A Whole-Woman Approach to Breast Cancer

Dr. Dixie Mills, the breast surgeon with whom I have collaborated at Deaconess Hospital, works closely with her breast cancer patients, helping them to make their own healing choices with regard to conventional medical treatment, complementary medicine, mind–body medicine, and social support. Dr. Mills's approach, which is balanced and compassionate, is a model for the treatment of breast cancer patients, with elements that address their needs for both emotional and physical healing. I will describe her approach because, with commitment and a willingness to network, you can create a program for yourself that includes the same elements.

From the moment of diagnosis, Dr. Mills's patients receive several gifts: her support, her orientation toward hope, and her regard for their autonomy. "I usually give a diagnosis over the phone," she remarked in a recent conversation. "I don't hang up until I have a real sense that someone is there with them, that their initial questions are answered, and that they have some hope." When she does meet with patients, she takes an hour or longer to discuss treatment options and to determine their sources of social support. She encourages the full involvement of husbands or significant others. And she offers them the option of contacting some of her other patients, who can speak to them about thriving and surviving with breast cancer.

Dr. Mills lays out possible courses of treatment, explaining the rationale and medical evidence to support various choices. In some cases, as in very early breast cancer, the number of choices may be fairly limited (i.e., either lumpectomy or mastectomy). In other cases, the range of choices, which involve adjuvant chemotherapy, hormonal therapy, radiation therapy, and combinations of these, are many and complex. After providing all the necessary information, she gives patients room to come to their own decisions, trusting their intelligence and intuition.

At the same time, Dr. Mills addresses complementary approaches, including nutrition and mind–body medicine. She introduces the patient to stress management, relaxation, and coping skills. She talks about the various forms of guided imagery and their usefulness during cancer treatment. During physical exams, she instructs the patient on deep breathing as an instant antidote to stress. She discusses the importance of diet, including low-fat eating and vitamin/mineral supplements, as well as exercise.

Aware of the importance of emotional expression in mind-body health, Dr. Mills has found a unique way to encourage it among her patients. Rather than making an overt suggestion, which could be misinterpreted, she honestly models emotional expression by being up-front about her own feelings. Though she is a calm and rational physician, she will also, at least momentarily, let her patients know that cancer makes her angry. She admits that she goes home and punches pillows to release the anger that builds up after seeing another woman—often a young woman—having to contend with this diagnosis. Her modeling appears to give some patients permission to acknowledge and express their own anger. Dr. Mills's patients know they can count on her. They feel her support, and it fosters optimism and a sense of control over their health and their fate.

A short time ago, with no fanfare whatsoever, Dr. Mills told me that a Harvard medical student recently conducted a statistical review of all her breast cancer patients—about 260 patients over the past seven years. After reviewing all follow-up medical records, the student was shocked to discover that only a half-dozen patients had died. I asked Dr. Mills whether she had seen a preponderance of early breast cancer patients, all of whom have a good prognosis for long-term survival. She said no, that her patients were fairly representative of breast cancer patients, including a mixture of women with early, moderately advanced, and advanced metastatic disease. Certainly, many of the 260 patients have been diagnosed in recent years, and it remains to be seen whether large numbers will be alive after five years (the benchmark for long-term recovery). However, the fact that only six patients have died over the course of seven years remains a remarkable finding.

Though Dr. Mills did not make this suggestion, I cannot help but wonder if her unique approach has something to do with her clinical results. Her patients benefit from her compassion and her respect for their choices, and many avail themselves of the mind-body techniques she exposes them to, either on their own or by participation in our programs at the Division of Behavioral Medicine.

Although there are few surgeons like Dr. Mills, you can adopt her approach by following these suggestions:

- Research your options for conventional and complementary medical care.
- Take charge of your own medical decisions, with the help and counsel of your physicians and specialists.

- Find health-care professionals—whether physicians, oncologists, nurses, psychiatrists, social workers, or psychotherapists—who are forthcoming and supportive, and who reinforce rather than undermine your fighting spirit.
- Join a group of breast cancer patients for therapy, support, or both.
- Join a mind-body or stress management group.
- Read about and practice mind-body medicine on your own.
- Educate yourself about nutritional approaches that may strengthen your defense against cancer, and do your best to make the needed dietary changes.

Mind-Body Groups for Women with Breast Cancer

Mind-body groups are ideal for women with breast cancer, and they are beginning to be formed throughout the country. Though not nearly as widespread as standard support groups, they are becoming more available. The benefits are unique, for they combine support with a panoply of coping skills and mind-body methods that generate optimism and healthy control. Ann Webster's groups at the New England Deaconess Hospital are fine examples of how this blend can empower women with breast cancer.

One of Ann Webster's patients, Allison, is a thirty-two-year-old woman diagnosed two years ago with breast cancer. In a recent conversation, Allison captured how, with the help of Dr. Webster's mind-body group, cancer became a positive turning point in her life.

The painful breakup of a five-year relationship occurred only a few months before she was diagnosed with an infiltrating ductal carcinoma of the breast. It was a particularly disturbing déjà vu, since Allison had survived a bout with Hodgkin's disease at the age of twenty-one. Apparently, the radiation treatments that helped cure her Hodgkin's disease had caused this breast cancer nine years later. Her doctors performed a mastectomy, and the return of cancer, coupled with the loss of her breast, left Allison depressed and furious. She wept through her initial phone consultation with Dr. Webster.

Once Allison entered the group, she glimpsed the possibility of transcendence—she did not have to wallow in her suffering. She could grieve her losses (which included the loss of child-bearing capacity due to chemotherapy—an occasional adverse effect), and get on with her life with the aid of relaxation and a completely new outlook. Though she was upset about the breakup of her relationship, she came to feel that her ex-boyfriend had not been the right man for her. "I grew and he didn't," she said. But she maintained a friendship with him, without lingering bitterness.

Allison described the positive tone of her group, a tone set by Dr. Webster. Certainly, she and her fellow participants would share their feelings, but they would expend much of their energy developing new coping "tools." "When we did bitch and moan, we were looking for solutions," she commented. Allison believes that the group changed her life, and here is how she explained that comment:

> In the past, I was aware of my negative patterns. But if you met me then, you'd see someone who always smiled and was always happy and was going a million miles an hour. Now, on the surface, I seem the same. But the change is internal. The negative thoughts and all the stuff that used to bug me beneath the surface no longer bugs me.
>
> This does not mean that I am stress-free 100 percent of the time. But I notice that when I start to feel anxious, I ask myself if I have meditated recently, or written out on paper what is bothering me. When I do these things, and stick with them, I can definitely see the correlation: on the inside, I am no longer upset by stresses that mean little in the scheme of things.

Cognitive work was especially important for Allison, including a clever concept taught to her by Dr. Webster: she'd place blue stickers on certain objects to remind her of her stress responses. "I stuck one smack in the middle of the steering wheel of my car. I put one on my computer at work and one on my telephone. These were places where I needed to remember that when I get stressed out, I can stop, take a deep breath, and choose how I wish to react."

Allison also restructured negative thoughts about her mastectomy. Now single, she worried how men would respond to scars from her reconstructive surgery. "I felt like damaged property," she said. But after much soul-searching and support, she was able to reframe these thoughts. "Right now, I feel like I am whole on the inside. And I know so many people who don't feel that way, people whose bodies are intact." Allison is still nervous about getting romantically involved, but she has little time to ruminate over these fears. She is too busy, what with a recent job promotion, her pursuit of spiritual practices, and a commitment to living joyfully in the moment.

A fascinating study by an expert in behavioral medicine for cancer offers insight into the health value of living joyfully in the moment. While at the Pittsburgh Cancer Institute, Sandra Levy, Ph.D., and her colleagues, including one of the country's leading breast cancer specialists, Marc Lippman,

M.D., followed the progress of thirty-six women with recurrent breast cancer over the course of seven years. Those who survived had something in common: at the start of the study, they had expressed more joy. This one factor—joy—was a more powerful predictor of survival than several medical factors that doctors rely on to determine prognosis.

Dr. Levy did not conclude that these women were joyful about their illness, a response that might have qualified them for a psychiatric evaluation. Rather, they managed to retain a capacity for joy *despite* their illness, which allowed them to maintain optimism and hope, two oft-cited factors in the psychobiology of healing.

Lifestyle Factors and Prevention

The most important lifestyle factors in the treatment and prevention of breast cancer are a low-fat diet and exercise, but other nutritional and environmental factors may also play a role.

A LOW-FAT DIET. There is no doubt that excess fat in our diets can increase estrogen levels, and estrogen is a known breast-cancer promoter. But the question of whether a high-fat diet really does contribute to breast cancer remains unresolved, although many population studies show correlations between fat intake and breast cancer incidence. The most commonly cited connection, mentioned earlier, is among Japanese women, who have a lower rate of breast cancer than women in the United States and whose fat intake is much lower. When these women move to the United States and their dietary habits become more Westernized—meaning they consume more fat—their breast cancer rates begin to rise. Specifically, the percentage of calories from fat in the diets of Japanese women ranges from 12 to 15 percent, while women in the United States have averaged about 40 percent.

However, recent findings from the Harvard School of Public Health, whose long-term follow-up of almost 90,000 nurses has been led by Walter Willet, M.D., and his colleagues, cast some doubt on the fat–breast cancer hypothesis. They found no significant differences in the breast cancer rates among women with high-fat diets and women with lower-fat diets. But the one sticking point that Dr. Willet has acknowledged is the question of what constitutes an actual low-fat diet. As it happened, few nurses in the study had truly low-fat diets, at least according to many nutritional experts. The lower-fat subjects had an intake of 32 percent, which may not have been low enough to create an appreciable difference in breast cancer rates. Indeed, in rat studies, reduced rates of breast cancer are not observed until their dietary fat intake goes below 20 percent.

Until further clarification is available, it makes good sense to lower the fat in your diet, whether you have breast cancer or wish to prevent the disease. As Dr. Susan Love writes in her book, "Overall, it seems likely, from the material in the various studies, that fat consumption and calorie intake do have some effect on your vulnerability to breast cancer. While there isn't nearly as solid proof as there is with smoking and lung cancer, the data are strong enough to make it worthwhile to seriously consider cutting back your animal fat consumption—especially when you consider that animal fat has been proven to be a factor in many other illnesses, and nothing good has ever been shown about high animal fat consumption, except perhaps that it tastes good." Consult chapter 9 for my "eating transitions" approach to cutting fat in your diet.

VITAMINS. There is also some evidence that women with a high intake of fruits and vegetables rich in beta carotene, vitamin E, and vitamin C have a reduced risk of cancer. But there is as yet scant evidence specifically to support the use of vitamin supplements for the prevention of breast cancer. The one exception is vitamin A pills, which the Harvard School of Public Health researchers have shown, in their study of nurses, reduced the risk of breast cancer among those women with a low intake of vitamin A from food sources. But remember, don't take more than 10,000 IU of vitamin A. The food sources of vitamins A, C, and E are essential for a healthy diet that lowers fat and prevents heart disease, so there are many other reasons to eat lots of fresh fruits and vegetables. Some studies suggest a lower incidence of breast cancer in women with an adequate intake of the mineral selenium, which is present in many antioxidant and multivitamin/multimineral preparations.

SOY PRODUCTS. Asian women who eat a lot of soy-based products—including tofu, miso, and tempeh—excrete estrogen at a relatively higher rate. They also have a lower risk of breast cancer. The link has not been proven, but these soy products do contain phytoestrogens, weak estrogens that may protect against breast cancer by blocking estrogen receptors on the cells from being overstimulated by internal estrogens. Soy products have many other health benefits, so if you happen to like them, increasing your intake might not be a bad idea.

ALCOHOL. Dr. Willet of the Harvard School of Public Health has conducted what many consider the definitive study on the role of alcohol in breast cancer risk. After tracking those 90,000 nurses over four years, he found that women who consumed substantial amounts of beer, wine, and hard liquor had an increased risk of breast cancer. Women who consumed zero to two drinks a week had no increased risk of breast cancer; three to nine drinks a week drove up risk 30 percent; and more than nine drinks increased risk by 60 percent. Younger women appear to be most affected. If you are concerned about breast cancer risk—particularly if you have a family history—try to limit your alcohol intake to only a few drinks per week.

EXERCISE. Leslie Bernstein and her colleagues at the University of Southern California's North Cancer Center studied over a thousand women, and found that moderate but regular physical activity can reduce a woman's risk of developing premenopausal breast cancer by as much as 60 percent. Women who received the greatest benefits were those who had borne children and those who were physically active in their teens and early twenties. Women who exercised for four hours or more a week had the most striking reduction. But even as little as two to three hours of weekly exercise was found to be beneficial. Consult chapter 9 for guidelines for a modest exercise program.

Risk Factors
The following list breaks down breast cancer risk factors, including those that are biological, nutritional, behavioral, and environmental.

Identified Risk Factors

- Family history: Risk is lower among those with no history of the disease among close relatives.
- Age at onset of menstruation: Risk is lowest among those who start menstruating late.
- Age at first pregnancy: Risk is lowest among those who have their first child by the age of twenty and who have a greater number of pregnancies.

Possible Risk Factors

- Breast-feeding: There may be some protective effect for those who breast-feed.
- Dietary factors: High-fat diets, high alcohol intake, or a need for certain vitamins or fiber may present risks.
- Environmental factors: Pollution or electromagnetic fields may be risk factors.
- Hormones: Hormones from birth-control pills or used as replacement therapy may pose a risk.

Probable Risk Factor Modifier

- Moderate regular physical activity, even two or three hours a week, is associated with a significantly lower breast cancer risk.

Healing the Feminine Soul: Gynecologic Cancers

*E*ach year in the United States, over 120,000 women are diagnosed with cancers of the reproductive system, which includes the ovaries, endometrium, vagina, and cervix. With regard to lifestyle factors in the prevention of these cancers, there is less evidence than there is for breast cancer. However, some studies suggest that both a low-fat diet and exercise may have positive roles in the prevention and treatment of gynecologic cancers.

Unlike tumors affecting most other organs, gynecologic cancers strike at the feminine soul. Often, the treatment involves hysterectomy—complete or near-complete removal of internal reproductive organs. When a woman's ovaries are removed, an instant surgical menopause occurs. Some women use HRT to relieve hot flashes and other symptoms, but others cannot because it may promote recurrences of cancer. As with menopause or tamoxifen-induced hot flashes, eliciting the relaxation response is recommended for the hot flashes that occur after surgical menopause.

In many cases of gynecologic cancer, the complications go beyond physical symptoms: the patient feels that she has lost part of her female identity. At the same time that a woman with gynecologic cancer undergoes surgery, chemotherapy, and radiation, she can embark on a process of healing the feminine soul. This process may or may not contribute to physical improvements, but it is invaluable nonetheless.

Emotional distress may cause hormonal and immunologic imbalances that favor the growth of gynecologic cancers. Several studies of cervical cancer support this hypothesis. Earlier pioneers in research on cancer and the mind, Dr. A. H. Schmale and Dr. Howard Iker from the University of Rochester, studied sixty-eight women before a biopsy to determine the presence or absence of cervical cancer. The researchers were able to predict which patients had cancer with 73 percent accuracy, based on one single factor: whether the patient evidenced feelings of hopelessness. Karl Goodkin, M.D., Michael Antoni, Ph.D., and their colleagues at the University of Miami evaluated seventy-three women awaiting workup for an abnormal Pap smear. They discovered that patients with advanced disease had more life stress, and had reacted to that stress with hopelessness.

This is not to suggest a simplistic equation between hopelessness and gynecologic cancer. Rather, experts in PNI and cancer believe that chronic hopelessness may be one factor, along with others, that could promote malignant growth before and after the appearance of a tumor. As we await more studies, it is safe to say that any approach we develop to resolve chronic feelings of hopelessness is worthwhile, since it is a state that is surely harmful to our psychological if not our physical health.

One of my patients with ovarian cancer, Samantha, was indeed feeling hopeless just before she was diagnosed. Samantha, thirty-five at the time, had been married to Kenneth for five years, and they had adopted a son. Literally on the eve of their second adoption, her husband informed her that he wanted a divorce. She suspected he was having an affair, which Kenneth denied. (She later discovered that she had indeed been correct.) Samantha's grief and anger were so enormous she could barely express them; she was in a state of shock. There had been few signs of impending trouble; none, at least, that she had been able to read. Five months after their divorce was finalized, she was diagnosed with a malignant tumor on one of her ovaries.

Ovarian cancer can be difficult to treat because it is so often caught late in the game; obvious symptoms may not be apparent early on. But Samantha's tumor was caught at a sufficiently early stage to give her doctors reason to believe that she could fully recover. Nevertheless, it would be a struggle. Right away, she had to have a complete hysterectomy. I was introduced to Samantha after her diagnosis but before her surgery, and she was terrified. I was able to accompany her into the operating room to offer moral support and a few methods she could use to elicit the relaxation response before and after surgery.

After her surgery, I continued to work with Samantha. Despite her enormously tough life circumstances—she was suddenly a single mother and a woman with cancer—I saw evidence of her fighting spirit, and I encouraged every life-affirming impulse that arose as we worked together. She had good support from her parents, and she relied upon them. We talked a great deal about her ex-husband and the shock and pain of his betrayal. But mostly, we focused on Samantha's strengths. I let her know that I believed she had the strength to get on with her life, as long as she did not succumb to self-blame. Her anger was her therapeutic ally; without it, she might have lapsed into despair. With her emotional resources, her son, and the support of her parents, Samantha was able to rebuild, a process that included a new home, a new job, and a new awareness of living in the moment.

Samantha was also helped by mind-body techniques, including a self-styled visualization she practiced whenever she was stressed by her illness or difficulties in her personal life. Right after her divorce, but before her cancer diagnosis, Samantha had joined with a friend—another divorced woman—for a weeklong Hawaiian vacation. It was a carefree escape, a time for her to put aside the pain, let down her hair, relax, and enjoy herself unabashedly. Later, after her diagnosis and during the many rapid changes and demands of her present life, Samantha would sometimes lie quietly and imagine herself back on the beach in Hawaii, soaking in the sun and the blissful sense of freedom.

In recent years, Samantha has experienced some turbulent changes, including the loss of a long-term live-in relationship, and the death of her beloved mother, who she had spent several years caretaking during the mother's own bout with cancer. But she feels she's been tested by fire and made all the stronger because of it. Samantha has had much grieving to do, but she continually rises to each new challenge and retains her energy and humor. Being a single parent certainly presents her with new challenges, but she has managed to flourish, with a recent job promotion as a strong confirmation to herself that she is a survivor.

And Samantha is a survivor, in every respect. Her ovarian cancer has not recurred, and she recently passed the five-year benchmark for recovery.

Some women with gynecologic cancers, particularly those with ovarian cancer, are made aware by their doctors of an unfavorable prognosis. While mind-body medicine supports fighting spirit, optimism, and a sense of control, there may come a point in the process when a patient shifts from a position of fighting to one of acceptance. When this occurs—or should occur—is an entirely individual decision. No one—not a doctor, a therapist, or a loved one—ought to tell a cancer patient when she should keep fighting or when she should surrender and accept the inevitability of death. I support my patients' deepest intuitions about this process. Patients may also shift back and forth in what therapist Robert Chernin Cantor calls "the resistance-surrender cycle." This, too, is normal, and if you have advanced cancer it helps to allow that natural rhythm to unfold.

When and if you do come to accept death, and to stop fighting in terms of a medical remission or cure, the instinct for healing does not have to die. For as Michael Lerner points out, healing in the broadest sense is not synonymous with curing. I have had many patients who continued to heal—emotionally and spiritually—long after they ceased striving for a medical cure.

One of the most critical cognitive and emotional shifts I encourage among women with gynecologic cancers is the recognition of their emotional wholeness and—if this has meaning for the patient—spiritual completeness. The loss of reproductive organs, particularly among pre-menopausal but also among postmenopausal women, can be enormously difficult. Women who've suffered these losses can benefit by honoring and expressing their grief. But they can also recognize that the feminine soul is indomitable—it can't be cut or burned or poisoned out. The removal of female organs of reproduction does not entail the removal of one's womanhood. Recognition of this reality may, however, require therapeutic work, including relaxation and a deep inner attunement. Some women (I think of Samantha) have not only retained their sense of themselves as women, they have gone a step further. They have come into their own as women.

I would never suggest that this process of grief and positive transformation is easy; only that it is possible. If you have been diagnosed with a gynecologic or breast cancer, I hope that you can seize this possibility, and thus retain your hope, your energy, your creative fire—your fighting spirit.

Sixteen

• • • • •

SOOTHING THE HURT:
ENDOMETRIOSIS AND
PELVIC PAIN

*E*ndometriosis, a condition in which the tissue lining inside the uterus appears elsewhere in a woman's pelvis, is all too common; an estimated five million women are affected. The condition, which occurs during the reproductive years and is partly driven by estrogen, is the second leading cause of infertility and is a terrible source of pain for countless numbers. Hysterectomy, once the first-line treatment, has been replaced by less radical treatments, such as laser surgery and hormones that can cause side effects. Mainstream medicine helps many women with endometriosis, but there remains no surefire cure. Endometriosis is a major cause of pelvic pain, although many women with chronic pelvic pain have no evidence of endometriosis.

Mind-body medicine can soothe the hurt of endometriosis and of chronic pelvic pain that has other causes. Behavioral approaches have solid track records in the treatment of pain, and endometriosis and pelvic pain are no exception. But why would mind-body medicine be effective for these specific conditions? Emotional stress may be a contributor to endometriosis and pelvic pain; uncovering and resolving sources of stress may promote healing. And sophisticated new studies suggest that pain signals can become programmed into our central nervous system, which helps to explain the clinical observation that people who change their mind-set about pain can indeed change their experience of pain. Mind-body medicine rarely eliminates the discomfort of endometriosis and pelvic conditions, but it can substantially alter pain perception and ease the despair among sufferers.

Endometriosis: Causes and Treatments

The endometrium, the tissue lining the uterus, normally stays within the uterine cavity. For reasons unknown, this tissue sometimes migrates outside the uterus and begins growing on other pelvic organs, causing adhesions that are the source of pain. Although most endometrial lesions latch onto the side walls of pelvic organs, they can occasionally migrate to the bowel or other organs outside the pelvis. In some instances, endometriosis develops underneath visible tissues, causing pain that mystifies surgeons who can't locate the source.

Generally speaking, the definitive way to diagnose endometriosis is through laparoscopy, a surgical procedure performed under general anesthesia in which a long rigid tube equipped with a periscopelike attachment is inserted into the pelvic cavity through a small incision. In rare instances, it can be detected through a pelvic exam, such as when lesions are present on the pelvic ligaments. The advent of laparoscopic procedures has revealed that endometrial lesions may be present in vast numbers of women, far more than report any symptoms.

Pelvic pain is the major symptom, although endometriosis can also cause cramping, abnormal menstrual cycles, and pain during intercourse. The pain of endometriosis can be debilitating, robbing women of energy and enthusiasm, particularly when activities such as sexual intercourse and exercise become difficult if not impossible. Infertility is a problem for about 30 percent of women with endometriosis.

What are the causes of endometriosis? Theories abound. One is that menstrual blood and endometrial tissues flow backward through the fallopian tubes to pelvic tissues, where these deposits begin to grow. Another is that endometriosis is congenital, developing from embryonic genital tissues in the pelvis that never migrated to the uterus. These embryonic cells become stimulated when girls start having their periods, and that is when lesions develop and pain starts. The congenital theory is backed up by the fact that endometriosis does tend to run in families, so there may be a hereditary factor.

But none of these theories has been proven. We do know that estrogen promotes endometrial overgrowth in susceptible women, but the question of why some women are susceptible is still unanswered. However, the fact that many of today's women are putting off child bearing and having more menstrual cycles may explain the increasing incidence of endometriosis, because women who don't get pregnant and nurse have higher circulating estrogen levels.

Although too little research has explored the question in depth, some experts do believe that stress may contribute to the progression and symptoms of endometriosis. It is often called "the working women's disease" for two reasons: first, its prevalence is greater among women who delay child bearing, often as they pursue careers; second, because the stress associated with work may be a common aggravating factor in symptomatic endometriosis. Neils H. Lauersen, M.D., Ph.D., is Clinical Professor of Obstetrics and Gynecology at New York Medical College and an endometriosis expert. Here is what he had to say about the role of stress:

> I'm a gynecologist, a specialist in women's health issues, a scientist who weighs and measures the minutiae of laboratory research before making an informed decision, but I am also a pragmatist and a humanitarian. I see who suffers from what and I set about to help them in an efficient and compassionate manner. And so I notice that nearly 95 percent of endometriosis patients are women under extreme stress who work or have worked.
>
> As part of treating the person, not the symptoms, we must examine the external influences—physiological and psychological—that create changes in her health.

Lauersen is not a New Age acolyte who believes that stress is the sole cause of endometriosis, nor is he a Neanderthal who believes that the condition is some form of comeuppance for women who ought to stay at home. He is a mainstream physician who recommends conventional treatments—including hormonal agents and surgery—in addition to stress management, nutritional changes, and sound health practices. Although he believes that stress contributes to the condition, he does not argue a simplistic cause-effect relationship, nor does he view women's professional advancements over the past decades as anything but a boon to women and our society. But the layering on of women's multiple roles, and society's ambivalence or outright hostility about our advances, have certainly introduced new pressures and challenges into our lives. These pressures and challenges will compromise our physical health unless we find creative new ways to adapt.

The biological mechanisms that explain how our stressful lives may contribute to endometriosis are not clear, but recent studies provide an intriguing clue. One investigation showed that women with symptomatic endometriosis had autoantibodies against their own tissues. Scientists have also uncovered evidence that macrophages—immune cells that engulf foreign invaders—can turn against endometrial tissue. This raises the question posed by a 1987 paper in the journal *Obstetrics and Gynecology*: "Is endometriosis an autoimmune disease?" If the answer turns out to be yes—even a qualified yes—then it is conceivable that stress contributes to endometriosis by causing a disturbance in our immune systems, leading them to attack our own tissues and generate endometrial overgrowth.

Among the most startling hypotheses is that early emotional, sexual, and physical abuse is a contributor to chronic pelvic pain. Research by Andrea J. Rapkin, M.D., of the UCLA School of Medicine, one of the country's leading experts on pelvic pain, has indeed shown a high incidence of early abuse among these patients. Whether early or ongoing abuse is a specific factor in endometriosis has not been clarified, but its role in chronic pelvic pain—which is so frequently caused by endometriosis—is becoming more widely accepted.

Of course, once endometriosis causes chronic pain, the pain itself is a source of stress. Women with severe pain from endometriosis often hop from doctor to doctor looking for effective treatments, and sometimes they endure multiple surgeries in their search for solutions. The pain can be disabling, and without sufficient relief such women can readily become depressed, if not downright hopeless. This particular vicious cycle, common in all forms of chronic pain, may actually worsen physical conditions underlying the pain, such as inflammation, autoimmunity, constriction of blood flow, and muscular tensions.

Here's another mystery of this condition: the location or extent of endometriosis seems to have little relation to the degree of pain, or to the presence of pain at all. Some women have extensive lesions and no pain; others have minimal disease and unrelenting pain. Though we don't understand why, stress and emotions could be pivotal in determining how pain is processed and perceived. Considering the potential role of stress, depression, and psychological traumas in endometriosis and pelvic pain, it is no wonder that mind-body medicine has much to offer women with this condition.

Though it has no magic bullet, mainstream medicine does have many effective treatments and options for women with endometriosis. Hormonal drug treatments include Danazol, which stops ovulation by blocking the surge of luteinizing hormone and inhibiting receptors in endometrial lesions. The main problem with Danazol, an often effective remedy, is its masculinizing side effects: hair growth and a deepening of the voice. The FDA has recently approved a group of drugs called GnRH agonists, which produce an artificial menopause, stopping the hormonal stimulation that feeds the growth of endometrial lesions. These costly drugs include Lupron and Synarel, but they cause side effects that mimic natural menopause—hot flashes, vaginal drying, and bone loss. These side effects will generally subside when the drugs are stopped, so some women find themselves in an on-again, off-again relationship with these agents, which do work pretty well to reduce endometrial lesions and the pain associated with them. Birth-control pills can also be effective for some patients.

Surgery can be quite effective for the removal of endometrial lesions without having to perform a hysterectomy. Such procedures are performed by laparoscopy, or by a more recent technical advance called pelviscopy (also known as operative laparoscopy). These methods allow for the diagnosis and removal of endometrial lesions without a long incision. Pelviscopy can remove these lesions, as well as any cysts or adhesions, through electrocautery (burning) or a laser. When these more conservative methods are unsuccessful, because the patient is still in pain, surgeons move up a ladder of increasingly invasive procedures. A complete hysterectomy, including removal of the ovaries, is considered the last resort.

Pelvic Pain: Mysteries and Consequences

Many women with chronic pelvic pain have no endometriosis, or if they do, their endometrial lesions do not appear to be the primary cause of their pain. Chronic pelvic pain can be a mystery, although a range of causal factors and underlying conditions in addition to endometriosis has been noted, including uterine fibroids, pelvic inflammatory disease (PID), infections, ovarian cysts, or adhesions from past surgeries or other causes. But often no clear cause can be identified.

As Andrea J. Rapkin has written, "Epidemiologic studies have highlighted a relationship between psychological factors such as depression, personality disorders, and physical and sexual abuse, and chronic pain states." Dr. Rapkin has shown a prevalence of these factors in chronic pelvic pain. My own clinical experience bears this out—pelvic-pain patients frequently report an abuse history, ongoing abuse in current relationships, extreme stress, and feelings of despair. I find that these patients often respond extremely well to cognitive and behavioral therapies.

My colleague at the Deaconess Hospital, Margaret Caudill, M.D., Ph.D., is Director of General and Specialty Programs in Harvard Medical School's Division of Behavioral Medicine. She directs the division's mind-body groups for people with chronic pain, and I strongly recommend her book

Managing Pain Before It Manages You, which offers a superb, user-friendly overview of mind-body medicine for chronic pain. Dr. Caudill has also treated many women with pelvic pain, most of whom have had multiple surgeries. She has come to believe that answers to the mysteries of chronic pelvic pain do not even lie in the pelvis. Rather, they lie in the central nervous system—the brain.

"Most people do not realize that a lot of chronic pelvic pain is really caused by an abnormality that may be set off from an original lesion or inflammation," said Dr. Caudill in a recent conversation. "But then through some quirk we still don't fully understand, the problem is perpetuated in the spinal cord and the brain, so you can remove an ovary, then another ovary, then the uterus, then the cervix, and you still have pain." She has seen patients whose pelvic pain endures even after they've had every pelvic organ removed. The problem, apparently, must reside in pain pathways in the central nervous system.

Although her explanation is quite technical, it can be summed up rather simply. Initial lesions, adhesions, or inflammations may traumatize our pain nerves. When they regenerate, they continue to fire abnormally, as if the source of pain were still present, even after that source has been removed (e.g., when surgery is performed to take out lesions or entire organs). A volley of pain messages continues to be received by the brain, and the person's experience of pain endures. It is also possible that psychological traumas (such as early sexual abuse) are remembered by the nervous system, causing a long-lasting alteration in the way women experience pain.

Pain specialists are uncovering more evidence to support Dr. Caudill's theory, which applies primarily to patients whose chronic pain is not relieved after every conceivable treatment has been tried. But the ramifications may be crucial for pain patients and their doctors. If the problem lies in the central nervous system, the solution, or at least one viable option, may also lie in the central nervous system. If we can change our mind-set about pain, we may be able to reprogram some of the pain messages that perpetuate our suffering. These findings also mean that some surgical procedures are unnecessary, if not counterproductive. We know that 30 percent of the hysterectomies performed for chronic pelvic pain fail to relieve adequately the suffering that afflicts these women.

Women with chronic pelvic pain should have careful diagnostic workups to determine whether clear causes can be identified. Before turning to surgery, other options should be considered, including mind-body medicine, which has no side effects. I have been encouraged by my experiences with pelvic-pain patients who have obtained significant relief, reduced their reliance on pain medication, and avoided major pelvic surgery.

The most effective mind-body treatments for chronic pain enable women to:

- Reestablish a sense of control over their pain and their lives.
- Reduce or resolve aggravating sources of stress and conflict.
- Complete unfinished emotional business.
- Develop a repertoire of coping skills they rely upon when pain interferes with their ability to function and enjoy themselves.

Mind-Body Relief for Pelvic Pain

Mind-body clinicians have shown that their methods work extremely well in the treatment of chronic pain. Dr. Caudill has published a study of 109 patients who participated in her ten-session program, which combines relaxation, pain monitoring, cognitive approaches, and nutritional and exercise education. One year after completing her program, Dr. Caudill's patients made 36 percent fewer visits to the doctor. With specific regard to chronic pelvic pain, Dr. Caudill has found that her patients' symptoms rarely disappear, but they are substantially better able to manage their pain. I have had the same experience, using similar methods. And I have often observed significant reductions in the pain experienced by women with endometriosis. In the following section, I present the key elements of a program you can apply for the management and alleviation of pelvic pain from endometriosis and other causes. (You may also apply many of these methods for other kinds of chronic pain, whether caused by headaches, backaches, arthritis, fibromyalgia, or any other disorder.)

Keeping a Pain Diary

Monitoring pain is an effective way to raise awareness of the triggers and consequences of your pain, and it is a first step toward taking control of your pain. I recommend Dr. Caudill's "pain diary" method:

- Designate an actual diary or notebook for this purpose.
- Record your pain levels in the diary three times a day at regular intervals (e.g., morning, noon, and bedtime).
- Describe the situation or activity that corresponds in time to each

rating. For instance, were you working, watching TV, talking to a friend?

- Rate your pain sensations, which refers to the physical aspects of your pain, such as achiness, stabbing, burning, tightness, or other sensations: 0 = no pain; 1–9 = ranges in degree of pain; 10 = the worst possible pain.
- Also rate your pain distress, which refers to your perception of pain, and is a measure of the emotional suffering you experience, such as frustration, anger, anxiety, sadness, and so on: 0 = no distress; 1–9 = ranges in degree of distress; 10 = the worst possible distress.

Start by keeping this pain diary for one week, then analyze the results. Search for patterns associated with your pain. They may be simple physical associations, such as an increase in pain when you get up in the morning, start eating, and so on. Also notice any correlations between emotional states, stressful events, or certain relationships and the onset of pain.

Be on the lookout for discrepancies between your ratings of your pain sensations and pain distress. You may find—as many patients do—that your distress numbers are frequently higher than your pain sensation numbers. What's the significance? It means that your pain perception, and your emotional suffering, go well beyond your physical sensations. At these times, your suffering about pain is a predominant factor in your pain experience. The purpose of the exercise is to separate your perceptions from your actual sensations, until you are fully aware of the gaps. When your pain sensations rate a three but your distress about pain is a seven, you know it is time to quiet your overanxious mind. When you do, it becomes easier to adopt thoughts such as: "Maybe I can live with this level of pain." "Perhaps by reducing my distress I can relieve some of my pain."

Emotional suffering around pain may feed back into pain processing centers in your nervous system, thus perpetuating your physical pain sensations. Therefore, it helps to remember that modifying your relentlessly negative thoughts and feelings about pain is one strategy to reduce pain itself!

Transforming Your Pain Perspective
Women with chronic pelvic pain and endometriosis often engage in negative "self-talk" that reinforces their helplessness and hopelessness. "I'll never get over this pain." "I'm miserable and it will never change." "This pain is going to ruin my life." We can be so convincing with negative self-talk that we drive ourselves into a state of hysteria or utter despair. Use your pain

diary as a launchpad for transforming your pain perspective. You can continue this process by putting your negative thoughts about pain to the test, using the cognitive restructuring method described in chapter 5.

Women with chronic pain are certainly unhappy about their condition, and there is no reason to deny the feelings. But the negative voices feed despair just as surely as estrogen feeds endometriosis. The misery becomes fixed when women have mentally resigned themselves to a terrible fate. The way out of this trap is a reasoned grasp of reality. More often than not, conventional or complementary medicine has options they can pursue. Women with pelvic pain are never beyond relief, resolution, and healing, even when the pain cannot be completely cured.

Here are several examples of how to restructure hopeless thoughts about endometriosis and pelvic pain: "I feel bad today, but there are many avenues I can pursue to feel better tomorrow." "I am so upset about this pain that I am making it worse. I need to provide myself with some distractions." "There are many strategies I can employ right now to feel better."

Dr. Caudill also suggests that women pay attention to physical cues that reveal the link between their perceptions and their pain. In other words, notice your pain sensations—when you are aware that you're engaging in negative self-talk. Does your pain get worse after you've hit yourself with a barrage of hopeless thoughts about your pain? Then, as you gradually begin to question and replace negative voices, do you notice a change? Do you experience fewer pain sensations after you talk to yourself about practical strategies or hopeful signs?

Cecilia, a patient of mine with searing pain from endometriosis, had been put on narcotic analgesics by her physician. After she committed herself to cognitive restructuring—radically transforming her pain perspective— Cecilia began to experience a surprising degree of relief. Within a matter of weeks, she was able to replace the narcotic medications with a few daily tablets of over-the-counter ibuprofen.

As you change your perspective about pain, don't counter negative self-talk by berating or cajoling yourself with Pollyanna positivism. The purpose is not to push yourself into positive thinking, but to counter the irrational excesses of the mind with rationality and compassion for yourself. It also helps to discover constructive steps that tend to reduce your distress about pain, and perhaps even the pain itself. Chronic pain is a chronic stressor, and when it worsens you may feel that your day of work or your evening of leisure is ruined. Every time you can reverse a slide into helpless or hopeless reactions, you win a small victory over chronic pain. So be systematic in your search for strategies that help. You may need to call a friend, luxuriate in a hot bath, take an anti-inflammatory, practice guided imagery or yoga, write out your frustration in your diary, or write out your cognitive distortions about pain so you can restructure them. Over time, these moment-to-moment strategies accumulate into a meaningful and often effective program for pain management, one that works because it entails one fundamental shift: the pain no longer has control over you, you have control over the pain.

Quieting Pain with Relaxation and Imagery

Eliciting the relaxation response is a tried-and-true method for pain management. As with cognitive restructuring, regular relaxation is not some magical cure-all, but it is another critical step toward gaining control over pelvic pain, or, for that matter, any form of chronic pain. I recommend that you practice relaxation techniques on a regular basis, twice a day if possible. But it also helps enormously to practice a mini-relaxation whenever chronic pain arises to cloud your consciousness or decimate your quality of life. In a matter of minutes, you can regain some control over pain and your experience of pain. When the pain is severe, and you are in a position to take fifteen to twenty minutes alone in a room, practice any method for eliciting the relaxation response, using the audiotapes if you find them helpful.

Women with pelvic pain often benefit from breath focus, meditation, or autogenic training. Gentle yoga can be particularly helpful if it does not cause too much additional discomfort. Moving and stretching—getting the energy flowing through your body—can offer pain relief over time. Use your own instincts about body-based meditations, including progressive muscle relaxation and body scan. Try them out; if they help to heal alienation from your body, and they bring about sensations of calm and tranquility, stick with them. If they foster an awareness of pain sensations that you find disturbing, or that only increase your anxiety, don't feel obliged to practice these methods.

GUIDED IMAGERY: I have found guided imagery to be a most useful method for women with chronic pelvic pain. The imagery tapes you can order by referring to Appendix B will take you on mental expeditions to places and scenes that, for most of us, generate a sense of tranquility and safety, releasing the grip of anxiety on our minds and bodies. But you can also develop your own visualizations that directly address your pelvic pain.

Here is one imagery exercise, taught to me by Margaret Ennis, M.A., that has helped my patients with chronic pain. Imagine a soothing, healing stream of blue light. Allow this light to enter through the top of your head, spreading through the inside of your head, then moving slowly down through each segment of your body—your neck, shoulders, chest, arms, abdomen, pelvis, and legs. Let the light fill your body with its soothing energy. Notice if there is any part of your body that seems to resist the entrance of the blue light. Simply observe this process; don't force it. Be mindful of your physical sensations as the healing blue light fills your body.

After practicing this imagery, Hope, who suffered with pelvic pain, described her images as she tried to allow blue light into her pelvis. She saw her pelvis as being red hot, and it resisted the blue light just as fire resists being put out by a puff of wind. Hope was astonished by how clear, specific, and revealing her imagery was, and it gave her insight into her pain experience. During later practices, she was able to let some of the blue light into her pelvis, and she found that the intensity of her pelvic pain would subside.

Perhaps the most dramatic and creative use of imagery occurred for Betsy, a patient with endometriosis that caused intense pelvic pain throughout most of her days. Tests showed that both of Betsy's fallopian tubes were blocked by lesions. She entered one of my mind-body groups, where she learned to elicit the relaxation response through a variety of methods. During one group session, we were practicing a simple meditation when Betsy, as she later revealed, spontaneously went into a visualization of her own creation, as if she were directing a movie in her mind but with no idea where the inspiration was coming from.

Betsy imagined herself outside a beautiful medieval church. A tiny monk exited the church, took her by the hand, and led her inside. He escorted her through the winding corridors of this mystical temple, until they came to a room where he had her lie down upon a table. There she saw a group of diminutive parishioners—all women—dressed in elaborate costumes of gold and lace. The women surrounded her on the table, and they began to massage her abdomen with sweetly aromatic oils and herbal preparations. They worked gently on her uterus and her fallopian tubes. Betsy allowed herself to sink into the sensations of warmth and pleasure generated by their loving hands. After they finished, the monk returned and led her back outside of the church.

When Betsy finally opened her eyes, she shared her experiences with us. She said she felt wonderful, and it was obvious—she was glowing. From that point on, Betsy deliberately returned to this visualization every time she meditated, seeing the monk and allowing the women to gently and expertly massage her reproductive organs, eliciting sensations of warmth and tranquility.

Within a few weeks of starting this practice, Betsy noticed her pain subsiding. She switched from prescription narcotics to over-the-counter analgesics. Several months later, a tubogram revealed that one of Betsy's fallopian tubes was fully open for the first time in ten years.

Margaret Caudill also recommends a "safe place" visualization for women with endometriosis and pelvic pain. To practice this approach, create an image of a place of peace and solace, a place where you feel safe and free. Draw upon your memories of such a place, or simply upon your imagination. It does not matter how you conjure this place, as long as it makes you feel safe. Sit quietly, and start with an "induction," a simple breath focus meditation or mini-relaxation. Then transport yourself to this safe place in your mind, and focus on senses. What do you see, hear, feel, taste, smell, and touch? If you are by a seashore, smell the ocean and hear the rolling roar of the waves. If you are in a forest, smell the pines, feel the crackle of twigs under your feet, see the play of light on green leaves. Stay in your safe place, soaking in the sensations and feelings, for about twenty minutes. Monitor how you feel, including your pain sensations, after you're finished.

MINDFULNESS: Mindfulness can also help women with pelvic pain, but it requires commitment. As practiced by Margaret Caudill, and by Jon Kabat-Zinn, Ph.D., perhaps the country's leading practitioner of mindfulness meditation, it involves a moment-to-moment awareness of the pain. Though it may seem paradoxical, it can help enormously to focus on your pain, without obsessive attention but with calm equanimity and a gentle allowance of sensations into consciousness. Many people with chronic pain employ strategies of pain avoidance, which can work, but they can also backfire. The mental effort it takes to avoid or repress the experience of pain can sometimes be more exhausting and debilitating than the pain itself.

As part of a mindful approach to pain, Dr. Caudill recommends that you "allow yourself simply to observe the pain and the feelings you may have, such as fear and anger, without running away from those feelings or the sensations. And say to yourself, 'Oh, yes, that's my pain and that's my anger.' " As you sit quietly, practicing mindfulness, keep coming back to a focus on your breath while letting your pain, and your thoughts about pain, flicker in and out of consciousness. You may notice the pain increasing in intensity. That is very common at first, and it helps to remind yourself that your awareness of pain cannot, in and of itself, make your actual pain worse. If you can sit through this heightened awareness, you'll notice frequent fluctuations in your experience of pain, how it ebbs and flows and changes quality.

I don't recommend mindfulness for every pelvic-pain patient. If it causes you excessive anxiety, move to another relaxation technique. But Jon Kabat-Zinn has shown that a vast number of pain patients can maintain a mindfulness practice, and that it very effectively helps them to manage pain and the distress associated with pain.

Steven Levine captures one commonsense reason why a strategy of mindfulness, as opposed to one of avoidance, can ease the suffering of people with chronic pain. What happens when we send hate into a part of the body in pain? What happens when we ostracize that part, isolating it from the rest of ourselves because we can't stand the messages it sends? Does that promote healing? Does that ease the suffering? Then ask yourself: What happens if I stop ostracizing that part of my body? What if I sent compassion and mercy into that part? What if I took time to focus the loving energies of my heart into the part of my body that holds so much suffering? Could that promote healing? Even if it doesn't stop the physical pain, might it not ease the emotional pain that builds as we isolate and fear a part of our own being?

Abuse, Anger, and Emotional Healing

As discussed earlier, Dr. Andrea Rapkin and others as well have helped to establish the prevalence of emotional, physical, and sexual abuse in the life histories of women with chronic pelvic pain. The complex interactions of memories, emotions, and physical pain signaling processes are not well understood. But there does appear to be a nexus of connections that, we believe, will eventually be uncovered by psychiatrists, neuroscientists, and pain specialists. Until then, women suffering with chronic pelvic pain can benefit by exploring these issues.

Both Dr. Caudill and I have found that many patients with a history of abuse suffer from posttraumatic stress disorder (PTSD), a psychological condition of ongoing distress that lingers from a past trauma. Dr. Caudill has observed an intriguing connection between their PTSD and their chronic pain: "I have frequently talked with these patients, and their descriptions of their pain mirror the effects of the psychological trauma they've experienced. They feel out of control. They hurt all the time. They say that nobody believes them."

In some instances, says Dr. Caudill, these patients can change their perception of pain signals by grappling directly with the early abuse in a thera-peutic context. It also helps when these patients can bolster their current social support systems so that they feel less isolated and less desperate. Re-lieving their desperateness to "get rid of the problem" may prevent unnec-essary surgeries that can, in some instances, make matters worse.

Obviously the fact that many women with pelvic pain have histories of abuse does not mean every such patient has an abuse history, and we know that some women searching for past events to explain current symptoms can get into trouble by believing in memories that are not real (the so-called false memory syndrome). Although the complex issues of recovered memo-ries are beyond the scope of this chapter, suffice it to say that you should proceed with care in this realm. Don't let anyone—friend, sibling, or thera-pist—tell you that you *must* have been abused. On the other hand, if you have clear memories, or sensations and images that you do not understand, seek qualified help from a mental health professional. If you have suffered abuse, dealing with the trauma and the emotions associated with that trauma can be psychologically and physically healing.

Even without an abuse history, many women with endometriosis and pelvic pain have stress, sorrow, and anger about circumstances of the past or present. Here again, psychotherapy is the best context for exploring and resolving these issues. But self-care is important, too. I strongly recommend the "Pennebaker" method of uncensored writing, described in chapter 8 (see page 161–64). Work through feelings about traumas or stressful events from childhood, the recent past, or your current life. Write out your deep-est thoughts and feelings about your pain—how it has affected your life and relationships. As you continue to write, allow yourself to move from cathar-sis to insight to action. Look for connections between your pain and various life events or stressors; then plan strategies that will enable you to manage your pain effectively.

Explore any anger you have about your pain. Many of my endometriosis and pelvic-pain patients are mad at surgeons, doctors, and hospitals for undertreating or overtreating their pain, and especially for removing organs they are no longer sure had to be removed. (The persistence of pain after surgery is a common cause of immense anger.) Other women may be angry at people in their lives who have hurt or betrayed them, blaming those people for their suffering. Therapy and journaling offer safe, healthy outlets for raw anger, including the sheer frustration about having to live with pain. But Margaret Caudill emphasizes that people who stake out a fixed position of blame—who can't stop being furious at people or institutions they feel have caused or worsened the pain—give away their power to manage their own pain. "It helps to ask yourself where is your responsibility to deal with your own pain," she has commented.

Dr. Caudill encourages women stuck in blaming anger to do their best to let it go. One reason they have trouble doing so, she suggests, is that giving up blame toward others is to somehow turn the finger of accusation back toward themselves. If it's not someone else's fault, it must be their own. Such black-and-white thinking is both distorted and hurtful. If you find yourself in this trap, here is one way to reframe your thinking: *The fact that your pain may not be someone else's fault does not mean that it is your fault.*

Eventually, it helps to move through anger toward acceptance of your pain and of your own responsibility for reducing it. Doing so does not entail self-blame; it entails a full recognition of your own power to change and to heal.

Moving Beyond Pain

I have seen much evidence that mind-body medicine can help women to better manage, and in some instances to resolve, endometriosis and pelvic pain. In some cases, the actual pain does not lessen significantly, but the woman is no longer emotionally or spiritually hobbled by the pain. I am reminded of an old 1970s routine by comedian Robert Klein, who described the hilarious absurdities of a visit to the dentist. At one point, he captured how nitrous oxide, the "laughing gas" used for pain, manages to be effective. Its magic does not lie in its ability to narcotize physical discomfort. "You still feel the pain," he explained, "but you don't give a ----!"

For some women who use mind-body methods, the experience may be comparable. They still feel the pain, but it no longer messes up their lives. As Margaret Caudill says, "It's pretty rare for my patients to have their pain miraculously disappear. But the early sessions of my groups are often amazing, because you would not know that these were pain patients. The transformation occurs surprisingly quickly, and it is so exciting. They are sitting there with their pain, but they are laughing and joking and carrying on as if they had no pain."

One of Dr. Caudill's pelvic-pain patients, Whitney, thirty-four, was first diagnosed with pelvic inflammatory disease (PID), but a later laparoscopy revealed endometriosis. She was desperate for relief, and her surgeon took out first one ovary, then the other, and eventually she had a complete hysterectomy. But her pain still persisted. She continued to go for physical evaluations, and new diagnoses kept being offered, including interstitial cystitis.

Like a substantial number of pelvic-pain patients, Whitney had a past history of abuse. She was also stressed by her financial circumstances, and by a relationship with a man made more difficult by her pain, which sometimes caused intercourse to be incredibly uncomfortable. There were times when she needed to say no but could not, because she wanted to please him. Meanwhile, her doctors and family members did not validate her pain, tagging her with that invidious old label, "hysteric."

Whitney was referred to one of Dr. Caudill's groups, where she learned all of the pain management methods described in this chapter. Relaxation and mindful walking helped, and Whitney began to control her own experience of pain. Dr. Caudill also validated her pain, and taught her assertiveness skills that empowered her to say no to sex when she did not feel like it. Given her abuse history, this ability to assert her needs and rights in a present-day relationships appears to have had a healing effect.

Whitney's pelvic pain has not completely gone away; nor has her anger at the surgeries she has endured, which may or may not have been necessary. But she is able to enjoy life again—to function at a level that makes her feel good about herself. She laughs with Dr. Caudill about the chronicity of her condition, saying, "I know, I know, Dr. Caudill. I have pelvic hyper-algesia!"

When you embark on a mind-body program for the management of endometriosis and/or pelvic pain, do so with hope but without illusions. Don't expect early miracles, because a lapse into disappointment or self-blame could make matters worse. Move forward with as much gentleness, patience, and self-compassion as you can muster, and you will shift the balance of power in your struggle with pain.

Seventeen

◆ ◆ ◆ ◆ ◆ ◆

SELF-ESTEEM IS A WOMEN'S HEALTH ISSUE

*W*omen's health issues are at the forefront of our cultural consciousness as never before. Media coverage of these concerns has reached a high-water mark, and it's about time. Activists have urged more research on women's health, and their efforts are bearing fruit with the federal government and at research institutions nationwide. Medical empowerment and self-care strategies are being advocated and practiced by increasing numbers of women. Books on women's health offer guidance through the medical maze and a variety of alternative treatments for every conceivable condition.

Yet for a long time, something crucial has been missing from the cultural equation on women's health. We have been rightly urged to take charge of our medical care, and we've been encouraged to treat our conditions with a spate of vitamins, herbs, and other alternatives such as acupuncture and homeopathy. But we have *not* been educated about how to utilize the most subtle yet powerful—and empowering—health-care system at our command: our own minds.

It has taken a long time, but the notion that mind-body treatments are frivolous additions to the medical armamentarium is finally being debunked. The old characterizations of mind-body medicine as soft, New Age, unscientific, or outright flaky are dying hard, as studies reveal how effective—*and* how cost-effective—these treatments can be for chronic pain, high blood pressure, arthritis, heart attack recovery, immune dysfunctions, and other disorders. And we now know that the most common women's health conditions can be successfully treated with mind-body medicine. The old dichotomy between mainstream and mind-body medicine is finally being overcome, and women are benefiting from fortuitous combinations of these two powerful and often complementary systems of healing.

Herbert Benson, M.D., has contributed enormously to the integration of mind-body medicine into the mainstream, a process that remains slow but steady. His work has helped to convince many scientists that there is no contradiction between these two approaches: a calm mind lays the foundation for a healing body. The biochemistry of healing can no longer be said to proceed without the orchestration of the brain, which produces an astonishing array of chemicals that influence every organ and bodily system, including our hearts, glands, tissues, and immune cells. Our work at Harvard Medical School's Division of Behavioral Medicine at the Deaconess Hospital, and at the Mind/Body Medical Institute, has shown that women's reproductive organs are certainly not exempt from this mind-body relationship. Indeed, the connections are so intimate that mind-body practices have proven their mettle in the treatment of many disorders or symptoms that affect only women.

The medical use of the relaxation response has endured, because its benefits simply cannot be ignored. Even the use of prayer and other spiritual practices, once deemed to have no place in medicine, is being accepted, because, as Dr. Benson and enlightened physicians such as Larry Dossey have shown, meditation and prayer can have powerfully positive physiologic effects. It does not matter how you explain this phenomenon, because it's not necessary to embrace any theology to acknowledge the physical changes that occur.

The relaxation response carries enormous benefits for women, helping them to cope with conditions ranging from PMS to breast cancer. But it also lays the groundwork for a deeper exploration of the mind-body connection, one that has special meanings and applications for women. Once we've achieved some peace of mind, we can finally get in touch with our needs, assess our conflicts, experience our bodies—thinking and feeling with clarity and purpose.

What many women discover is that they have not felt entitled to care, because they've been living too long with shame about their bodies or themselves. Though we still don't understand every physiological linkage between mind and body, it is becoming clear that shame and low self-esteem can erode our healing abilities. Of course, the opposite is also true: self-esteem promotes health and healing. The "mechanisms" behind this relationship are many: women with self-esteem are better able to take charge of their medical care, procuring skilled and responsive doctors, following leads for effective treatments, demanding information and involvement in every decision. But we're also learning that women's self-esteem may bolster internal healing processes of the body. Such women not only have inner calm, but the healthy sense of control that I have come to view as a litmus test of mind–body health.

That is why I believe self-esteem to be a health issue, on a par with diet, exercise, and early detection of disease. Mind–body techniques are gateways to wellness, but in my experience they are most effective when they open doors to self-acceptance and self-worth. For instance, we know that social support is a major contributor to the prevention of, and recovery from, most chronic and life-threatening diseases. Women who lack self-esteem may not be able to procure the kind of support they need to remain healthy or to heal. Nor will they feel entitled to express their emotions, or assert their rights in the home or the workplace or the hospital. In differing ways, research by David Spiegel, Lydia Temoshok, Steven Greer, and James Pennebaker all strongly suggest that expressing emotions can promote healing processes in the body.

Put differently, our willingness to take care of our needs, based on a bedrock of self-worth, sends a message not only to people we love and interact with; it sends a message to our own bodily systems, a message that appears to strengthen our resistance and our resilience. As demonstrated by the body of research cited in this book, it's now quite apparent that the message is received by our reproductive systems; such research has demonstrated the benefits of mind–body medicine for women with PMS, hot flashes caused by natural or artificial menopause, breast cancer, and infertility, among other conditions.

But mind–body medicine is, indeed, just a gateway to self-esteem for women. We must "go the extra mile" and be certain to use these techniques not as disconnected remedies—as if they were pills—but rather as integrated attempts to uncover our real selves and build our self-worth. As a therapist, I never dictate what kind of lives women must lead in order to feel good about themselves. There should be no politically correct recipes for career, family, and creative pursuits that bolster self-esteem.

Consider the case of Linda, a forty-five-year-old nurse with a nimble mind and sparkly personality, who suffered every month with bouts of PMS and terrible mood swings. From an early age, Linda's parents had inculcated her with caretaking behaviors. The oldest of four children, Linda was obliged to watch over her younger siblings when her parents were both working. As so often happens, Linda was a terrific surrogate parent, and she got kudos for her abilities—kudos that gradually transformed into a label ("You're such a great helper!") and a powerful expectation: Linda's life's work should, of course, center around her wonderful caretaking skills. Her parents encouraged her to become a nurse, and the rest was history. After she married and had two children, Linda assumed the same role in her own family—the rock of support with boundless energy for fulfilling everyone else's desires.

It was Linda's symptoms that finally prompted her to consider the need for change. Her deeper explorations, helped along by mind-body methods, led Linda to realize that she was indeed a wonderful caretaker, but that was not all she was. She had always loved to write, but had never pursued writing because she had so little time in the spaces between caretaking her patients and her own children. So she began to write poems and short stories. This required Linda to insist on time for herself, which was tough to do with a hard working husband and two young children. But she found the time, and made certain she was left in quiet solitude to pursue her writing. Eventually, one of her short stories was published in a literary journal.

In time, Linda's PMS improved and her mood swings were no longer so dramatic. She still loved nursing, and she did not have to quit to create balance and harmony in her life. By honoring her creative urges, and taking time for herself, Linda forged that proper balance, which had a positive influence on her work, her family life, and, she believes, her own biology.

Linda's story shows that self-esteem means honoring the self. When we care for every sparkling facet of ourselves—the professional, the parent, the lover, the wife, the friend, the artist, the adventurer—we uplift our self-esteem and physical well-being. To honor these "selves," relaxation is a first step, paving the way to heightened awareness. But then we need to make a firm commitment to caring for ourselves, to living out our potentialities. In *Honoring the Self,* psychologist Nathaniel Branden, Ph.D., writes what amounts to a covenant that we can make with ourselves to maintain this commitment:

> To honor the self is to be willing to think independently, to live by our own mind, and to have the courage of our perceptions and judgments.
>
> To honor the self is to be willing to know not only what we think but also what we feel, what we want, need, desire, suffer over, are frightened or angered by—and to accept our right to experience such feelings. The opposite of this attitude is denial, disowning, repression—self-repudiation.

To honor the self is to preserve an attitude of self-acceptance—which means to accept what we are, without self-oppression or self-castigation, without any pretense about the truth of our own being, pretense aimed at deceiving either ourselves or anyone else.

To honor the self is to live authentically, to speak and act from our innermost convictions and feelings.

To honor the self is to refuse to accept unearned guilt and to do our best to correct such guilt as we may have earned.

To honor the self is to be committed to our right to exist, which proceeds from the knowledge that our life does not belong to someone else's expectations. To many people, this is a terrifying responsibility. To honor the self is to be in love with our own life, in love with our own possibilities for growth and experiencing joy, in love with the process of discovering and exploring our distinctively human potentialities.

I like Dr. Branden's covenant, which speaks particularly eloquently to women. It also speaks to the qualities we need when we interface with mainstream medicine: a commitment to our right to exist, to preserve an attitude of self-acceptance, and to speak and act from our innermost convictions and feelings. I also believe, based on the mind-body research presented here, that we honor the body when we honor the self, supporting our innate capacities for self-repair and regeneration. Women who live out their true identity, without shame or apology, are nourishing the life of the mind and the body.

Appendix A

♦ ♦ ♦ ♦ ♦ ♦ ♦

REFERENCES AND

SUGGESTED READINGS

1. *Women, Stress, and Mind–Body Medicine*

Beeson, P. B. "Age and sex associations of 40 autoimmune diseases." *American Journal of Medicine* 96,5 (1994): 457–62.

Benson, H., E. M. Stuart, and staff of the Mind/Body Medical Institute. *The Wellness Book: The Comprehensive Guide to Maintaining Health and Treating Stress-Related Illness.* New York: Carol Publishing, 1992.

Deckro, J., A. Domar, and G. Deckro. "Clinical applications of the relaxation response in women's health." *NAACOG's Clinical Issues in Perinatal and Women's Health Nursing* 4 (1993): 311–19.

Hatcher, R. *Contraceptive Technology 1984–85.* New York: Irvington Publishers, 1984.

Hoffman, E. *Our Health, Our Lives.* New York: Pocket Books, 1996.

Kiecolt-Glaser, J. K., and R. Glaser. "Stress and immune function in humans." In R. Ader, D. L. Felten, and N. Cohen, eds., *Psychoneuroimmunology,* 2nd ed., pp. 849–67. San Diego: Academic Press, 1991.

Levy, S. M., R. B. Herberman, M. Lipman, and T. D'Angelo. "Correlation of stress factors with sustained depression of natural killer cell activity with predicted prognosis in patients with breast cancer." *Journal of Clinical Oncology* 5,3 (1987): 348–53.

Lipton, R. B., and W. F. Stewart. "The epidemiology of migraine." *European Neurology* 34 Supplement 2 (1994): 6–11.

Loftus, T. "Psychogenic factors in anovulatory women; behavioral and psychoanalytic aspects of anovulatory amenorrhea." *Fertility and Sterility* 13 (1962): 20.

Morse, D. *Women Under Stress.* New York: Van Nostrand Reinhold, 1982.

Northrup, C. *Women's Bodies, Women's Wisdom: Creating Physical and Emotional Health and Healing.* New York: Bantam Books, 1994.

Piotrowski, T. "Psychogenic Factors in Anovulatory Women." *Fertility and Sterility* 13 (1962): 11.

Sapolsky, R. M. *Why Zebras Don't Get Ulcers.* New York: Freeman and Co., 1994.

Semler, T. C. *All About Eve: The Complete Guide to Women's Health and Well-Being*. New York: HarperCollins, 1995.

Speroff, L., R. Glass, and R. Kase. *Clinical Gynecologic Endocrinology and Infertility*. Baltimore: Williams and Wilkins, 1989.

Steinem, G. *Revolution from Within: A Book of Self-Esteem*. Boston: Little, Brown, 1993.

Suter, D., and N. Schwartz. "Glucocorticoids suppress the responsiveness of the pituitary to LHRH." *Endocrinology* 117 (1985): 849.

Swartzman, L. C., R. Edelberg, and E. Kemmann. "Impact of stress on objectively recorded menopausal hot flushes on flush report bias." *Health Psychology* 9 (1990): 529–45.

Weil, A. *Spontaneous Healing*. New York: Alfred A. Knopf, 1995.

Wolf, N. *The Beauty Myth*. New York: Anchor Books, 1992.

2. The Relaxation Response and Other Coping Skills

Beary, J. F., and H. Benson. "A simple psychophysiologic technique which elicits the hypometabolic changes of the relaxation response." *Psychosomatic Medicine* 36 (1974): 115–20.

Benson, H. *Your Maximum Mind*. New York: Times Books, 1987.

Benson, H., and M. Klipper. *The Relaxation Response*. New York: Avon, 1976.

Caudill, M., et al. "Decreased clinic use by chronic pain patients' response to behavioral medicine intervention." *Clinical Journal of Pain* 7 (1991): 305–10.

Domar, A., and H. Benson. "Application of behavioral medicine techniques to the treatment of infertility." In M. Seibel, ed., *Technology and Infertility*. New York: Springer, 1993.

Domar, A., L. Everett, and M. Keller. "Preoperative anxiety: Is it a predictable entity?" *Anesthesiology Analgesia* 69 (1989): 763–67.

Domar, A., J. H. Irvin, R. Friedman, and D. Mills. "The effect of relaxation training on tamoxifen-induced hot flashes." Paper presented at the annual meeting of the Society of Behavioral Medicine, San Diego, March 1995.

Domar, A., J. Noe, and H. Benson. "The preoperative use of the relaxation response with ambulatory surgery patients." *Journal of Human Stress* 13 (1987): 101–17.

Dreher, H. *The Immune Power Personality: 7 Traits You Can Develop to Stay Healthy*. New York: Dutton Books, 1995.

Goodale, I., A. Domar, and H. Benson. "Alleviation of premenstrual symptoms with the relaxation response." *Obstetrics and Gynecology* 75 (1990): 649–55.

Hoffman, J. W., H. Benson, P. A. Arns, et al. "Reduced sympathetic nervous system responsivity associated with the relaxation response." *Science* 215 (1982): 190–92.

Irvin, J. H., A. Domar, C. Clark, P. C. Zuttermeister, and R. Friedman. "The effects of relaxation response training on menopausal symptoms." In press, *Journal of Psychosomatic Obstetrics and Gynecology*.

Jacobs, G., P. Rosenberg, R. Friedman, J. Matheson, A. Peavy, A. Domar, and H. Benson. "Multifactor treatment of chronic sleep-onset insomnia using stimulus control and the relaxation response." *Behavioral Modification* 17 (1993): 498–508.

Kaplan, S. H., S. Greenfield, and J. E. Ware. "Assessing the effects of physician-patient interactions on the outcomes of chronic disease." *Medical Care* 27, Supplement 3 (1989): S110–27.

Kiecolt-Glaser, J. K., R. Glaser, E. C. Strain, et al. "Modulation of cellular immunity in medical students." *Journal of Behavioral Medicine* 9 (1986): 5–21.

Kobasa, S. O. "Commitment, control, and challenge: The winning combination for a long and happy life." In E. Padus, et al., eds., *Your Emotions and Your Health*. Emmaus, Pa.: Rodale Press, 1986.

———."Stressful life events, personality and health: An inquiry into hardiness." *Journal of Personality and Social Psychology* 37 (1979): 1–11.

Kobasa, S. C., S. Maddi, and S. Kahn. "Hardiness and health: A prospective study." *Journal of Personality and Social Psychology* 42 (1982): 168–77.

Lehmann, J. W., I. L. Goodale, and H. Benson. "Reduced pupillary sensitivity to topical phenylephrine associated with the relaxation response." *Journal of Human Stress* 12 (1986): 101–4.

Leserman, J., et al. "Nonpharmacologic intervention for hypertension: Long-term follow-up." *Journal of Cardiopulmonary Rehabilitation* 9 (1989): 316–24.

Mandle, C., A. Domar, D. Harrington, J. Leserman, E. Bozadjian, R. Friedman, and H. Benson. "The use of the relaxation response in alleviating pain and anxiety in patients undergoing femoral arteriograms." *Radiology* 174 (1990): 737–40.

Mikulas, W. L., and M.G.T. Kwee, eds. "Meditation, self-control, and personal growth." In *Psychotherapy, Meditation, and Health: A Cognitive-Behavioral Perspective*. London and The Hague: East-West Publications, 1990.

Shapiro, D., and M.G.T. Kwee, eds. "Meditation, self-control, and control by a benevolent other: Issues of content and context." In *Psychotherapy, Meditation, and Health: A Cognitive-Behavioral Perspective*. London and The Hague: East-West Publications, 1990.

3. Roads to Relaxation

Achterberg, J. *Imagery in Healing*. Boston: New Science Library, 1985.

Benson, H., J. Beary, and M. Carol. "The relaxation response." *Psychiatry* 37 (1974): 37.

Borysenko, J. *Minding the Body, Mending the Mind*. Reading, Mass.: Addison-Wesley, 1987, p. 2.

Dossey, L. *Healing Words: The Power of Prayer and the Practice of Medicine*. New York: HarperCollins, 1994.

Goldstein, J., and J. Kornfield. *Seeking the Heart of Wisdom: The Path of Insight Meditation*. Boston: Shambhala, 1987.

Jacobson, E. *You Must Relax*. New York: McGraw-Hill, 1962.

Kabat-Zinn, J. *Full Catastrophe Living: Using the Wisdom of Your Body and Mind to Face Stress, Pain and Illness*. New York: Delacorte, 1991.

———. "An outpatient program in behavioral medicine for chronic pain patients based on the practice of mindfulness meditation." *General Hospital Psychiatry* 4 (1982): 33.

———. *Wherever You Go, There You Are: Mindfulness Meditation in Everyday Life, Meditation for Daily Living*. New York: Hyperion, 1994.

LeShan, L. *How to Meditate.* Boston: Little, Brown and Co., 1974.

O'Brien, P. *Yoga for Women.* New York: HarperCollins, 1995.

Rossman, M. L. *Healing Yourself: A Step-by-Step Program for Better Health Through Imagery.* New York: Walker, 1987.

Schultz, J. H., and W. Luthe. *Autogenic Therapy.* 6 vols. New York: Grune and Stratton, 1969.

Sheikh, A. A., ed. *Imagination and Healing.* Farmingdale, N.Y.: Baywood, 1984.

Tobias, M. *Complete Stretching.* New York: Random House, 1992.

4. Mini-Relaxations: The Perfect Portable Stress Managers

Benson, H., E. M. Stuart, and staff of the Mind/Body Medical Institute. *The Wellness Book: The Comprehensive Guide to Maintaining Health and Treating Stress-Related Illness.* New York: Carol Publishing, 1992.

Hendler, S. S. *The Oxygen Breakthrough.* New York: Pocket Books, 1989.

5. Catching the Nasty Mind: Cognitive Restructuring

Beck, A. T. *Cognitive Therapy and Emotional Disorders.* New York: International Universities Press, 1976.

Borysenko, J. *Guilt Is the Teacher, Love Is the Lesson.* New York: Warner Books, 1990.

Burns, D. D. *The Feeling Good Handbook: Using the New Mood Therapy in Everyday Life.* New York: William Morrow, 1989.

Meichenbaum, D. *Cognitive-Behavioral Modification: An Integrative Approach.* New York: Plenum Press, 1977.

Peterson, C., and M.E.P. Seligman. "Explanatory style and illness." *Journal of Personality* 55 (1987): 237–65.

Peterson, C., M.E.P. Seligman, and G. E. Vaillant. "Pessimistic explanatory style is a risk factor for physical illness: A thirty-five-year longitudinal study." *Journal of Personality and Social Psychology* 55 (1988): 23–27.

6. Healing Through Self-Nurturance

Brody, R. "The sweet science of smell." *American Health* 5 (May) 1986: 55–60.

Ironson, G., T. Field, and F. Scafidi, et al. "Massage therapy is associated with enhancement of the immune system's cytotoxic capacity." *International Journal of Neuroscience,* 1995.

Katcher, A. H., et al. "Comparison of contemplation and hypnosis for the reduction of anxiety and discomfort during dental surgery." *American Journal of Clinical Hypnosis* 27 (1984): 14–21.

Leibowitz, S. "Brain neurotransmitters and drug effects on food intake and appetite: Implications for eating disorders." In Walsh, ed., *Eating Behavior in Eating Disorders.* Washington, D.C.: American Psychiatric Press, 1988.

Moen, P., D. Dempster-McClain, and R. M. Williams. "Social integration and longevity: An event history analysis of women's roles and resilience." *American Sociological Review* 54 (1989): 635–47.

————. "Successful aging: A life course perspective on women's multiple roles and health." *American Journal of Sociology* 97(6) (1992): 1612–38.

Montagu, A. *Touching: The Human Significance of the Skin.* New York: Harper and Row, 1978.

Moos, R. H., and G. F. Solomon. "Psychologic comparisons between women with rheumatoid arthritis and their non-arthritic sisters I. Personality test and interview rating data." *Psychosomatic Medicine* 27 (1965): 135–49.

————. "Psychologic comparisons between women with rheumatoid arthritis and their non-arthritic sisters II. Content analysis of interviews." *Psychosomatic Medicine* 27 (1965): 150–64.

Ornstein, R., and D. Sobel. *Healthy Pleasures.* Reading, Mass.: Addison-Wesley, 1989.

Rider, M. S., J. W. Floyd, and J. Kirkpatrick. "The effect of music, imagery, and relaxation on adrenal corticosteroids and the reentrainment of circadian rhythms." *Journal of Music Therapy* 22(1) (1985): 46–58.

Solomon, G. F., et al. "Early experience and immunity." *Nature* 220 (1968): 821–22.

Solomon, G. F., M. E. Kemeny, and L. Temoshok. "Psychoneuroimmunologic aspects of human immunodeficiency virus infection." In R. Ader, D. L. Felton, and N. Cohen, eds., *Psychoneuroimmunology II.* New York: Academic Press, 1991.

Solomon, G. F., L. Temoshok, A. O'Leary, and J. Zich. "An intensive psychoimmunologic study of long-surviving persons with AIDS." *Annals of the New York Academy of Sciences* 496 (1987): 647–55.

7. Reaching Out to Friends and Family

Berkman, L. F., et al. "Emotional support and survival after myocardial infarction." *Annals of Internal Medicine* 117 (1992): 1003–9.

Berkman, L. F., and S. L. Syme. "Social networks, host resistance, and mortality: A nine-year follow-up study of Alameda County residents." *American Journal of Epidemiology* 109 (1979): 186–204.

Gjerdingen, D. K., et al. "The effects of social support on women's health during pregnancy, labor and delivery, and the postpartum period." *Family Medicine* 23 (July 1991): 370–75.

House, J. S., K. R. Landis, and D. Umberson. "Social relationships and health." *Science* 241 (1988): 540–45.

Kiecolt-Glaser, J. K., et al. "Negative behavior during marital conflict is associated with immunological down-regulation." *Psychosomatic Medicine* 55 (1993): 395–409.

Lee, K. A., and C. A. Rittenhouse. "Health and perimenstrual symptoms: Health outcomes for employed women who experience perimenstrual symptoms." *Women and Health* 19 (1992): 65–78.

Maunsell, E., et al. "Social support and survival among women with breast cancer." *Cancer* 76 (1995): 631–37.

Moen, P., D. Dempster-McClain, and R. M. Williams. "Successful aging: A life course perspective on women's multiple roles and health." *American Journal of Sociology* 97(6) (1992): 1612–38.

Montero, I., et al. "Social functioning as a significant factor in women's help-seeking behavior during the climacteric period." *Social Psychiatry and Psychiatric Epidemiology* 28 (August 1993): 178–83.

Ney, P. G., et al. "The effects of pregnancy loss on women's health." *Social Science and Medicine* 38 (May 1994): 1193–1200.

Spiegel, D., J. R. Bloom, H. C. Kraemer, and E. Gottheil. "Effect of psychosocial treatment on survival of patients with metastatic breast cancer." *Lancet* 2 (1989): 888–91.

Wolf, S., and J. G. Bruhn. *The Power of Clan.* New Brunswick, N.J.: Transaction Publishers, 1993.

8. *Women's Anger, Women's Joy: Emotional Expression*

Bower, S. A., and G. Bower. *Asserting Yourself.* Reading, Mass.: Addison-Wesley, 1976.

Greer, S., and T. Morris. "Psychological attributes of women who develop breast cancer: A controlled study." *Journal of Psychosomatic Research* 19 (1975): 147–53.

Gross, J. "Emotional expression in cancer onset and progression." *Social Science and Medicine* 28(12) (1989): 1239–48.

Lerner, H. G. *The Dance of Anger: A Woman's Guide to Changing the Patterns of Intimate Relationships.* New York: Harper and Row, 1985.

Levy, S. M., J. Lee, C. Bageley, and M. Lippman. "Survival hazards analysis in first recurrent breast cancer patients: Seven-year follow up." *Psychosomatic Medicine* 50 (1988): 520–28.

Pennebaker, J. W. *Opening Up: The Healing Power of Confiding in Others.* New York: William Morrow and Co., 1990.

———. "Putting stress into words: Health, linguistic, and therapeutic implications." *Behavioral Research and Therapy* 31 (1993): 539–48.

Pennebaker, J. W., and S. Beall. "Confronting a traumatic event: Toward an understanding of inhibition and disease." *Journal of Abnormal Psychology* 95 (1986): 274–81.

Pennebaker, J. W., K. Kiecolt-Glaser, and R. Glaser. "Disclosure of traumas and immune function: Health implications for psychotherapy." *Journal of Consulting and Clinical Psychology* 56 (1988): 239–45.

Temoshok, L. "Biopsychosocial studies on cutaneous malignant melanoma: Psychosocial factors associated with prognostic indicators, progression, psychophysiology, and tumor-host response." *Social Science and Medicine* 20(8) (1985): 833–40.

9. *Mindful Eating, Modest Exercise*

Alpha-Tocopherol, Beta Carotene Cancer Prevention Study Group. "The effect of vitamin E and beta carotene on the incidence of lung cancer and other cancers in male smokers." *New England Journal of Medicine* 330 (1994): 1029–35.

Bernstein, L., B. E. Henderson, R. Hanisch, J. Sullivan-Halley, and R. K. Ross. "Physical exercise activity and reduced risk of breast cancer in young women." *Journal of the National Cancer Institute* 86 (1994): 1403.

Bisbind, M. S. "Nutritional deficiency in the etiology of menorrhagia, cystic mastitis, premenstrual syndrome, and treatment with vitamin B complex." *Journal of Clinical Endocrinology and Metabolism* 3 (1943): 227–334.

Blot, W. J., J.-Y. Li, P. R. Taylor, et al. "Nutrition intervention trials in Linxian, China: Supplementation with specific vitamin/mineral combinations, cancer incidence, and disease-specific mortality in the general population." *Journal of National Cancer Institute* 85 (1993): 1483–92.

Brody, J. "Vitamin E greatly reduces risk of heart disease, studies suggest." *New York Times,* 20 May 1993, p. A1.

———. Making the case for antioxidants." *New York Times,* 20 April 1994, p. C11.

Brown, J. D. "Staying fit and staying well: Physical fitness as a moderator of life stress." *Journal of Personality and Social Psychology* 60 (1991): 555–61.

Butler, E. B., and E. McKnight. "Vitamin E in the treatment of primary dysmenorrhea." *Lancet* 1 (1955): 844–47.

Butterworth, C. E., et al. "Improvement in cervical dysplasia associated with folic acid therapy in users of oral contraceptives." *American Journal of Clinical Nutrition* 35 (1982): 73.

Colbin, A. *Food and Healing.* New York: Ballantine Books, 1988.

Cooper, K. *The Aerobics Program for Total Well-Being.* New York: Bantam Books, 1985.

deVries, H. A. "Tranquilizer effect of exercise: A critical review." *Physician and Sports Medicine* 9 (1981): 47–55.

Frisch, R. E., G. Wyshak, N. Albright, et al. "Lower lifetime occurrence of breast cancer and cancer of the reproductive system among former college athletes." *American Journal of Clinical Nutrition* 45 (1987): 328.

Griest, J. H., M. H. Klein, R. R. Eischens, J. Faris, A. S. Gurman, and W. P. Morgan. "Running as a treatment for depression." *Comparative Psychiatry* 53 (1979): 20–41.

Hunter, D. J., et al. "A prospective study of the intake of vitamins C, E, and A and the risk of breast cancer." *New England Journal of Medicine* 329(4) (July 1993): 234–40.

Landau, R. S., et al. "The effect of alpha tocopherol in premenstrual symptomatology: A double-blind trial." *Journal of the American College of Nutrition* 2 (1983): 115–23.

London, S. J., et al. "Carotenoids, retinol, and vitamin E and risk of proliferative benign breast disease and breast cancer." *Cancer Causes and Control* 3(6) (November 1992): 503–12.

Martin-Moreno, J. M., et al. "Dietary fat, olive oil intake and breast cancer risk." *International Journal of Cancer* 58(6) (September 1994): 774–80.

Milunsky, A., et al. "Multivitamin/folic acid supplementation in early pregnancy reduces the prevalence of neural tube defects." *Journal of the American Medical Association* 262 (1989): 2847–52.

O'Neill, M. "So it may be true after all: Eating pasta makes you fat." *New York Times,* 8 February 1995, p. A1.

Romney, S. L., et al. "Plasma, vitamin C and uterine cervical dysplasia." *American Journal of Obstetrics and Gynecology* 151(7) (1985): 976–80.

Roth, G. *When Food Is Love.* New York: Dutton, 1990.

Thayer, R., and J. R. Newman. "Exercise is the best strategy for changing a bad mood, raising energy, and reducing tension." *Journal of Personality and Social Psychology* 67(5) (November 7, 1994): 910–25.

Willett, W. C., et al. "Dietary fat and fiber in relation to risk of breast cancer. An 8-year follow-up." *Journal of the American Medical Association* 268 (October 21, 1992): 2037–44.

Willett, W. C., and D. J. Hunter. "Vitamin A and cancers of the breast, large bowel and prostate: Epidemiologic evidence." *Nutrition Reviews* 52 (part 2) (February 1994): S53–59.

10. The Storm Before the Calm: PMS

Abplanalp, J. M., L. Livingston, R. M. Rose, and D. Sandwisch. "Cortisol and growth hormone responses to psychological stress during the menstrual cycle." *Psychosomatic Medicine* 39 (1977): 158–77.

Abraham, G. E. "Nutritional factors in the etiology of the premenstrual tension syndromes." *Journal of Reproductive Medicine* 28 (1983): 446–64.

Collins, A., P. Eneroth, and B. Landgren. "Psychoneuroendocrine stress responses and mood as related to the menstrual cycle." *Psychosomatic Medicine* 47 (1985): 512–27.

Goodale, I., A. Domar, and H. Benson. "Alleviation of premenstrual symptoms with the relaxation response." *Obstetrics and Gynecology* 75 (1990): 649–55.

Horrobin, D. F. "The role of essential fatty acids and the prostaglandins in the premenstrual syndrome." *Journal of Reproductive Medicine* 28 (1983): 465–68.

Kirkby, R. J. "Changes in premenstrual symptoms and irrational thinking following cognitive-behavioral coping skills training." *Journal of Consulting and Clinical Psychology* 62(5) (1994): 1026–32.

Lark, Susan. *PMS Self-Help Book*. Santa Monica, Calif.: Forman Publishing, 1984.

London, R. S., et al. "Evaluation and treatment of breast symptoms in patients with premenstrual syndrome." *Journal of Reproductive Medicine* 28 (1983): 503–8.

Marinari, K. T., A. I. Leshner, and M. P. Doyle. "Menstrual cycle status and adrenocortical reactivity to psychological stress." *Psychoneuroendocrinology* 1 (1976): 213–18.

Prior, J. "Conditioning exercise decreases premenstrual symptoms: A prospective, controlled 6-month trial." *Fertility and Sterility* 47 (1987): 402.

Semler, T. C. *All About Eve: The Complete Guide to Women's Health and Well-Being*. New York: HarperCollins, 1995.

Siegel, J., J. Johnson, and I. Sarason. "Life changes and menstrual discomfort." *Journal of Human Stress* 5 (1979): 41–46.

Steiner, M., et al. "Fluoxetine in the treatment of premenstrual dysphoria." *New England Journal of Medicine* 332 (June 8, 1995): 1529–34.

Woods, N. F., and G. K. Dery. "Stressful life events and perimenstrual symptoms." *Journal of Human Stress* 8 (1982): 23–31.

Woods, N. F., A. Most, and G. D. Longenecker. "Major life events, daily stressors and perimenstrual symptoms." *Nursing Research* 34 (1985): 263–67.

11. *Reclaiming Your Life: Infertility*

Benedek, Therese, et al. "Some emotional factors in infertility." *Psychosomatic Medicine* 15(5) (1953): 485–98.

Boivin, J. "The relationship between treatment distress and embryo quality in predicting pregnancy rate with in vitro fertilization (IVF)." Paper presented at the meeting of the American Society for Reproductive Medicine. Seattle, Washington, October 7–12, 1995.

Domar, A. D. "Cognitive-behavioral approaches in the treatment of infertility." In A. Kuczmierczyk and A. Reading, eds., *Handbook of Behavioral Obstetrics and Gynecology*. New York: Plenum Press, in press.

————. "A behavioral medicine program for infertility." Paper presented at conference, The Treatment of Infertility: Bigger Issues, Better Solutions, September 14–15, 1995. Paris, France.

————. "Infertility and women's health." In H. Benson and E. Stuart, eds., *The Wellness Book*, pp. 304–20. New York: Carol Publishing, 1992.

Domar, A., and H. Benson. "Application of behavioral medicine techniques to the treatment of infertility." In M. Seibel, ed., *Technology and Infertility*. New York: Springer, 1993.

Domar, A., A. Broome, P. Zuttermeister, M. Seibel, and R. Friedman. "The prevalence and predictability of depression in infertile women." *Fertility Sterility* 58 (1992): 1158–63.

Domar, A. D., and J. H. Irvin. "The clinical application of behavioral medicine to women's health issues." Paper presented at the annual meeting of the Society of Behavioral Medicine. Boston, April 13–16, 1994.

Domar, A., and M. Seibel. "The emotional aspects of infertility." In M. Seibel, ed., *Infertility: A Comprehensive Text*, pp. 23–35. E. Norwalk, Conn.: Appleton-Lange, 1989.

Domar, A., M. Seibel, and H. Benson. "The mind/body program for infertility: A new behavioral treatment approach for women with infertility." *Fertility Sterility* 53 (1990): 246–49.

Domar, A. D., P. C. Zuttermeister, and R. Friedman. "Stress and female infertility I: Cognitive-behavioral treatment of distress." 1996, submitted for publication.

Domar, A. D., P. C. Zuttermeister, and R. Friedman. "Stress and female infertility II: The relationship between distress and conception." 1996, submitted for publication.

Domar, A., P. Zuttermeister, and R. Friedman. "The psychological impact of infertility: A comparison with patients with other medical conditions." *Journal of Psychosomatic Obstetrics and Gynecology* 14 (1993): 45–52.

Domar, A., P. Zuttermeister, M. Seibel, and H. Benson. "Psychological improvement in infertile women following behavioral treatment: A replication." *Fertility and Sterility* 58 (1992): 144–47.

Mahlstedt, P. "The psychological component of infertility." *Fertility and Sterility* 43 (1985): 335–46.

Menning, B. "The emotional needs of infertile couples." *Fertility and Sterility* 34 (1980): 313–19.

Seibel, M. M., and M. L. Taymor. "Emotional aspects of infertility." *Fertility and Sterility* 37 (1982): 137–45.

Thiering, P., et al. "Mood state as a predictor of treatment outcome after in vitro fertilization/embryo transfer technology (IVF/ET)." *Journal of Psychosomatic Research* 37 (1993): 481–91.

Wasser, S. K., G. Sewall, and M. R. Soules. "Psychosocial stress as a cause of infertility." *Fertility and Sterility* 59 (March 1993): 685–89.

12. Calming the Womb: Miscarriage and Difficult Pregnancy

Arck, P. C., et al. "Stress-triggered abortion: Inhibition of protective suppression and promotion of tumor-necrosis factor alpha (TNF-alpha) release as a mechanism triggering resorptions in mice." *American Journal of Reproductive Immunology* 33(1) (January 1995): 74–80.

Blau, A., et al. "The psychogenic etiology of premature births." *Psychosomatic Medicine* 25 (1963): 201.

Grim, E. R. "Psychological investigation of habitual abortion." *Psychosomatic Medicine* 24 (1962): 369–78.

Huisjes, H. *Spontaneous Abortion.* New York: Churchill Livingstone, 1984.

Lapple, M. "Stress as an explanatory model for spontaneous abortions and recurrent spontaneous abortions." *Zentralblatt Fur Gynakologie.* (in German) 110 (1988): 325.

Myers, R. "Maternal anxiety and fetal death." In L. Ziochella and P. Pancheri, eds., *Psychoneuroendocrinology in Reproduction.* New York: Elsevier, 1979.

Weil, R. J. "The problem of spontaneous abortion." *American Journal of Obstetrics and Gynecology* 73 (1957): 322.

Weil, R. J., and C. Tupper. "Personality, life situation, communication: A study of habitual abortion." *Psychosomatic Medicine* 22(6) (1960): 448–55.

13. Minding the Change: Menopause

Aldercreutz, H. "Dietary phyto-oestrogens and the menopause in Japan." *Lancet* 339 (1992): 1233.

Aloia, J. F., et al. "Prevention of involutional bone mass by exercise." *Annals of Internal Medicine* 89(3) (1978): 351–58. Washington, D.C.: Consensus Development Conference on Osteoporosis, National Institutes of Health, 1989.

Colditz, G. A., et al. "The use of estrogens and progestins and the risk of breast cancer in postmenopausal women." *New England Journal of Medicine* 332 (June 15, 1995): 1589–93.

Freedman, R. R., and S. Woodward. "Behavioral treatment of menopausal hot flashes: Evaluation by ambulatory monitoring." *American Journal of Obstetrics and Gynecology* 167 (1992): 436–39.

Germaine, L. M., and R. R. Freedman. "Behavioral treatment of menopausal hot flashes: Evaluation by objective methods." *Journal of Consulting and Clinical Psychology* 52 (1984): 1072–79.

Greenwood, S. *Menopause Naturally: Preparing for the Second Half of Life*. Volcano, Calif.: Volcano Press, 1992.

Hunter, M., R. Battersby, and M. Whitehead. "Relationships between psychological symptoms, somatic complaints and menopausal status." *Maturitas* 8 (1986): 217–28.

Irvin, J. H., A. Domar, C. Clark, P. C. Zuttermeister, and R. Friedman. "The effects of relaxation response training on menopausal symptoms." In press, *Journal of Psychosomatic Obstetrics and Gynecology*.

Kronenberg, F., and J. A. Downey. "Thermoregulatory physiology of menopausal hot flashes: A review." *Canadian Journal of Physiological Pharmacology* 65 (1986): 1312–24.

Lark, S. M. *The Menopause Self-Help Book*. Berkeley, Calif.: Celestial Arts, 1992.

Northrup, C. *Women's Bodies, Women's Wisdom*. New York: Bantam Books, 1994.

Ornish, D. *Dr. Dean Ornish's Program for Reversing Heart Disease*. New York: Random House, 1991.

Prince, R., et al. "Prevention of postmenopausal osteoporosis: A comparative study of exercise, calcium supplementation, and hormone replacement therapy." *New England Journal of Medicine* 325(17) (1991): 1189–1204.

Shaver, J.L.F. "Beyond hormonal therapies in menopause." *Experimental Gerontology* 29(3–4) (1994): 469–76.

Sheehy, G. *The Silent Passage*. New York: Random House, 1991.

Stevenson, D. W., and D. J. Delprato. "Multiple component self-control program for menopausal hot flashes." *Journal of Behavior Therapy and Experimental Psychiatry* 14(2) (1983): 137–40.

Swartzman, L. C., R. Edelberg, and E. Kemmann. "Impact of stress on objectively recorded menopausal hot flushes on flush report bias." *Health Psychology* 9 (1990): 529–45.

———. "The menopausal hot flush: Symptom reports and concomitant physiological changes." *Journal of Behavioral Medicine* 13 (1990): 15–30.

14. Fat Is a Mind-Body Issue: Eating Disorders

Agras, W. S. "Nonpharmacologic treatments of bulimia nervosa." *Journal of Clinical Psychiatry* 52, Supplement (October 1991): 10.

Fairburn, C. G., and G. T. Wilson, eds. *Binge Eating: Nature, Assessment and Treatment*. New York: Guilford Press, 1993.

Fairburn, C. G., R. Jones, R. C. Peveler, S. J. Carr, R. A. Solomon, M. E. O'Connor, J. Burton, and R. A. Hope. "Three psychological treatments for bulimia nervosa." *Archives of General Psychiatry* 48 (1991): 463–69.

Goleman, D. "Eating disorder rates surprise the experts." *New York Times*, 4 October 1995, p. C11.

Hirschmann, J. R., and C. H. Munter. *Overcoming Overeating*. New York: Fawcett Colombine, 1989.

Rodin, J. *Body Traps: Breaking the Binds That Keep You from Feeling Good About Your Body*. New York: William Morrow and Co., 1992.

Wilfley, D. E., et al. "Group cognitive-behavioral therapy and group interpersonal psychotherapy for the nonpurging bulimic individual: A controlled comparison." *Journal of Consulting and Clinical Psychology* 61(2) (1993): 296–305.

Wilson, G. T., and C. G. Fairburn. "Cognitive treatments for eating disorders." *Journal of Consulting and Clinical Psychology* 61(2) (1993): 261–69.

15. *From Trauma to Transformation: Breast and Gynecologic Cancers*

Antoni, M. H., and K. Goodkin. "Host moderator variables in the promotion of cervica neoplasia—I. Personality facets." *Journal of Psychosomatic Research* 3 (1988): 327–81.

Buell, P. "Changing incidence of breast cancer in Japanese-American women." *Journal of the National Cancer Institute* 51 (1973): 1479–83.

Burnish, T. G., et al. "Behavioral relaxation techniques in reducing distress of cancer chemotherapy patients." *Oncology Nursing Forum* 10 (1983): 32–35.

Domar, A. D., J. H. Irvin, R. Friedman, and D. Mills. "The effect of relaxation training on tamoxifen-induced hot flashes." Paper presented at the annual meeting of the Society of Behavioral Medicine, San Diego, March 1995.

Dreher, H. *Your Defense Against Cancer.* New York: HarperCollins, 1994.

Fawzy, F. I., N. W. Fawzy, C. S. Hyun, R. Elashoff, D. Guthrie, J. L. Fahey, and D. L. Morton. "Effects of an early structured psychiatric intervention, coping and affective state on recurrence and survival six years later." *Archives of General Psychiatry* 50 (1993): 681–89.

Goodkin, K. "Stress and hopelessness in the promotion of cervical epithelial neoplasia to invasive squamous cell carcinoma of the cervix." *Journal of Psychosomatic Research* 30 (1986): 67–76.

Greer, S., and T. Morris. "Psychological attributes of women who develop breast cancer: A controlled study." *Journal of Psychosomatic Research* 19 (1975): 147–53.

Greer, S., T. Morris, and K. W. Pettingale. "Psychological response to breast cancer: Effect on outcome." *Lancet* 2 (1979): 785–87.

Greer, S., T. Morris, K. W. Pettingale, and J. Haybittle. "Mental attitudes toward cancer: An additional prognostic factor." *Lancet* 1 (1985): 750.

———. "Psychological response to breast cancer and fifteen-year outcome." *Lancet* 1 (1990): 49–50.

Gruber, B. L., N. R. Hall, S. P. Hersh, and P. Dubois. "Immune system and psychologic changes in metastatic cancer patients while using ritualized relaxation and guided imagery." *Scandinavian Journal of Behavioral Therapy* 17 (1988): 24–46.

Lerner, M. *Choices in Healing: Integrating the Best of Conventional and Complementary Approaches to Cancer.* Cambridge, Mass.: MIT Press, 1994.

LeShan, L. *Cancer as a Turning Point.* New York: Dutton Books, 1989.

Levy, S., et al. "Perceived social support and tumor estrogen progesterone receptor status as predictors of natural killer cell activity in breast cancer patients." *Psychosomatic Medicine* 52 (1990): 73–85.

Levy, S. M., R. B. Herberman, M. Lippman, and T. D'Angelo. "Correlation of stress factors with sustained depression of natural killer cell activity with predicted prognosis in patients with breast cancer." *Journal of Clinical Oncology* 5(3) (1987): 348–53.

Levy, S. M., J. Lee, C. Bagley, and M. Lippman. "Survival hazards analysis in first recurrent breast cancer patients: Seven year follow-up." *Psychosomatic Medicine* 50 (1988): 520–28.

Love, S. M. *Dr. Susan Love's Breast Book*. 2nd ed. Reading, Mass.: Addison-Wesley, 1995.

McConnell, K. P., et al. "The relationship between dietary selenium and breast cancer." *Journal of Surgical Oncology* 5(1) (1980): 67–70.

Redd, W. H. "Management of anticipatory nausea and vomiting." In J. C. Holland and J. H. Rowland, eds., *Handbook of Psychosocial Oncology: Psychological Care of Patients with Cancer*. New York: Oxford University Press, 1989.

Rosenberg, L., et al. "Breast cancer and alcoholic beverage consumption." *Lancet* 1 (1982): 267.

Runowicz, C. D., and D. Haupt. *To Be Alive: A Woman's Guide to a Full Life After Cancer*. New York: Henry Holt and Co., 1994.

Scherg, H. "Psychosocial factors and disease bias in breast cancer patients." *Psychosomatic Medicine* 49 (1987): 302–12.

Schmale, A. H., and H. Iker. "Hopelessness as a mediator of cervical cancer." *Social Science and Medicine* 5 (1971): 95–100.

Spiegel, D. *Living Beyond Limits*. New York: Times Books, 1993.

———. "Psychosocial interventions and cancer: Letters." *Advances* 8(1) (1992): 2–4.

Spiegel, D., J. R. Bloom, H. C. Kraemer, and E. Gottheil. "Effect of psychosocial treatment on survival of patients with metastatic breast cancer." *Lancet* 2 (1989): 888–91.

Temoshok, L., and H. Dreher. *The Type C Connection: The Behavioral Links to Cancer and Your Health*. New York: Random House, 1992.

Temoshok, L., B. W. Heller, R. W. Sagebiel, M. S. Blois, D. M. Sweet, R. J. DiClemente, and M. L. Gold. "The relationship of psychosocial factors to prognostic indicators in cutaneous malignant melanoma." *Journal of Psychosomatic Research* 29 (1985): 139–54.

Walker, L. G., and O. Eremin. "Psychoneuroimmunology: A new fad or the fifth cancer treatment modality?" *American Journal of Surgery* 170 (July 1995): 2–4.

Wirsching, M., H. Stierlin, F. Hoffman, G. Weber, and B. Wirsching. "Psychological identification of breast cancer patients before biopsy." *Journal of Psychosomatic Medicine* 26 (1982): 1–10.

16. Soothing the Hurt: Endometriosis and Pelvic Pain

Caudill, M. *Managing Pain Before It Manages You*. New York: Guilford Press, 1994.

Domar, A. "Psychological aspects of pelvic examinations: Individual needs and physician involvement." *Women's Health* 10 (1985): 75–90.

Domar, A., R. Friedman, and H. Benson. "Behavioral therapies in the treatment of pain." In C. Warfield, ed., *The Anesthesiologist's Guide to Pain Management*. New York: McGraw-Hill, 1992.

Fukaya, T., H. Hoshiai, and A. Yajima. "Is pelvic endometriosis always associated with chronic pain? A retrospective study of 618 cases diagnosed by laparoscopy." *American Journal of Obstetrics and Gynecology* 169 (1993): 719–22.

Gleicher, N. "Is endometriosis an autoimmune disease?" *Obstetrics and Gynecology* 70 (July 1987).

Lauersen, N., and C. DeSwann. *The Endometriosis Answer Book: New Hope, New Help.* New York: Rawson Associates, 1988.

Rapkin, A. J. "Adhesions and pelvic pain: A retrospective study." *Obstetrics and Gynecology* 68 (1986): 13–15.

———. "Pelvic visceral pain in women." *ASP Newsletter*, September–October 1995, pp. 4–61.

Rapkin, A. J., L. D. Kames, L. L. Darke, F. M. Stampler, and B. D. Naliboff. "History of physical and sexual abuse in women with chronic pelvic pain." *Obstetrics and Gynecology* 76 (1990): 90–96.

Reiter, R. C. "A profile of women with chronic pelvic pain." *Clinical Obstetrics and Gynecology* 33 (1990): 130–36.

Appendix B

♦ ♦ ♦ ♦ ♦ ♦ ♦

ORGANIZATIONS
AND RESOURCES

Mind-Body Medicine

The Division of Behavioral Medicine at the Deaconess Hospital in Boston, which includes our clinical mind-body programs, can be reached at this address:

Division of Behavorial Medicine
Deaconess Hospital
1 Deaconess Road
Boston, MA 02215
(617) 632-9530

The Mind/Body Medical Institute, headed by Herbert Benson, M.D., is our research, training, and educational arm. You can order relaxation audiotapes from the institute, including tapes with guided imagery exercises from:

Mind/Body Medical Institute
Deaconess Hospital
Attention: Tapes
1 Deaconess Road
Boston, MA 02215

The following tapes can be ordered by writing to the above address. (Each tape is

$10. No tax or postage fee is required. Please make checks payable to the Mind/Body Medical Institute.)

- Basic Relaxation Exercise/Mindfulness Meditation (female voice)
- Basic Relaxation Response Exercise (male voice)
- Advanced Relaxation Response Exercise (female voice)
- Guided Visualization with Ocean Sounds/Breath and Body Awareness (female voice)
- Relaxation Exercise/Mountain Stream Mental Imagery
  This tape, narrated by Dr. Domar, includes on side 1 breathing techniques leading into a body scan relaxation. Side 2 offers a guided imagery exercise in which you walk through a forest to a mountain stream.
- Relaxation Response Extended Session/Mental Imagery (Beach Scene)
  Also narrated by Dr. Domar. The first side, extended to forty minutes, includes a long body scan relaxation and

a guided visualization of taking a warm, comfortable bath. This side was created to be especially useful to people undergoing medical, surgical, or dental procedures. Side 2 offers body scan and guided imagery of exploring a sandy beach on a summer day.

- A Gift of Relaxation/Garden of Your Mind (female voice)
Side 2 incorporates imagery of a lovely garden, one you have visited or that you create in your mind. Both sides include positive affirmations.
- Tuning In to Your Body, Tuning Up Your Mind (female voice)
Includes relaxation exercises practiced standing, sitting, or lying down.
- An Introduction to the Relaxation Response/A Special Time for You (female voice)
- Body Scan Relaxation with Ocean Sounds (female voice)
- Relaxation Exercises I and II (female voice)
Side 1 includes a progressive muscle relaxation exercise; side 2 includes a body scan relaxation and ends with a brief, peaceful visualization.
- Relaxation Response Exercise Tape (male voice)
Side 1 offers instruction on eliciting the relaxation response during exercise. Side 2 has nondistracting music that can be used for relaxation during exercise once the first side is no longer needed.
- Rest in Gratitude/Healing Light (female voice)
Gentle body scan and guided imagery.
- Safe Place/Pain Visualization (female voice)
Progressive muscle relaxation and comforting imagery designed for people with chronic pain.
- Basic Yoga Stretching Exercises/Stretching and Balancing Exercises (female voice)
- Body Scan, Breathing, and Autogenic Exercises (male voice)

The Mind/Body Medical Institute has established a number of affiliates, each of which offers a variety of clinical mind-body programs to the public. The following list includes the hospitals or medical centers where these affiliates have already been established:

Mercy Hospital and Medical Center
Stevenson Expressway at King Drive
Chicago, IL 60616
(312) 567-2600

Memorial Healthcare System
7500 Beechnut, Suite 321
Houston, TX 77074
(713) 776-5020

Morristown Memorial Hospital
The Rehabilitation Institute
95 Mt. Kemble Avenue
Morristown, NJ 07962
(201) 971-4575

Riverside Methodist Hospital
3535 Olentangy River Road
Columbus, OH 43214
(614) 566-4050

Baptist Hospital, Inc.
2000 Church Street
Nashville, TN 37236
(615) 284-6463

St. Peter's Medical Center
254 Easton Avenue
New Brunswick, NJ 08901
(908) 745-8528

Other Mind-Body Organizations

The Fetzer Institute
9292 West KL Avenue
Kalamazoo, MI 49009
(616) 375-2000

The Fetzer Institute supports mind-body research and publishes *Advances: The Journal of Mind-Body Health.*

Academy for Guided Imagery
P.O. Box 2070
Mill Valley, CA 94942
(415) 389-9324

Dr. Martin Rossman's academy offers teaching and training in guided imagery.

The Center for Cognitive Therapy
The Science Center
Room 754
3600 Market Street
Philadelphia, PA 19104
(215) 898-4102

The American Self-Help Clearinghouse
St. Clares–Riverside Medical Center
25 Pocono Road
Denville, NJ 07834
(201) 625-7101

Contact this organization for information and referrals to support groups for various illnesses.

Mind-Body Health Sciences, Inc.
393 Dixon Road
Boulder, CO 80302
(303) 440-8460

Dr. Joan Borysenko's organization.

Stress Reduction Clinic
University of Massachusetts Medical
  Center
Worcester, MA 01655
(508) 856-1616

Dr. Jon Kabat-Zinn's clinic offers an eight-week mind-body program and a limited number of five-day residential programs to meet the needs of people who live beyond commuting distance.

American Holistic Medical Association
4101 Lake Boone Trail
Suite 201
Raleigh, NC 27607
(919) 787-5181

Institute for Noetic Sciences
475 Gate Five Road
Suite 300
Sausalito, CA 94965
(415) 331-5650

Women to Women
One Pleasant Street
Yarmouth, ME 04096
(207) 846-6163

Dr. Christiane Northrup's Center for Women's Health is a gynecologic practice with a strong emphasis on holistic and mind-body medicine.

National Institute for the Clinical
  Application of Behavioral Medicine
Box 523
Mansfield Center, CT 06250
(203) 456-1153

Society of Behavioral Medicine
103 South Adams Street
Rockville, MD 20850
(301) 251-2790

Arthritis

The Arthritis Foundation
P.O. Box 19000
Atlanta, GA 30326
(800) 283-7800

Breast Cancer

National Alliance of Breast Cancer
  Organizations
1180 Avenue of the Americas
New York, NY 10036
(212) 719-0154

Y-ME National Breast Cancer
  Organization
212 West Van Buren Street
Chicago, IL 60607
(312) 986-8228
Toll-free hotline: (800) 221-2141

Komen Alliance
Susan G. Komen Foundation
Occidental Tower
5005 LBJ Freeway
Suite 370
Dallas, TX 75244

Cancer Care, Inc./National Cancer Care
  Foundation
1180 Avenue of the Americas
New York, NY 10036
(212) 211-3300

Cancer in General

National Cancer Institute
Office of Cancer Communications
Building 31, Room 10A16
Bethesda, MD 20892
Cancer Information Services:
(800) 4-CANCER
Evenings: (800) 638-6694

Dial (800) 4-CANCER for information
as well as the Physician's Data Query
(PDQ) service, which provides you with a
printout of available clinical trials of
experimental treatments.

American Cancer Society
1599 Clifton Road NE
Atlanta, GA 30329-4251
(404) 320-3333

The National Coalition for Cancer
  Survivorship
1010 Wayne Avenue
5th Floor
Silver Spring, MD 20910
(301) 585-2616

Commonweal Cancer Help Program
P.O. Box 316
Bolinas, CA 94924
(415) 868-0970

Commonweal holds regular retreats for
individuals with cancer.

The Wellness Community
2200 Colorado Avenue
Santa Monica, CA 90404
(310) 453-2200

Chronic Pain

American Chronic Pain Association
P.O. Box 850
Rocklin, CA 95677
(916) 632-0922

Eating Disorders

National Association of Anorexia
  Nervosa and Associated Disorders
P.O. Box 7
Highland Park, IL 60036
(708) 831-3438

American Anorexia/Bulimia Association
418 East 76th Street
New York, NY 10022
(212) 734-1114

National Eating Disorders Organization
445 East Granville Road
Worthington, OH 43085
(614) 436-1112

Overeaters Anonymous, Inc.
World Service Office
P.O. Box 44020
Rio Rancho, NM 87174
(505) 891-2664

Endometriosis

Endometriosis Association
8585 North 75th Place
Milwaukee, WI 53223
(800) 992-ENDO

General Gynecological Problems

American College of Obstetricians and
Gynecologists Resource Center
409 12th Street NW
Washington, DC 20024-2188
(202) 638-5577

National Women's Health Network
514 10th Street NW, Suite 400
Washington, DC 20004

National Women's Health Resource
Center
2440 M Street NW, Suite 325
Washington, DC 20037

Heart Health

American Heart Association
(800) AHA-USA-1, or look for your
local chapter of the AHA in the
phone book

National Heart, Lung, and Blood
Institute
Information Center
P.O. Box 30105
Bethesda, MD 20824-0105
(301) 251-1222

Hysterectomy

Hysterectomy Educational Resources and
Services
(HERS Foundation)
422 Bryn Mawr Avenue
Bala Cynwyd, PA 19004
(610) 667-7757

Infertility

RESOLVE, Inc.
National Headquarters
1310 Broadway
Somerville, MA
(617) 623-1156
Helpline: (617) 623-0744

American Society for Reproductive
Medicine
1209 Montgomery Highway
Birmingham, AL 35216-2809
(205) 978-5000

National Committee on Adoption
1930 17th Street NW
Washington, DC 20009
(202) 328-1200

Lupus

The Lupus Foundation of America
1717 Massachusetts Avenue NW
Washington, DC 20026
(800) 558-0121

Menopause

North American Menopause Society
c/o University Hospitals of Cleveland
Department of OB/GYN
11100 Euclid Avenue
Cleveland, OH 44106
(216) 844-3344

National Osteoporosis Foundation
2100 M Street NW
Suite 602
Washington, DC 20037
(202) 223-2226

National Institute on Aging Information
Center
P.O. Box 8057
Gaithersburg, MD 20892-8057
(800) 222-2225

Mental Health

Depression Awareness, Recognition and
Treatment
D/ART Program
National Institute of Mental Health
5600 Fishers Lane
Room 15C-05
Rockville, MD 20857
(301) 443-4513

National Foundation for Depressive
Illness
2 Pennsylvania Plaza
New York, NY 10121
(800) 248-4344

Anxiety Disorders Association of
America
6000 Executive Blvd.
Suite 513
Rockville, MD 20852-4004
(301) 231-9350

American Psychological Association
750 1st Street NW
Washington, DC 20002
(202) 336-5500

Miscarriage

A.M.E.N.D.
4324 Berrywick Terrace
St. Louis, MO 63128
(314) 487-7528

Provides one-on-one support among
parents coping with miscarriage, stillbirth,
or the loss of newborn infants.

SHARE
Pregnancy and Infant Loss Support, Inc.
St. Joseph's Health Center
300 First Capitol Drive
St. Charles, MO 63301
(314) 947-6164

Offers referrals to support groups nationwide and other helpful information.

PMS

National PMS Society
P.O. Box 11467
Durham, NC 27703
(919) 489-6577

Premenstrual Syndrome Action
P.O. Box 9326
Madison, WI 53715
(608) 274-6688

Premenstrual Syndrome Program
40 Salem Street
Lynnfield, MA 01940
(617) 227-6992

Pregnancy and Delivery

U.S. Department of Health and Human
 Services
National Maternal and Child Health
 Clearinghouse
8201 Greensboro Drive
Suite 600
McLean, VA 22102
(703) 821-8955, ext. 254

National Association of Child-Bearing
 Centers
3123 Gottschall Road
1518 Perkiomenville, PA 18074
(215) 234-8068

Index

♦ ♦ ♦